APPLIED BAYESIAN STATISTICAL STUDIES IN BIOLOGY AND MEDICINE

APPLIED BAYESIAN STATISTICAL STUDIES IN BIOLOGY AND MEDICINE

Edited by

M. Di Bacco,
Università di Bologna

G. D'Amore,
Università di Firenze

F. Scalfari,
Polo Universitario Asti Studi Superiori

Kluwer Academic Publishers
Boston/Dordrecht/London

Distributors for North, Central and South America:
Kluwer Academic Publishers
101 Philip Drive
Assinippi Park
Norwell, Massachusetts 02061 USA
Telephone (781) 871-6600
Fax (781) 871-6528
E-Mail <kluwer@wkap.com>

Distributors for all other countries:
Kluwer Academic Publishers Group
Post Office Box 322
3300 AH Dordrecht, THE NETHERLANDS
Telephone 31 78 6576 000
Fax 31 78 6576 474
E-Mail <orderdept@wkap.nl>

Electronic Services <http://www.wkap.nl>

Library of Congress Cataloging-in-Publication

Di Bacco, M./ D'Amore, G./ Scalfari, F.
Applied Bayesian Statistical Studies in Biology and Medicine
ISBN-13:978-1-4613-7946-1 e-ISBN-13:978-1-4613-0217-9
DOI: 10.1007/978-1-4613-0217-9

Printed on acid-free paper.

Contents

Contributing Authors

F. Bartolucci, Istituto di Scienze Economiche, Università di Urbino, Urbino, Italy.

F. Bertolino, Dipartimento di Matematica, Università di Cagliari, Cagliari, Italy.

M. Bolzan, Dipartimento di Statistica, Università di Padova, Padua, Italy.

A. Brogini, Dipartimento di Statistica, Università di Padova, Padua, Italy.

A. Capotorti, Dipartimento di Matematica e Informatica, Università di Perugia, Perugia, Italy.

G. D'Amore, Laboratori di Antropologia, Dipartimento di Biologia Animale e Genetica, Università di Firenze, Florence, Italy.

J. Deely, Department of Statistics, Purdue University, West Lafayette, IN, USA

F. De Santis, Dipartimento di Statistica, Probabilità e Statistiche Applicate, Università di Roma "La Sapienza", Rome, Italy.

M. Di Bacco, Dipartimento di Scienze Statistiche, Università di Bologna, Bologna, Italy.

S. Fagundes Leite, Istituto di Anatomia e Istologia Patologica, Divisione di Ricerca sul Cancro, Università di Perugia, Perugia, Italy.

P. Frederic, Dipartimento di Scienze Statistiche, Università di Bologna, Bologna. Italy.

F. Lad, Department of Mathematics and Statistics, University of Canterbury, Christchurch, New Zealand/Aotearo.

D. V. Lindley, "Woodstock", Quay Lane, Minehead, TA24 5QU, UK.

A. Mira, Dipartimento di Economia, Università dell'Insubria, Varese, Italy.

A. J. O'Malley, Department of Health Care Policy, Harvard Medical School, Boston, MA, USA.

E. Pacciani, Soprintendenza ai Beni Archeologici della Toscana, Florence, Italy.

M. Perone Pacifico, Dipartimento di Statistica, Probabilità e Statistiche Applicate, Università di Roma "La Sapienza", Rome, Italy.

S. Pezzulli, Department of Meteorology, The University of Reading, Early Gate P.O. Box 243, Reading, RG6 6BB, UK.

A. Ratto, Dipartimento di Matematica, Università di Cagliari, Cagliari, Italy.

A. Rinaldi, Dipartimento di Studi Geoeconomici, Linguistici, Statistici, Storici per l'Analisi Regionale, Università di Roma "La Sapienza", Rome, Italy.

L. Scaccia, Dipartimento di Scienze Statistiche, Università di Perugia, Perugia, Italy.

J. Shoemaker, Department of Biostatistics and Bioinformatics, Duke University Medical Center, Durham, NC, U.S.A.

D. Slanzi, Dipartimento di Statistica, Università di Padova, Padua, Italy.

Foreword

It was written on another occasion* that "It is apparent that the scientific culture, if one means production of scientific papers, is growing exponentially, and chaotically, in almost every field of investigation". The biomedical sciences *sensu lato* and mathematical statistics are no exceptions. One might say then, and with good reason, that another collection of bio-statistical papers would only add to the overflow and cause even more confusion. Nevertheless, this book may be greeted with some interest if we state that most of the papers in it are the result of a collaboration between biologists and statisticians, and partly the product of the Summer School "Statistical Inference in Human Biology" which reaches its 10th edition in 2003 (information about the School can be obtained at the Web site http://www2.stat.unibo.it/eventi/Sito%20scuola/index.htm).

This is rather important. Indeed, it is common experience – and not only in Italy – that encounters between statisticians and researchers are sporadic and hasty. This is not the place to justify this statement, which may sound too severe, as this preface would become much too long. It is sufficient to point out that very often whoever introduces young biologists and medical doctors to inductive reasoning about "data" either does not have a real interest in the concrete and specific meaning of the data or – if interested – does not have a solid statistical background. In other words, he is usually a "theoretical" statistician or a biological or medical "technician". Naturally there are many places where things are different. Yet we are convinced that biologists and doctors are generally encouraged to look on statistical "tools"

* Preface to "Probability and Bayesian Statistics in Medicine and Biology". BARRAI, I. COLETTI, G., DI BACCO, M. Eds. Giardini Editorie Stampatori in Pisa, Pisa, 1992.

as laboratory instruments, without worrying about how they function; it is merely enough to learn how to draw a response from them – the "black boxes" of which de Finetti spoke in a context not very different from the current one. One may ask then: do biologists and doctors also need to be statisticians and, vice versa, do statisticians need to be doctors or biologists? Obviously this would be expecting the impossible. Yet one may expect the two kinds of scientists to collaborate, and not only work together as if in an assembly line. In this way, the statistician would know the empirical hypothesis before the "data" are produced, would understand their meaning, and would hear what is said about the hypothesis in a broad discussion among experts. This should suffice to arouse his interest in the research proposal or – even better – for him to be fascinated by it. On the other hand, in their regular meetings with the statisticians (which would remove the "terrifying formulae", again the words of de Finetti), the doctors and biologists would learn the essentials of the statistical tools most suitable to interrogate the data; tools that can neither say "yes" nor "no", nor "++" nor anything else, but can only help the user to reason, to infer, coherently. However, what we have just written will be found among the many "reflections" of Professor Lindley that begin this volume (and we suspect that those reflections will upset the tranquil sleep of many statisticians).

Therefore, this volume provides examples of collaboration – we use the noun in the full sense in which we used the corresponding verb – between statisticians and non-statisticians, and this also holds for those papers in which the latter might not appear as co-authors. Naturally our examples are not perfect paradigms of such collaboration: at times, the formulae seem terrifying and it might have been better to write something more accessible to the non-statistician. On the other hand, the description of the concrete problem is at times rather hasty. Yet statisticians and non-statisticians await the revocation of the "biblical command" «*confundamus ibi linguam eorumut, ut non audiat unusquisque vocem proximi sui*» ("confuse their language, they may not understand one another's speech") (Gen. 11.7). We hope the revocation arrives soon. However, in the present hour, as tragedy follows numerous other tragedies, we are even more presented with the need to ask that each man learn to understand reasons of the other.

April, 2003 The Editors

Acknowledgments

The Editors express their sincere thanks to Professor Franco Giannessi (Università di Pisa) for his encouragement and suggestions, and to Dr. Giovanna Filippini (Università di Bologna) for her active cooperation. The Editors are all indebted to Università degli Studi di Bologna, Polo Universitario Asti Studi Superiori, Associazione per lo Sviluppo Scientifico e Tecnologico di Asti, Fondazione Cassa di Risparmio di Asti, Regione Piemonte, for their financial support. Then, sincere thanks to Laila Lucarelli Company (Pisa) for the final typing of the manuscripts.

Finally, the Editors want to express their special thanks to Kluwer Publishing Company for their unfailing cooperation.

Summaries of the papers

D. V. LINDLEY. *Some reflections on the current state of statistics.*

Paraphrasing the Author's words, the paper dwells upon a topic "where experience may be more important than originality". Therefore, he says something about how he views statistics today. In our opinion, the chief points of his reflections are:

- statistics is the study of uncertainty and to study uncertainty coherently the only tool we have is coherent probability;
- however, in the statistical world, it is necessary to integrate probability and utility: really "the pinnacle of the Bayesian achievement is the maximum expected utility";
- Exploratory Data Analysis is useful – necessary, indeed – because when statisticians "encounter a new, small world they have first to find their way around it before they can make their formal structure".

F. BARTOLUCCI, A. MIRA AND L. SCACCIA. *Answering two biological questions with a latent class model via MCMC applied to capture-recapture data.*

The Authors propose a Bayesian model with latent classes for capture-recapture data. Through two applications, the first concerning a sample of snowshoe hares and the second a sample of diabetics in a small Italian town, they show how the proposed approach can be used to obtain credibility intervals for the size of a closed-population. To estimate the model, they use the Reversible jump MCMC algorithm and the Delayed Rejection strategy to improve the efficiency.

F. BERTOLINO AND A. RATTO. *On the Bayesian inference of the Hardy-Weinberg equilibrium model.*

The Authors study the classical problem of testing whether a given population is in Hardy-Weinberg equilibrium. Some variants, including the case of numerous consanguineous matings and the Bernstein disequilibrium model, are also studied.

A. BROGINI, M. BOLZAN AND D. SLANZI. *Identifying a Bayesian Network for the problem "Hospital and families: the analysis of patient satisfaction with their stay in hospital".*

The Authors intend to research and describe variables, indicators and their relationships associated with the discomfort, suffering and quality of assistance that families deal with when a family member must make use of certain welfare services, such as hospitalisation. Indeed, such events take on different characteristics depending on the demographic, epidemiological, social, health and economic typology of the patient and the family involved. The data used for this analysis were selected from the Multiscope Survey on the Family "Aspects of daily life" carried out by ISTAT 1998. The problem appears as a complex system and the Authors use a Bayesian Network as the statistical model. A Bayesian Network is a graphical representation of a multivariate joint probability distribution over the domain of interest, which exploits the dependencies between the variables of the system. This method provides the advantage of a formal probabilistic model, presented in an easily viewed form, together with the availability of efficient computational methods. The Authors concentrate on the Bayesian approach with the goal of identifying the most probable Bayesian Network, given a complete database, for an understanding of the whole behaviour of the social system.

A. CAPOTORTI AND S. FAGUNDES LEITE. *Reliability of GIST diagnosis based on partial information.*

The focus is on the diagnosis of gastrointestinal stromal tumors (GISTs), for which a new and reliable phenotypic marker (the KIT protein CD117) has recently been introduced. The Authors attempt to determine consistent bounds for predictive values when the available information is extremely uncertain, either because it comes from different sources or because it is not fully detailed. The methodology is that of "embedding" the problem in a coherent setting, i.e. the class of conditional probabilities that agree with the available information is sought and it is used to perform an optimization procedure to compute the probabilistic bounds for the statements relevant to evaluation of the "goodness" of the diagnostic process.

J. DEELY. *Comparing two groups or treatments - a Bayesian approach.*

Two practical statistical problems involving the comparison of two treatments or populations are discussed. The first problem compares the cholesterol levels of two groups of people and the second problem compares a new treatment to a control at the interim in a clinical trial. A Bayesian approach is used to compute quantities which have practical significance. For problem one, this quantity is the posterior probability that the mean level of one group is larger than that of the other group by some specified amount. For problem two, the predictive probability that the new treatment will be sufficiently better than the control at the end of the experiment is computed.

F. DE SANTIS AND M. PERONE PACIFICO. *Two experimental settings in clinical trials: predictive criteria for choosing the sample size in interval estimation.*

Two experimental settings are considered in which sample size determination is the central issue. The first setting is concerned with choosing the appropriate number of statistical units to consider in a clinical trial comparing the effects of two alternative therapies for the treatment of pelvic cancer. The second experimental problem is concerned with estimating the effect of a drug used to maintain remission in acute leukemia on the expected lifetime of the patients. From a statistical point of view, both problems can be formalized as problems of optimal sample size determination in the context of interval estimation of a quantity of interest. The Authors propose the use of Bayesian methods, which are particularly suitable to incorporate pre-experimental information in the analysis and to deal with potential nuisance parameters.

P. FREDERIC, G. D'AMORE AND E. PACCIANI. *Attributing a paleoanthropological specimen to a prehistoric population: a Bayesian approach with multivariate B-spline functions.*

Human bones (a cranial vault) were recovered near Ancona (central Italy) during archaeological excavations. The aim of the present work is to attribute this paleoanthropological specimen with uncertain sex and chronology to a prehistoric population. The attribution was obtained following the Bayesian paradigm: the priors were assigned taking into account the reliability of the combined information on morphological features and some absolute chronological data; multivariate B-spline functions were used to elicit likelihood functions using data for the alternative populations.

F. LAD. *An example of the subjectivist statistical method for learning from data: Why do whales strand when they do?*

This is a didactic article on the application of the operational subjective statistical method, designed for readers who are not familiar with the motivation for and practice of subjective Bayesian statistics. The substantive scientific issue concerns the timing of whale strandings with respect to the phase of the lunar month, a very controversial question among marine zoologists. Technical analysis of historical whale stranding data is preceded by a discussion of the foundations of subjective statistical analysis. A simpler example of a statistical problem in cattle breeding then displays the general form of applied analysis that uses Bayes' theorem. The whale stranding data are derived from records kept in the New Zealand Whale Stranding Data Base. The statistical analysis focuses on the computation of predictive distributions for the lunar date of the next stranding that cohere with viewpoints supported by differing zoological theories.

A. J. O'MALLEY. *Development and communication of Bayesian methodology for medical device clinical trials.*

The Author describes newly proposed methods for the analysis and design of medical device clinical trials of medical devices, with particular application to coronary-artery stents. Trials of medical devices often compare outcomes associated with the new device to the expected outcomes associated with approved devices. Bayesian hierarchical regression models are used to model the multivariate mixed outcome data, and to compute related inferences. Bayesian methodology is also used to evaluate the statistical power and the optimal sample size for historically-controlled clinical trials.

S. PEZZULLI. *An adaptive SIR algorithm for Bayesian multilevel inference on categorical data.*

Sample data from different groups of individuals are often collected and simultaneously investigated. The fundamental hypothesis, in this case, is that the groups are similar and can be considered as stochastic variations of the same human population. The multinomial hierarchy is a Bayesian model that can be used when the data consist of the frequency composition of the individuals with respect to some set of alternative features. Here a method to fit this model is introduced and two problems are discussed. The first deals with colour-blindness data from North East India, resulting in a rather clear difference between Caucasian and Mongoloid populations. In the second problem, the allele frequencies of loci TH01 and FES are investigated in ten Italian subpopulations. Forensic practice currently uses such data; it is shown how the method can have an impact on forensic identification procedures.

A. RINALDI, E. PACCIANI AND M. DI BACCO. *Age at death diagnosis by cranial suture obliteration: a Bayesian approach.*

The effectiveness of cranial suture obliteration for diagnosis of the age at death is a widely discussed problem. However, there are some doubts about the statistical procedures currently used to support both the favorable and the critical viewpoint. Here this problem is discussed using the tools of Bayesian statistical decision theory. The Authors diagnose the age on the basis of the suture obliteration stage in 198 skulls of individuals of known age at death, and to model the corresponding distribution they build an appropriate hierarchical model. Comparison of the results of this diagnosis with the corresponding true ages of the individuals taken from the Registry Office suggests that suture obliteration is a rather rough indicator of the age at death.

J. SHOEMAKER AND A. RINALDI. *Bayesian estimation of restriction fragment length from electrophoretic analysis.*

Lengths of restriction fragments are usually estimated from their electrophoretic mobility. The basis of the estimation is the inverse relationship between length of the fragment and the distance it travels in a gel. Some methods have been developed and are commonly used for this estimation process, but they are purely descriptive and do not allow one to build the usual confidence intervals. The Authors approach this problem according to the Bayesian framework and propose a solution which allows one to evaluate the lengths in a probabilistic perspective.

Chapter 1

SOME REFLECTIONS ON THE CURRENT STATE OF STATISTICS

D. V. Lindley*

"Woodstock", Quay Lane, Minehead, TA24 5QU, UK. E-mail:thombayes@aol.com

Despite the kind invitation from Professor Di Bacco, it was not possible for me to give some lectures at the Summer School on Bayesian methods in biology and medicine, but I have much pleasure in accepting his second invitation to write an introductory note to this book. Approaching eighty, it is not sensible to pretend that anything I say is new; rather let me turn to a topic where experience may be more important than originality, and say something about how I view statistics today.

I am often asked, as are other statisticians, what is meant by the subject of statistics. My view is that we should take the question very seriously, especially when it is put by a lay person, if only because we all have a responsibility to society and, for society adequately to judge us, its members must be properly informed about what we can do. There are many of my professional colleagues who do not appear to agree with me. I say 'appear' on the basis that there are few contributions from statisticians that try to inform people, without their expertise, what they are doing. There are text books but they are trying to teach the tyro to be a statistician, which is different from the informed view that I have in mind. Thus my first criticism of contemporary statistics is that we do not pay enough attention to public relations. Here is a little example that arose recently in Britain. Hospitals throughout the country were assessed for quality by several criteria, one of which took into account deaths as a result of a particular, surgical operation. Now it is well-known that, in default of external influences, such deaths will occur in a Poisson process so that there will naturally be a variation, from hospital to hospital, of about two standard deviations either side of the mean, and that the deviation is the square root of the mean. The assessment of the

* For correspondence: thombayes@aol.com

hospitals showed about this amount of variation yet, when it was seen that the better hospitals had death rates 50% above the worst, efforts were made to correct the imbalance; corrections that were totally unnecessary because there was just Poisson at work. Statisticians ought to have educated responsible people doing such assessments into the idea of natural variation and perhaps the mysteries of the square-root rule. Yet we do not; we explore our hierarchical models and shun the exposure to everyday phenomena, whereas we ought to be doing both. There is an addendum to this tale. If the variation is truly Poisson, and successive years are independent, those 'bad' hospitals will, in any case, appear to get better next year. Then the administrators can point with pride to how effective their remedial measures appear to have been, without mentioning the deterioration in the 'top' hospitals.

Returning to the question of what is meant by statistics, my reply is essentially that it is the study of uncertainty. In the hospital example, there is uncertainty about the numbers of deaths that will arise as a result of the surgery. Many people, including some statisticians, think of the subject as being concerned primarily with data but data are means of reducing uncertainty about quantities, like parameters, and to effect this reduction we need also to consider the data uncertainty. Also there are data that are of no concern to a statistician, such as the measurements of a building, and it is only when uncertainty enters that statistics may become relevant. Sometimes the questioners are already modestly knowledgeable; for example, they may be technologists who are seeking advice about the treatment of their data, when the question may be altered to ask what is meant by Bayesian statistics. This is more difficult to answer but the essence is conveyed by saying that, in the Bayesian view, ali uncertainties are described in terms of probability. Probability is the language of uncertainty. Many questioners have come across expressions like " significant at 5%" , when one can point out that this is a statement of uncertainty but surprisingly is <u>not</u> expressed in terms of an assertion, in the form of probability, about the quantity that is uncertain, the significant effect. Although probability is present in the significance test, it concerns the data, were the effect absent, not the effect. We laugh at lawyers and others who commit the prosecutor's fallacy, failing to distinguish between $p(A / B)$ and $p(B / A)$, but frequentist statisticians are, in the Bayesian view, just as prone to the error, with A effect and B data.

Identifying uncertainty with probability is rarely adequate as an answer because lay persons have an inadequate understanding of probability, thinking of it simply as a number between 0 and 1 that describes how likely it is that the uncertain event be true. If that was all probability was, there would be no reason to get excited about it. There is more, much more, because probabilities combine in two different ways: by addition under some circumstances, and by multiplication in others. It is these two rules of combination that make probability assume the importance that it has. There are few concepts in this world that can combine in two distinct ways to produce another example of the concept. Even human beings cannot do it, at least not until recently with artificial fertilization. The important point about the two rules is that they connect uncertainties together. In fact, if the connection is not according to the rules, a Dutch book could be made against you, there will be the possibility of your losing money for sure and you can be made to look foolish. It is the two rules that ensure the uncertainty statements made by a Bayesian statistician form a coherent whole. Indeed, it is this coherency that characterizes the Bayesian position. There is nothing in the Bayesian canon that says what your uncertainties, or beliefs, might be; it only requires that, whatever they are, they cohere and form a logical whole. The Bayesian thesis is for the Christian, the Muslim and the agnostic. There is one group for whom it is not: the fundamentalists, whether Christian or Muslim. The reason is that they attach zero uncertainty to the idea that a text is ever false. As a result, they can never take heed of evidence because prior zero will have posterior zero, whatever the evidence. This follows by our favourite coherency result, Bayes rule, and were fundamentalists to take note of evidence, they would be illogical.

I have so far talked about uncertainty but if we go back to our founding fathers it can be seen that there is more to be said. These founders are, for me, Harold Jeffreys, Bruno de Finetti, Frank Ramsey and Jimmie Savage. (Of course, there are other candidates, like Laplace, but these four set the wheels in motion in the last century.) Both Jeffreys and de Finetti developed probability as the coherent appreciation of uncertainty, but Ramsey and Savage looked at the world rather differently. Their starting point was not the concept of uncertainty but rather decision-making in the face of uncertainty. They thought in terms of action, rather than in the passive contemplation of the uncertain world. Coherence for them was not so much a matter of how your beliefs hung together but of whether your several actions, considered collectively, made sense. They came to the same conclusions as the thinkers, in demonstrating the necessity of the rules of probability, but they went further in showing that, to be coherent, the consequences of your actions had to be assessed in terms of utility and that, properly done, implied the best act was that of maximum expected utility (MEU), the expectation incorporating the necessary probability. MEU is, in my view, the pinnacle of the Bayesian achievement, in that it tells us how to behave in the face of uncertainty. It is the only sensible way for a single decision-maker to act. Let me qualify that remark. The approaches of the founding fathers, and the subsequent developments, are all in terms of a single person, or group of persons acting as a social unit. It does not apply when two, or more, decision-makers are in conflict. We desperately need another Ramsey to provide a coherent system for peoples with different utilities and probabilities, when in conflict. All we seem to have are negative results, like Arrow's theorem. As Bayesians, we should do well to remind ourselves of this important limitation to our paradigm, though comfort can be had from the fact that the frequentists are equally restricted.

If one looks today at a typical statistical paper that uses the Bayesian method, copious use will be made of probability, but utility, or MEU, will rarely get a mention. Do they arise anywhere in this book? You do get mention of loss functions but employment of these can easily lead to incoherence and, even when they are sensibly used, they are typically of standard forms like quadratic loss. When I look at statistics today, I am astonished at the almost complete failure to use utility. Here we have in MEU the only coherent method of acting, yet we rarely employ it or use one of its twin ideas. Probability is there but not utility. This failure has to be my major criticism of current statistics; we are abandoning our task half-way, producing the inference but declining to explain to others how to act on that inference. The lack of papers that provide discussions of utility is another omission from our publications.

It has already been emphasized that probability tells us how our uncertainties, beliefs and inferences hang together, or cohere, but it does not say what those beliefs should be. It is the same with utility; I can value Beethoven and abhor rock, whereas you can do the opposite, the difference showing itself in our contrasting utilities concerning what CD to buy. One aspect of this flexibility in both probability and utility reveals itself in our performance of probability calculations without paying much attention to what the numbers are that go into them. Bayes rule, yes; but the prior, oh assume a normal. Why? Rao-Blackwell theorem, yes; but for the best estimate use quadratic loss. Why? I put it to you that Bayesians have paid too little attention to the actual numbers that ultimately have to go into the calculations. We have not interrogated our clients to find what they think, and then incorporated their knowledge into our analysis. An analogy may be helpful. We are like geometers who prove wonderful theorems but never bother with how the lengths and angles are to be measured; that task being left to surveyors, often thought of as second-class citizens in comparison with pure mathematicians. We ought not to neglect our measurements. My view is that there should be co-operation between statisticians and experimental psychologists to help people express their beliefs and preferences in the appropriate forms. Suppose that a clinical trial is to be conducted to assess the effectiveness of a new drug. The clinicians will have opinions about how good the drug might be. How do we help them express their valuable judgements in the necessary form of probability? A drug to relieve one illness is expensive; another for a different illness is cheap. How do we justify the expense? How do we assess the utilities associated with the cures? Surely we do not have to use our normals and quadratics in these days of powerful computing methods but can instead use values that reflect reality more accurately. The general standard of technical excellence of the papers in our statistical journals, and those presented at conferences like this, seems high. Now that good computing techniques have been developed, we can escape the strait-jacket of mathematical analysis and handle more realistic and complicated situations. We are not restricted to the exponential family and conjugate priors. But we still have the problem of assessing the numerical values of the probabilities and utilities to be inserted into our calculations. Incidentally, these numbers are not those of the statistician, but of our client, the scientist or technologist. Our task is to help them describe their views in the appropriate form that coherence may be achieved.

At the beginning of this essay, our poor communication with the layman was mentioned. Another aspect of this concerns the teaching of our subject, especially at the elementary level. I was asked recently to review what I was given to understand was the most popular text in the USA for a first course in statistics. It was beautifully produced, had excellent, realistic examples and clearly expounded the performance of elementary, statistical procedures like the *t*-test. (With a flat prior, this will do for a Bayesian; but why flat?) But where was the probability? The book, being based on frequency ideas, did not make as much use of probability as a Bayesian would, but still there was very little about it. Worse still, conditional probability barely got a mention. (I was told it was thought too difficult for the students.) To a Bayesian, all probability is conditional, for any uncertainty depends both on the uncertain quantity and on the conditions under which that uncertainty is being assessed. This almost complete omission of the basic tool of statistics is surely disastrous for the students' proper appreciation of their uncertain world. What the book did was to instruct students in the manipulation of data so that they could perform the simpler procedures. It did this very well, but it did not, in my view, help them to think about what they were doing. They would be able to use statistical packages but not think about the relationship between the package and reality. The book was American but British texts are broadly similar. The primary function of education is to help people to reason and think. I am not convinced that statisticians are helping people to do this.

A criticism that has been levelled against some of the points that have been made in this essay, is that much statistical work is not involved with the formal apparatus of probability and utility, but instead uses what has come to be called exploratory data-analysis (EDA). That is perfectly correct; we can go a long way without the Bayesian apparatus. But what is the purpose of

EDA ? My answer is that it is a necessary part of the manipulation of the data so that one can insert sensible numbers into the formal apparatus. In the example of the hospitals above, preliminary plots of the data are essential to establish that the Poisson model is reasonable. Ideal Bayesians have their probabilities and utilities ready for any aspect of the world that they encounter. Real Bayesians have to work in what Savage termed 'small worlds', so that when they encounter a new, small world, they have first to find their way around it before they can make their formal structure. This is the function of EDA.

I hope that the tone of this essay is not too churlish. Excellent work is being done in statistics now that we are really taking notice of the computer revolution. It is perhaps at the level of contact with outsiders that our defects emerge. Let us also not forget that the Bayesian paradigm enables us to think coherently about the uncertain world we live in and to act coherently in that world.

Chapter 2

ANSWERING TWO BIOLOGICAL QUESTIONS WITH A LATENT CLASS MODEL VIA MCMC APPLIED TO CAPTURE-RECAPTURE DATA

F. Bartolucci,[1] A. Mira[2*] and L. Scaccia[3]

Istituto di Scienze Economiche, University of Urbino, Italy[1]; Dipartimento di Economia, University of Insubria, Italy[2]; Dipartimento di Scienze Statistiche, University of Perugia, Italy[3]

1. INTRODUCTION

A well-known method for estimating the size, N, of a certain population is the *capture-recapture* method (for a review see Yip *et al.*, 1995a and Schwarz and Seber, 1999). The first motivations to the development of these methods arose in biology where researchers were interested in estimating the number of animals of a certain species (see, for instance, Schnabel, 1938, and Darroch, 1958). Subsequently, this methodology was also applied in medical and social contexts where it is important to estimate the number of subjects with a certain disease or in a particular situation (Yip *et al.*, 1995b).

A typical capture-recapture study consists in capturing and somehow marking subjects at different occasions so that a *capture configuration*, $\mathbf{r} = (r_1 \quad \cdots \quad r_J)^T$, may be associated to each subject captured at least once, where J is the number of capture occasions (or *lists*) and r_j is equal to 1 if the subject has been captured at the j-th occasion and 0 otherwise. The population is estimated on the basis of the resulting data that may be arranged in an *incomplete* contingency table with, at most, $2^J - 1$ not empty cells, as the entry corresponding to the subjects never captured is systematically empty. Estimation is usually carried out through a conditional

* For correspondence: antonietta.mira@unica.it

maximum likelihood approach: the multinomial distribution is assumed for the (hypothetical) contingency table including also the missing cell, while the parameters of the model are estimated on the basis of the incomplete table (Sanathanan, 1972). Consequently, N is estimated as $n/[1-\hat{p}(\mathbf{0})]$, where $\hat{p}(\mathbf{0})$ is the estimated probability of the missing configuration and n is the sample size. Since a saturated model may not be used for these data, a variety of restricted models has been proposed. Many of these models are of the log-linear type (Fienberg, 1972; Darroch *et al.*, 1993), but a more recent approach is based on the Latent Class (LC) model; Agresti (1994) was one of the first to use the LC approach in this context. This model assumes that the population may be divided into k classes so that the subjects within each class have the same degree of "catchability" with respect to the same list. Moreover, given the latent class, the conditional probability of being captured in a certain list is independent of that of being captured in other lists. This allows to account for heterogeneity between individuals; furthermore, the parameters of the model may be easily interpreted. This model has also many variants as a finite-mixture version of the Rasch model (Lindsay *et al.*, 1991) that has been applied with success in the capture-recapture context by Bartolucci and Forcina (2001).

Bayesian literature on capture-recapture data has had some developments only in the last two decades. One of the first important contributions seems to be that of Castledine (1981) who developed a model in which capture probabilities may vary between sampling occasions and provided an approximation to the posterior distribution of N under the proposed model. His approach has been refined by Smith (1991) who derived the exact posterior distribution of N. Later, George and Robert (1992) dealt with Bayesian inference for several capture-recapture models, while Madigan and York (1997) proposed the use of a class of decomposable Bayesian graphical models which can incorporate covariates. More recent papers are those of Fienberg *et al.* (1999), who dealt with a continuous-trait version of the Rasch model, and Basu and Ebrahimi (2001) and Tardella (2002) who proposed alternative ways for dealing with population heterogeneity. However, we believe that Bayesian inference for the LC model, which represents one of the most sensible ways to account for hetorogeneity between individuals, can be successfully used for capture-recapture data. Thus, our aim is to develop this type of inference using Markov chain Monte Carlo (MCMC) methods (Tierney, 1994) for estimation purposes. In particular, we consider models with a varying number of latent classes and take advantage of the Reversible Jump (RJ) strategy (Green, 1995), which allows joint inference about the model and the parameters. The RJ algorithm has recently been employed in Bayesian log-linear models for estimating population size by King and Brooks (2001). We improve the efficiency of the estimators obtained via RJ by using the Delayed Rejection (DR) strategy (Tierney and Mira, 1999; Green and Mira, 2001).

From the MCMC output, we can easily obtain a point estimate as well as a credibility interval for N. Furthermore, as a result of the simulation, we also get the estimated probability of the number of classes, given the data at hand, and the estimated posterior distribution for the model parameters, conditional on the number of classes.

The paper is organized as follows. In Section 2 we illustrate the LC model and the prior distributions on the parameters that we shall use for inference. In Section 3 we present the MCMC estimation approach based on the RJ and the DR algorithm. Finally, in Section 4, we analyse two real data sets, the first concerning the number of snowshoe hares in a certain region and the second concerning cases of diabetes in Casale Monferrato, Italy.

2. BAYESIAN LATENT CLASS MODEL

The basic assumption of the LC model is that the population is made of k homogeneous classes, in the sense that the subjects in any class share the same probability of being caught in the J lists. So, the probability of the capture configuration $\mathbf{r}$ is given by

$$p(\mathbf{r}) = \sum_{c=1}^{k} \pi_c \lambda(\mathbf{r} \mid c), \tag{1}$$

where π_c is the weight of the latent class c and $\lambda(\mathbf{r} \mid c)$ is the conditional probability of $\mathbf{r}$ for the subjects in the same class that, under the assumption of *local independence*, is given by

$$\lambda(\mathbf{r} \mid c) = \prod_{j=1}^{J} \lambda_{j|c}^{r_j} (1-\lambda_{j|c})^{1-r_j}, \tag{2}$$

where $\lambda_{j|c}$ is the conditional probability of being caught at the j-th occasion; the latter parameters will be collected into the vector $\boldsymbol{\lambda}$ by letting the index j run faster than c. Note that the model above is invariant to permutation of the class labels ($c = 1,\dots,k$) therefore we adopt a unique labeling in which the π_c are in increasing order.

We assume the following prior distributions for the parameters of the model above:

- the number of latent classes, k, has Uniform distribution between 1 and k_{max};
- the vector $\boldsymbol{\pi} = (\pi_1 \quad \cdots \quad \pi_k)^T$ has Dirichlet distribution with parameter $\mathbf{v} = (v_1 \quad \cdots \quad v_k)^T$, restricted to the set $\pi_1 < \pi_2 < \cdots < \pi_k$;
- for any j and c, $\lambda_{j|c}$ has Beta distribution with parameters $\boldsymbol{\beta} = (\beta_1 \quad \beta_2)^T$.

Moreover, given the parameters, we assume that the frequencies of the hypothetical table, including also the missing cell, follow the multinomial distribution with parameters N and $\{p(\mathbf{r})\}$. According to Sanathanan (1972), this implies that the likelihood of the observed frequencies, collected in the column vector $\mathbf{y} = \{y(\mathbf{r}), \mathbf{r} \neq \mathbf{0}\}$, is

$$L(\mathbf{y} \mid \mathbf{p}) = \prod_{r \neq 0} \left[\frac{p(\mathbf{r})}{\sum_{r \neq 0} p(\mathbf{r})} \right]^{y(\mathbf{r})},$$

with $\mathbf{p} = \{p(\mathbf{r}), \mathbf{r} \neq \mathbf{0}\}$.

3. BAYESIAN ESTIMATION

Our main aim is estimating the posterior distribution of N. For this purpose, we construct a Markov chain that has the posterior distribution of interest as its unique stationary and limiting distribution. Since the number of latent classes is not a priori fixed, we use the RJ algorithm (Green, 1995) to construct such a Markov chain. At any step of the algorithm, a candidate move is proposed and accepted with a probability that preserves reversibility with respect to the target posterior. As we show in the remaining part of this section, some of the moves try to jump between models with a different number of latent classes; the others simply update the parameters within the current model and so are of standard Metropolis-Hastings type. In order to improve the efficiency of the algorithm, we adopt the DR strategy (Green and Mira, 2001) for the moves of the first type, that is, upon rejection of a candidate move, instead of retaining the same position as done in a standard Metropolis-Hastings algorithm, we attempt a second stage move whose acceptance probability is appropriately computed. This strategy leads to an algorithm that dominates the standard RJ in the sense of the Peskun ordering (Peskun, 1973); thus, all the resulting MCMC estimates have a smaller asymptotic variance.

3.1 Updating the parameters of the current model

When we do not change the number of latent classes, a Metropolis-Hastings step is performed to update the parameters of the model. As proposal distribution for the weights of the latent classes we use the distribution

$$\text{Dirichlet}\left(\sigma\frac{\boldsymbol{\pi}}{\min(\boldsymbol{\pi})}\right),$$

where $\boldsymbol{\pi}$ denotes the current value of the weights and σ is a positive constant suitably chosen. If the entries of the proposed parameter vector, $\boldsymbol{\pi}'$, are not in increasing order, such a vector is discarded and a new one is drawn. Then, $\boldsymbol{\pi}'$ is accepted with probability

$$\min\left\{1,\frac{L(\mathbf{y}\,|\,\mathbf{p}')p(\boldsymbol{\pi}'\,|\,k)q(\boldsymbol{\pi}\,|\,\boldsymbol{\pi}',k)}{L(\mathbf{y}\,|\,\mathbf{p})p(\boldsymbol{\pi}\,|\,k)q(\boldsymbol{\pi}'\,|\,\boldsymbol{\pi},k)}\right\},$$

where $\boldsymbol{p}'$ is the proposed vector of joint probabilities whose entries are computed according to (1), $p(\boldsymbol{\pi}\,|\,k)$ denotes the density of the prior distribution of $\boldsymbol{\pi}$ and $q(\boldsymbol{\pi}'\,|\,\boldsymbol{\pi},k)$ denotes that of the proposal distribution. Note that, because of the constraint $\pi_1<\pi_2<\cdots<\pi_k$, these densities are equal to $k!$ times the corresponding Dirichlet densities.

The conditional probabilities of being caught, $\lambda_{j|c}$'s, are updated independently. For any j and c, we propose $\lambda'_{j|c}$ from the distribution $\text{Beta}(\upsilon,\omega)$, where $\upsilon=\left[\lambda_{j|c}(\omega-2)+1\right]/\left(1-\lambda_{j|c}\right)$ and $\omega=\alpha+b\pi_c$, with $\alpha>1$ and $b>0$; note that υ and ω are chosen so that the proposal distribution has mode equal to the current value of $\lambda_{j|c}$ and variance proportional to $1/\pi_c$. The proposed $\lambda'_{j|c}$ is then accepted with probability

$$\min\left\{1,\frac{L(\mathbf{y}\,|\,\mathbf{p}')p(\lambda'_{j|c}\,|\,k)q(\lambda_{j|c}\,|\,\lambda'_{j|c},k)}{L(\mathbf{y}\,|\,\mathbf{p})p(\lambda_{j|c}\,|\,k)q(\lambda'_{j|c}\,|\,\lambda_{j|c},k)}\right\},$$

where $p(\lambda_{j|c} \mid k)$ again denotes the density of the prior distribution and $q(\lambda'_{j|c} \mid \lambda_{j|c}, k)$ that of the proposal distribution.

3.2 Changing the number of latent classes

Updating the value of k implies a change of dimensionality for the parameters of the model. The approach we follow consists in a random choice between splitting an existing latent class into two and combining two existing latent classes into one. Using the standard notation (see, for instance, Green, 1995), we denote the probabilities of these alternatives by b_k and $d_k = 1 - b_k$, respectively, where k is the current number of latent classes. Of course, $b_1 = 1$ and $b_{k_{\max}} = 0$; otherwise, we choose $b_k = d_k = 0.5$, for $k = 2,3,\ldots,k_{\max} - 1$.

The **combine proposal** consists in randomly choosing a pair of adjacent latent classes (c_1, c_2) that we try to merge into a new one, labelled $c*$, whose parameters are chosen as follows

$$\pi'_{c*} = \pi_{c_1} + \pi_{c_2}$$

$$\lambda'_{j|c*} = \lambda_{j|c_2}, \qquad j = 1,\ldots,J .$$

The **split proposal** starts by choosing a latent class c^* at random that we try to split into two new ones, labeled c_1 and c_2, augmenting k by 1. The corresponding parameters are chosen as follows. We generate u and $v_j, j = 1,\ldots,J$, from Beta (2,4) and Beta (1,1), respectively; then, we set

$$\pi'_{c_1} = \pi_{c*} u, \qquad \pi'_{c_2} = \pi_{c*}(1-u),$$

$$\lambda'_{j|c_1} = v_j, \qquad \lambda'_{j|c_2} = \lambda_{j|c*}, \qquad j = 1,\ldots,J .$$

Obviously, we need to check that the constraints on the weights are satisfied.

According to the RJ recipe, the acceptance probability for the split move is

$$\alpha_1(\{\pi,\lambda\},\{\pi',\lambda'\}) = \min(1, A_1),$$

where

$$A_1 = \frac{L(\mathbf{y}\,|\,\mathbf{p}')}{L(\mathbf{y}\,|\,\mathbf{p})} \times \frac{p(k+1)}{p(k)} \times (k+1) \frac{\left(\pi'_{c_1}\right)^{\nu_{c_1}-1} \left(\pi'_{c_2}\right)^{\nu_{c_2}-1}}{\pi_{c*}^{\;\nu_{c*}-1}}$$

$$\times \prod_{j=1}^{J} \frac{1}{B(\beta_1,\beta_2)} \left(\frac{\lambda'_{j|c_1} \lambda'_{j|c_2}}{\lambda_{j|c*}} \right)^{\beta_1-1} \left[\frac{\left(1-\lambda'_{j|c_1}\right)\left(1-\lambda'_{j|c_2}\right)}{1-\lambda_{j|c*}} \right]^{\beta_2-1}$$

$$\times \frac{d_{k+1}}{b_k} \times \left[f(u,2,4) \prod_{j=1}^{J} f\left(v_j,1,1\right) \right]^{-1} \times \pi_{c*}, \tag{3}$$

B (r,q) is the Beta function and *f (x,r,q)* denotes the Beta *(r,q)* density. The first two lines of (3) are the product of the likelihood ratio ant the prior ratio for the parameters of the model. The third line is the product of the proposal ratio and the Jacobian of the transformation from $(\boldsymbol{\lambda},\boldsymbol{\pi})$ to $(\boldsymbol{\lambda}',\boldsymbol{\pi}')$.

The acceptance probability for the combine move is $\min\left(1, A_1^{-1}\right)$, with some obvious adjustments in the expression for A_1.

3.2.1 Delayed Rejection strategy

When a rejection decision is taken in either a split or a combine move, instead of advancing the simulation time and retaining the same position, we make another attempt to move according to the DR strategy of Tierney and Mira (1999). This second attempt is done also in the case in which a split or a combine move is rejected due to mis-ordering of the weights. If at the first stage we rejected a combine move, at the second stage we try again to combine two classes but with a more "timid" move, that is we merge the latent class c_2, chosen at the first stage of the RJ, with the latent class 1, i.e. the one with the smallest weight. We then chose the parameters of the new latent class as follows

$$\pi''_{c*} = \pi_1 + \pi_{c_2}$$

$$\lambda''_{j|c*} = \lambda_{j|c_2}, \qquad j = 1,\ldots,J\,.$$

If, instead, at the first stage we rejected a split proposal, at the second stage we try again to split the latent class $c*$, chosen at the first stage, but now into the latent classes 1 and c_2. The corresponding parameters are chosen as at the first stage, namely as

$$\pi''_1 = \pi_{c*}\tilde{u}, \qquad \pi''_{c_2} = \pi_{c*}\left(1-\tilde{u}\right),$$

$$\lambda''_{j|1} = \tilde{v}_j, \qquad \lambda''_{j|c_2} = \lambda_{j|c*}, \qquad j = 1,\ldots,J,$$

but in this case, the random number $\tilde{u}$ is generated from Beta (1,8), while $\tilde{v}_j$, $j = 1,\ldots,J$, is still generated from Beta (1,1). As before we need to check that the constraints on the weights $\boldsymbol{\pi}''$ are satisfied.

Following Green and Mira (2000), the second stage proposal is then accepted with probability equal to

$$\alpha_2\left(\{\boldsymbol{\pi},\boldsymbol{\lambda}\},\{\boldsymbol{\pi}'',\boldsymbol{\lambda}''\}\right) = \min\left(1, A_2\right),$$

where

$$A_2 = \frac{L(\mathbf{y}\,|\,\mathbf{p}'')}{L(\mathbf{y}\,|\,\mathbf{p})} \times \frac{p(k+1)}{p(k)} \times (k+1) \frac{\left(\pi''_1\right)^{v_1-1}\left(\pi''_{c_2}\right)^{v_{c_2}-1}}{\pi_{c*}^{v_{c*}-1}}$$

$$\times \prod_{j=1}^{J} \frac{1}{B(\beta_1,\beta_2)} \left(\frac{\lambda''_{j|1}\lambda''_{j|c_2}}{\lambda_{j|c*}}\right)^{\beta_1-1} \left[\frac{\left(1-\lambda''_{j|1}\right)\left(1-\lambda''_{j|c_2}\right)}{1-\lambda_{j|c*}}\right]^{\beta_2-1}$$

$$\times \frac{d_{k+1}}{b_k} \times \left[f(\tilde{u},1,8)\prod_{j=1}^{J} f(\tilde{v}_j,1,1)\right]^{-1} \times \pi_{c*}$$

$$\times \frac{1-\alpha_1\left(\{\boldsymbol{\pi}'',\boldsymbol{\lambda}''\},\{\boldsymbol{\pi}^{\dagger},\boldsymbol{\lambda}^{\dagger}\}\right)}{1-\alpha_1\left(\{\boldsymbol{\pi},\boldsymbol{\lambda}\},\{\boldsymbol{\pi}',\boldsymbol{\lambda}'\}\right)} \qquad (4)$$

and $\{\boldsymbol{\pi}^{\dagger},\boldsymbol{\lambda}^{\dagger}\}$ represents the first stage proposal in the reverse path from $\{\boldsymbol{\pi}'',\boldsymbol{\lambda}''\}$ to $\{\boldsymbol{\pi},\boldsymbol{\lambda}\}$; this is given by

$$\pi^{\dagger}_{c*} = \pi''_{c_1} + \pi''_{c_2}$$

$$\lambda^{\dagger}_{j|c*} = \lambda''_{j|c_2}, \qquad j = 1,\ldots,J.$$

The last line in (4) is now the ratio between the rejection probabilities of the first stage moves (for the forward path at the denominator and for the hypothetical reverse path at the denominator).

The acceptance probability for the second stage combine move is $\min\left(1, A_2^{-1}\right)$, with some obvious adjustments in the expression for A_2 and with

$$\pi^{\dagger}_{c_1} = \pi''_{c*} u\,, \quad \pi^{\dagger}_{c_2} = \pi''_{c*}(1-u),$$

$$\lambda^{\dagger}_{j|c_1} = v_j, \qquad \lambda^{\dagger}_{j|c_2} = \lambda''_{j|c*}, \qquad j = 1,\ldots,J\,.$$

Green and Mira (2001) showed that this second stage acceptance probability preserves reversibility (and thus stationarity) of the Markov chain with respect to the posterior distribution of interest.

3.3 Inference from the MCMC output

At the end of the algorithm, we obtain a sample drawn from the joint posterior distribution of $(\boldsymbol{\pi} \;\; \boldsymbol{\lambda} \;\; k)$; we denoted this sample by $(\boldsymbol{\pi}^{(t)} \;\; \boldsymbol{\lambda}^{(t)} \;\; k^{(t)})$, t = 1,...,T, where T is the number of sweeps. From this output, we can estimate the posterior probability of k as the ratio between the number of times the algorithm visited the model with k latent classes and the total number of sweeps.

For any sweep t we also have that the ratio $n/(\mathbf{1}'\mathbf{p}^{(t)})$ is an estimate of the population size. Averaging these estimates across all the MCMC sweeps gives an "overall" point estimate of the population size, i.e.

$$\hat{N} = \frac{1}{T}\sum_{t=1}^{T}\frac{n}{\mathbf{1}'\mathbf{p}^{(t)}}\,.$$

Credibility intervals can also be easily obtained. Notice that overall estimates are calculated without choosing a specific number of latent classes and, in this sense, they take into account the uncertainty existing about the model. In addition, it is possible to obtain "with-in" model estimates, by averaging across the MCMC sweeps, conditional on fixed values of k.

Even if the focus of our analysis is on estimating the population size, evaluation of the marginal probability of appearing in any list can also be of interest; this is particularly useful when different capturing sources need to be compared on the basis of their effectiveness. Let λ_j denote such probability for the j-th list; a natural MCMC estimator for this quantity is

$$\hat{\lambda}_j = \frac{1}{T}\sum_{t=1}^{T}\sum_{c=1}^{k^{(t)}}\lambda^{(t)}_{j|c}\pi^{(t)}_c\,.$$

4. APPLICATIONS

The method for estimating the population size illustrated so far is applied to two different capture-recapture data sets. In the RJ sampler with DR, the following settings were used for previously unspecified constants: $k_{max} = 10$, $\nu = 1$, $\beta = 1$, $\sigma = 10$, a =2 and b =10. Simulation studies not reported here indicate that results are quite robust to reasonable perturbations of these values.

4.1 Rabbits Redux

The first data set refers to a population of snowshoe hares. The study reported by Cormack (1992) is based on J=6 consecutive trapping days. The data set has also been analysed by Agresti (1994). The data on the 68 observed animals are presented in Table 1. The 63 observable cells are given in the standard order 000001, 000010, 000011, ... by rows in the table.

Table 1. Results of capture-recapture of snowshoe hares and estimated probabilities of capture configurations (in italic).

-	4	4	2	3	4	1	1	5	2	0	1	0	1	0	0
9.7	*4.6*	*3.7*	*1.9*	*3.6*	*2.5*	*1.4*	*1.1*	*2.7*	*1.6*	*1.0*	*0.7*	*1.1*	*1.1*	*0.4*	*0.6*
6	1	3	1	3	3	0	1	0	2	0	1	0	2	0	1
4.2	*2.6*	*1.8*	*1.2*	*1.9*	*2.0*	*0.8*	*1.0*	*1.2*	*1.2*	*0.5*	*0.7*	*0.6*	*1.2*	*0.3*	*0.9*
3	1	2	0	2	0	0	1	1	0	1	0	1	0	0	0
2.8	*1.2*	*1.2*	*0.6*	*1.0*	*0.7*	*0.5*	*0.3*	*0.9*	*0.5*	*0.4*	*0.3*	*0.4*	*0.3*	*0.2*	*0.2*
0	1	1	0	0	0	0	0	0	0	0	0	0	0	0	2
1.1	*0.6*	*0.5*	*0.4*	*0.5*	*0.5*	*0.3*	*0.4*	*0.3*	*0.3*	*0.2*	*0.3*	*0.2*	*0.4*	*0.1*	*0.4*

The results reported here correspond to 100 000 sweeps of the MCMC algorithm, including a burn-in of 50 000 sweeps. The algorithm seems to mix well over the parameter space, with an acceptance rate of the split/combine move approximately equal to 15% at the first stage and to 20% at the second stage. A plot of the changes in k against the number of sweeps is presented in Figure 1(a) (for sake of clarity, data are plotted every 100 sweeps). It shows that the MCMC algorithm mixes well over k, excursions into very high values being short-lived. A useful check on the stationarity is given by the plot of the cumulative occupancy fractions for different values of k against the number of sweeps. This is presented in Figure 1(b), where it can be seen that the burn-in is more than adequate to achieve stability in the occupancy fractions.

Estimated posterior probabilities for k are given in Figure 1(c). It is immediately apparent that there are a number of competing explanations of the data which are tenable. The posterior for k favors 2 to 4 latent classes.

Agresti (1994) also found the ordinary LC model, as well as the quasi-symmetric model, with two classes to fit the data quite well. However, in our context, we do not need to choose a specific number of latent classes, and we can take into account the uncertainty existing about the model, overcoming the model-dependence problem of the classical approach.

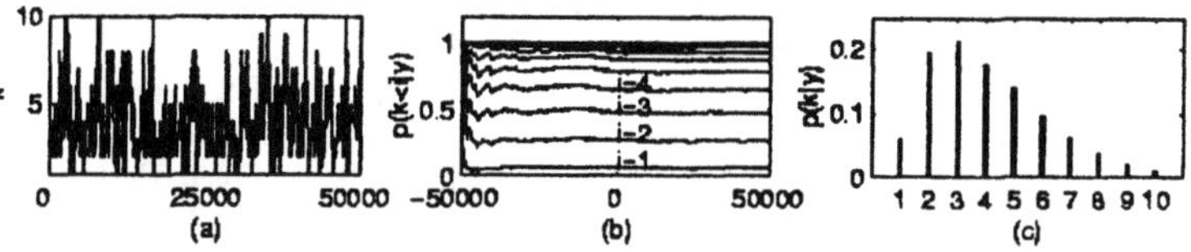

Figure 1. Example of trace of k for 50 000 sweeps after burn-in (a), cumulative occupancy fractions for complete run including burn-in (b) and posterior distribution of k (c).

Overall point estimates for the probability of each capture configuration are given in Table 1. Cellwise inspection reveals a good fit of the model to the observed data. Table 2 provides the posterior model probabilities for the a posteriori most probable models, together with the corresponding with-in model estimates and 95% credibility intervals for N. Overall estimates are also presented, as well as the results obtained by Agresti (1994) with different classical LC models. The overall estimate for N that we obtain is 77.7, suggesting that only 10 snowshoe hares were missed by all 6 trapping occasions. Agresti (1994) obtains a very similar result using a quasi-symmetric LC model with 2 classes. Our overall credibility interval is (72.2, 87.3), which is larger than the confidence interval found by Agresti (1994) for the quasi-symmetric model, but smaller than those he found for ordinary models with 2 or 3 latent classes. It is probably worthwhile to spend a few words on this result. Agresti (1994) stresses that for such sparse data, quite different models can appear to fit adequately yet can provide highly diverse point and interval estimates of N. Particularly with small sample sizes, a model selection procedure may suggest a model that is much simpler than the one that truly represents reality well, leading to confidence intervals for N that tend to be too narrow. We believe, therefore, that the overall credibility interval we estimated, properly reflecting our uncertainty on the "true" model, is not affected by this problem. For this reason it is not as "optimistic" as the one for the simple quasi-symmetric model. On the other side, it has the advantage of being narrower than the confidence intervals found by Agresti for models more complicated than the quasi-symmetric one.

The estimates of the probability of being caught at the j-th occasion are presented in Table 3. In the present case there are no relevant differences between the capture occasions, i.e. between the six consecutive trapping days, revealing that the captures were likely performed under the same conditions.

Table 2. Posterior model probabilities for most probable models, together with point and interval estimates of population size.

Model	Posterior probability	Estimate of N	95% CI
Bayesian latent class			
$k = 2$	0.192	79.0	(72.7, 89.0)
$k = 3$	0.211	78.3	(72.5, 87.8)
$k = 4$	0.176	78.0	(72.4, 87.9)
Model-averaged		77.7	(72.2, 87.3)
Classical latent class			
Quasi-symmetric, $k = 2$		77.3	(73.1, 84.9)
Ordinary, $k = 2$		85.2	(76.2, 104.0)
Ordinary, $k = 3$		81.3	(72.0, 103.6)

Table 3. Point and interval estimates of the probabilities of being caught at different occasions.

	$j = 1$	$j = 2$	$j = 3$	$j = 4$	$j = 5$	$j = 6$
λ_j	0.23	0.37	0.28	0.35	0.31	0.42
95% CI	(0.14,0.33)	(0.26,0.49)	(0.18,0.38)	(0.24,0.46)	(0.21,0.42)	(0.30,0.53)

4.2 Diabetes study

The data in Table 4 are taken from Bruno *et al.* (1994) and refer to 2069 cases of diabetes in a small town in northern Italy recorded in October 1988 on the basis of four different lists: (i) clinics (all patients diagnosed as diabetics by the local clinic and/or family physicians); (ii) hospitals (all patients discharged with a primary or secondary diagnosis of diabetes in all private and public hospitals in the region); (iii) prescriptions (a computerized list of insulin and hypoglycemic prescriptions); (iv) reimbursement (all patients who requested reimbursement for insulin and reagent strips). The same dataset is also analysed by Yip *et al.* (1995a), Biggeri *et al.* (1999), Fienberg *et al.* (1999) and Bartolucci and Forcina (2001).

Table 4. Data from prevalent cases of known diabetes for resident of Casale Monferrato, Piemonte, Italy, and estimated probabilities of capture configurations (in italic).

-	10	182	8	74	7	20	14	709	12	650	46	104	18	157	58
506.2	*8.9*	*179.4*	*8.3*	*72.2*	*7.1*	*27.6*	*12.8*	*708.3*	*16.8*	*649.2*	*45.0*	*102.2*	*18.0*	*155.1*	*58.2*

For this dataset, the MCMC algorithm mixes slightly slower than for the previous one. This is is due to the fact that now the cell counts are larger, the posterior densities under the different models are more picked and, therefore, it is slightly harder to jump from a model to another one. For this reason, we allowed for a longer burn-in: we run 200 000 sweeps of the algorithm and discarded the first 150 000 as burn-in. The slower mixing also determined a high autocorrelation in the MCMC output, with an *integrated autocorrelation time* (see Section 5) equal to 3118.2. In order to reduce this autocorrelation and, consequently, the variance of the estimates, we sub-sampled from the MCMC output and considered only one every 10 sweeps for estimating purpose. This reduced the integrated autocorrelation time to 311.5.

Looking at the changes in k (Figure 2(a)) and cumulative occupancy fractions (Figure 2(b)), it can be seen that the mixing is still satisfactory (with an acceptance rate of the split/combine move approximately equal to 4% at the first stage and to 8% at the second stage) and the algorithm eventually converges. For this dataset, the posterior density for k is more concentrated than for the previous one. The three most probable models, i.e. those with 3, 4 and 5 latent classes, have a total posterior density equal to 0.97. Moreover, models with 1, 2 and 10 latent classes are never visited. The most probable model seems to be the one with 3 latent classes. Notice that both Biggeri *et al.* (1999) and Bartolucci and Forcina (2001) consider models with only 2 latent classes. However, given the latent class, they allow for interactions between the different lists while we do not. This is likely the reason why we found models with a larger number of latent classes to fit the data better.

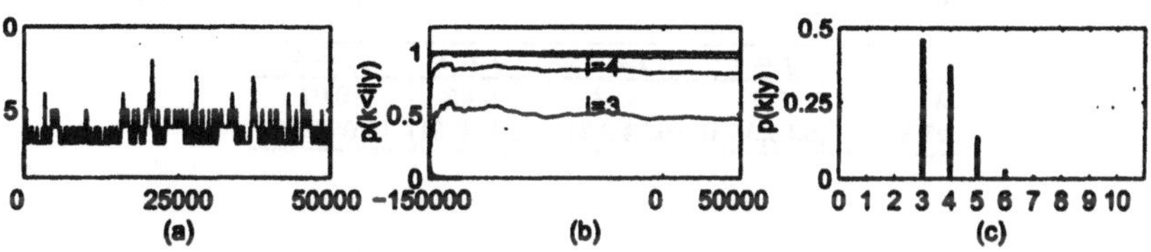

Figure 2. Example of trace of k for 50 000 sweeps after burn-in (a), cumulative occupancy fractions for complete run including burn-in (b) and posterior distribution of k (c).

Table 5 shows with-in model and overall estimates and credibility intervals for N, compared with the results obtained by Biggeri *et al.* (1999) and Bartolucci and Forcina (2001). Note that the with-in model estimates and credibility intervals are based on the whole MCMC run, without sub-sampling, to avoid the risk of calculating estimates on a too small number of runs.

Both the with-in model and the overall estimates of N we obtained are in between the one obtained by Bartolucci and Forcina (2001) and the one obtained by Biggeri *et al.* (1999). Moreover our credibility intervals include both the confidence intervals in Bartolucci and Forcina (2001) and in Biggeri *et al.* (1999). It is also interesting to notice that, as the number of latent classes considered increases, the estimate of N decreases and the credibility interval gets larger and larger.

Table 5. Posterior model probabilities for most probable models, together with point and interval estimates of population size.

Model	Posterior probability	Estimate of N	95% CI
Bayesian latent class			
$k = 3$	0.463	2616.0	(2275.5, 3154.0)
$k = 4$	0.370	2543.2	(2274.1, 3233.3)
$k = 5$	0.132	2534.3	(2269.1, 3355.3)
Model-averaged		2575.5	(2273.6, 3204.2)
Classical latent class			
Biggeri *et al.* (1999)		2696	(2502, 2950)
Bartolucci and Forcina (2001)		2403	(2280, 2585)

In Table 6 the estimated probabilities of being caught by the different lists are reported. For this dataset, a considerable heterogeneity between lists is evident. The list clinics in the one with the highest "catchability" followed by prescriptions, hospitals and reimbursements. This ordering of the lists with respect to their catchability is completely consistent with that found in Bartolucci and Forcina (2001).

Table 6. Point and interval estimates of the probabilities of being caught by the different lists.

	$j = 1$	$j = 2$	$j = 3$	$j = 4$
λ_j	0.69	0.18	0.45	0.07
95% CI	(0.55,0.78)	(0.14,0.21)	(0.35,0.51)	(0.05,0.08)

5. COMPARING DELAYED REJECTION AND STANDARD REVERSIBLE JUMP SAMPLER

In general, comparing the performance of MCMC samplers is not an easy task. Following Green and Mira (2001), we define 'performance' as the efficiency in estimating the expectation $E(\phi)$ of a given function ϕ on the state space, under the stationary distribution of the Markov chain. For our comparisons we focus on estimating the population size (this specifies indirectly the function ϕ).

There are two quantities to take into account when comparing the performance of the MCMC samplers: the running time R needed to obtain a fixed number of sweeps T plus a fixed number of burn-in steps, and the integrated autocorrelation time, $\tau=\sum_{k=-\infty}^{\infty}\rho_h$ where $\rho_h=\mathrm{Cov}[\phi(X_0),\phi(X_h)]/\sigma^2$, is the lag-$h$ autocorrelation, X_t being the value of the Markov chain at time t, and σ^2 is the variance of ϕ under the stationary distribution (assumed to be finite). The product of τ and R gives a reasonable measure of the efficiency of an MCMC algorithm: it estimates the running time needed to obtain the same precision in estimating $E(\phi)$ as from T independent draws from the stationary distribution.

In our comparison it is reasonable to believe the two codes developed are similarly efficient (and thus an average of the running times of a few simulations is a good estimate of R) since a two stage DR algorithm is compared with a one-stage algorithm (i.e. a standard RJ), which actually forms the first stage of the DR, therefore the DR code is a superset of the other.

To estimate τ we used Sokal's adaptive truncated periodogram estimator (Sokal, 1989), $\sum_{|h|\le M}\hat{\rho}_h$ where the window width M is chosen adaptively as the minimum integer such that $M\ge 3\hat{\tau}$. We used the fast Fourier transform to estimate the autocorrelations $\hat{\rho}_h$.

The value in the column named 'ratio' is the ratio of R times $\hat{\tau}$ for the standard RJ method and the DR algorithm. Thus values greater than one indicate how much more efficient the DR strategy is. We know that by the Peskun-Tierney theorem (Peskun, 1973; Thierney, 1998) the DR algorithm will always give smaller values of τ than a regular Metropolis-Hastings algorithm, for every function of interest ϕ.

Table 7 and 8 are obtained by averaging 10 simulations and refer to the examples studied in Section 4.1 and 4.2 respectively.

Typically, for a given number of steps, a DR algorithm has a running time which is larger than the corresponding one stage MCMC algorithm, since the DR strategy consists in trying harder to move away from the current position (and this takes simulation time). Still, in both tables the value in the column named ratio shows that the gain in terms of asymptotic efficiency due to the DR strategy more than compensates for the extra computational time needed to run the DR algorithm.

The high value of $\hat{\tau}$ in Table 8 has motivated the much larger sample size and burn-in used in Section 4.2 to draw our inference and the need for subsampling.

Table 7. Rabbits: T = 10 000 burn-in = 5 000

	no delay		delay		ratio
	R in hours	$\hat{\tau}$	R in hours	$\hat{\tau}$	
N	1.82	31.79	1.85	25.87	1.21

Table 8. Diabetes: T = 100 000 burn-in = 50 000

	no delay		delay		ratio
	R in hours	$\hat{\tau}$	R in hours	$\hat{\tau}$	
N	4.70	3134.8	4.83	2033.2	1.50

ACKNOWLEDGEMENTS

This work has been partially supported by the *"Progetti di eccellenza 2002/3"* founds granted by the University of Insubria, Varese, Italy.

REFERENCES

AGRESTI, A. (1994). Simple capture-recapture models permitting unequal catchability and variable sampling effort. *Biometrics 50*, 494-500.

BARTOLUCCI, F. AND FORCINA, A. (2001). The Analysis of Capture-Recapture Data with a Rasch-type Model allowing for Conditional Dependence and Multidimensionality. *Biometrics 57*,714-719.

BASU, S. AND EBRAHIMI, N. (2001). Bayesian capture-recapture methods for error detection and estimation of population size: hetorogeneity and dependence. *Biometrika 88*, 269-279.

BIGGERI, A., STANGHELLINI, E., MERLETTI, F. AND MARCHI, M. (1999). Latent class models for varying catchability and correlation among sources in capture-recapture estimation of the size of a human population. *Statistica Applicata 11*, 563-586.

BRUNO, G., BIGGERI, A., MERLETTI, F., LAPORTE, R., MCCARTHY, D. AND PAGANO, G. (1994). Applications of capture-recapture to count diabetes. *Diabetes Care* 17, 548-556.

CASTLEDINE, B. J. (1981), A Bayesian analysis of multiple-recapture sampling for a closed population, *Biometrika 68*, 197-210.

CORMACK, R. M. (1992). Interval estimation for mark-recapture studies of closed populations. *Biometrics* 48, 567-576.

DARROCH, J. N. (1958). The multiple-recapture census I. Estimation of a closed population. *Biometrika 45*, 343-359.

DARROCH, J. N., FIENBERG, S. E., GLONEK, G. F. V. AND JUNKER, B. W. (1993). A three-sample multiple-recapture approach to census population estimation with heterogeneous catchability. *Journal of the American Statistical Association 88*, 1137-1148.

FIENBERG, S. E. (1972). The multiple recapture census for closed populations and incomplete 2^k contingency tables. *Biometrika 59*, 591-603.

FIENBERG, S. E., JOHNSON, M. S. AND JUNKER, B. W. (1999). Classical multilevel and Bayesian approaches to population size estimation using multiple lists. *Journal of the Royal Statistical Society A 162*, 383-405.

GEORGE, E. I. AND ROBERT, C. P. (1992). Capture-recapture estimation via Gibbs sampling. *Biometrika 79*, 677-683.

GREEN, P. J. (1995), Reversible jump Markov chain Monte Carlo computation and Bayesian model determination. *Biometrika 82*, 711-732.

GREEN, P. J. AND MIRA, A. (2001), Delayed Rejection in Reversible Jump Metropolis-Hastings. *Biometrika 88*, 1035-1053.

KING, R. AND BROOKS, S. P. (2001). On the Bayesian analysis of population size. *Biometrika 88*, 317-336.

LINDSAY, B., CLOGG, C. AND GREGO, J. (1991). Semiparametric estimation in the Rasch model and related exponential response models, including a simple latent class model for item analysis. *Journal of the American Statistical Association 86*, 96- 107.

MADIGAN, D. AND YORK, J. C. (1997). Bayesian methods for estimation of the size of a closed population. *Biometrika 84*, 19- 31.

PESKUN, P. H. (1973). Optimum Monte Carlo sampling using Markov chains. *Biometrika 60*, 607-612.

SANATHANAN, L. (1972). Estimating the size of a multinomial population. *The Annals of Mathematical Statistics 43*, 142-152.

SCHNABEL, Z. E. (1938). The estimation of the total fish population of a lake. *American Mathematical Monthly 45*, 348-52.

SCHWARZ, C. J. AND SEBER, A. F. (1999). Estimating animal abundance: review III. *Statistical Science 14*, 427-456.

SMITH, P. J. (1991). Bayesian analyses for a multiple capture-recapture model. *Biometrika 78*, 399-407.

SOKAL, A. D. (1989). Monte Carlo methods in statistical mechanics: foundations and new algorithms. *Cours de Troisième Cycle de la Phisyque en Suisse Romande*, Lausanne.

TARDELLA, L. (2002). A new Bayesian method for nonparametric capture-recapture models in presence of heterogeneity. *Biometrika 89*, 807-817.

TIERNEY, L. (1994). Markov chains for exploring posterior distributions. *Annals of Statistics 22*, 1701-1762.

TIERNEY, L. (1998). A Note on Metropolis-Hastings kernels for general state spaces. *Annals of Applied Probability 8*, 1-9.

TIERNEY, L. AND MIRA, A. (1999). Some adaptive Monte Carlo methods for Bayesian inference. *Statistics in Medicine 18*, 2507-2515.

YIP, P. S. F., BRUNO, C., TAJIMA, N., SEBER, C. A. F., BUCKLAND, S. T., CORMACK, R. M., UNWIN, N., CHANG, Y.-F., FIENBERG, S. E., JUNKER, B. W., LAPORTE, R. E., LIBMAN, I. M. AND MCCARTY, D. J. (1995a). Capture-recapture and multiple-record systems estimation I: history and theoretical development. *American Journal of Epidemiology 142*, 1047-1058.

YIP, P. S. F., BRUNO, C., TAJIMA, N., SEBER, C. A. F., BUCKLAND, S. T., CORMACK, R. M., UNWIN, N., CHANG, Y.-F., FIENBERG, S. E., JUNKER, B. W., LAPORTE, R. E., LIBMAN, I. M. AND MCCARTY, D. J. (1995b). Capture-recapture and multiple-record systems estimation II: applications in human diseases. *American Journal of Epidemiology 142*, 1059-1068.

Chapter 3

ON THE BAYESIAN INFERENCE OF THE HARDY-WEINBERG EQUILIBRIUM MODEL

F. Bertolino* and A. Ratto
Department of Mathematics, University of Cagliari, via Ospedale 72, 09124 Cagliari, Italy.

1. INTRODUCTION

If we look through the literature concerning the genetic *equilibrium of Hardy-Weinberg*, hereafter H - We, then we have no difficulty to ascertain that the works which adopt a frequentist point of view are far more numerous than those which are carried out in a Bayesian perspective. A possible explanation for the limited interest shown by subjectivists towards those matters may well be the opinion that standard techniques are largely sufficient.

However, in this scenario two exceptions are present. Namely, the works of Pereira and Rogatko (1984) and of Lindley (1988), where, for the first time, it was pointed out that the Bayesian analysis of the H - We is affected by an ambiguity which is a direct implication of the *Borel-Kolmogorov paradox*, hereafter B - Kp, a fact which can lead to non-univocal inferential conclusions. Indeed, as a direct consequence of the B - Kp, conditioning a probability density function, hereafter *p.d.f.*, to a measure zero subset yields a result which depends on the parametrization of the sample model and on the specific limit procedure which is adopted.

After the above mentioned work of Lindley, the lack of specific methods to tackle the effects of the B - Kp has probably been the main reason why Bayesian statisticians have not devoted further efforts to study the H - We.

In our opinion, the analysis of the H - We is an interesting starting point for the development of a systematic method that can also be applied to

* For correspondence: bertolin@unica.it

several other classical statistical problems. However, the present paper will only be concerned with the analysis of the following two problems, both well-known to scientists working in genetics: *(i)* how can we test the hypothesis that a given population is in the *H – We? (ii)* if the population is in the *H - We*, how can we determine the *p.d.f.* of the allelic proportions?

We shall make the following two assumptions: an expert has provided us with some a priori information about the population, and a certain set of observations is available.

In order to evaluate the diversity between different inferential conclusions, we shall introduce a suitable *index of paradoxality*. In particular, our analysis of artificial, but realistic, data will show that the *B-Kp* may lead, in problem *(i)*, to relevant differences between inferential conclusions, even if the number of observations is large.

By contrast, the analysis of problem *(ii)* is much less infuenced by the *B-Kp*. In particular, the *p.d.f.*'s induced by different parametrizations of the model are not far from each other, even when the sample size n is small. Moreover, the differences tend to zero as $n \rightarrow \infty$.

To end this introduction, we also recall that other satisfactory Bayesian solutions which evidence the presence of the *B-Kp* in the *H-We* test are furnished in Pereira and Rogatko (1984) and Lindley (1988). Difficulties associated with this paradox are discussed in these papers.

For an elementary exposition of the *B-Kp*, see DeGroot (1986), p.171. Geometric techniques to compute *p.d.f.*'s, conditionally to measure null events, were developed in detail in Bertolino and Ratto (2002).

Our work is organized as follows. Section 2 analyzes the *H-We* which is assumed as the null hypothesis, while the alternative hypothesis is the departure from *H-We*. We consider two different disequilibrium models: the first is described by a Dirichlet distribution, the second is a particular *disequilibrium* model due to Bernstein. These examples show that the inferential conclusions, drawn by these two particular disequilibrium models, differ to some extent.

One of the main features of these examples is the dependency of the Bayes factor on the choice of the sample model parametrization, a fact which, as we stress again, will justify both the need for precaution and the introduction of a measure of paradoxality.

Section 3 contains final comments and remarks. An Appendix includes a summary of the basic ideas introduced in Bertolino and Ratto (2002).

2. THE HARDY-WEINBERG EQUILIBRIUM

For the sake of simplicity, we shall assume that, in a given population, a certain allele is present in two forms, say A and a. Let $t \in (0,1)$ be the proportion of the allele A in the population and $\mathbf{y} = (y_1, y_2, y_3)$ the vector of the proportions of the genotypes AA, Aa and aa, (Aa and aA are phenotypically indistinguishable). Note that the vector $\mathbf{y}$ belongs to the *simplex* $\mathcal{Y} = \{\mathbf{y} \in \mathbb{R}^3 : \Sigma_i y_i = 1, y_i > 0, \forall i\}$.

As it is well-known, we say that a *closed* population is in *H-We* if the following conditions hold: *(ci)* the matings are (genetically) random: $\Pr_{HW}\{A \cap A\} = t^2, \Pr_{HW}\{(A \cap a) \cup (a \cap A)\} = 2t(1-t), \Pr_{HW}\{a \cap a\} = (1-t)^2$ *(c2)* the genotypes AA, Aa and aa have the same fertility and there exists no selection against a particular genotype.

In particular, in the case of the *H-We*, vector $\mathbf{y}$ belongs to the curve $\gamma \subset \mathcal{Y}$ given by

$$\gamma : \{y_1 = t^2, y_2 = 2t(1-t), y_3 = (1-t)^2, t \in (0,1)\}. \tag{1}$$

In this notation, problem *(i)* of the Introduction, $\{H_0 : H-We,$ *versus* $H_1 : \overline{H}_0\}$ is equivalent to testing the system of hypotheses $\{H_0 : \mathbf{y} \in \gamma \text{ versus } H_1 : \mathbf{y} \notin \gamma\}$.

After discussion with some biologist, prior information about the population is available. We suppose that the biologist elicits the prior probability $\pi_0 = \Pr\{H_0\}$ of the hypothesis H_0; he also asserts that the proportions of the genotypes follow the Dirichlet law

$$(Y_1, Y_2) \sim \mathcal{D}(y_1, y_2 | \boldsymbol{\alpha}) = \frac{1}{B(\alpha_1, \alpha_2, \alpha_3)} y_1^{\alpha_1 - 1} y_2^{\alpha_2 - 1} (1 - y_1 - y_2)^{\alpha_3 - 1} \mathbf{1}_{\mathcal{Y}^*}(y_1, y_2) \tag{2}$$

where $\mathcal{Y}^*$ denotes the simplex $\mathcal{Y}^* = \{(y_1, y_2) \in \mathbb{R}^2 : y_1 + y_2 < 1, y_j > 0, \forall j\}$ and $\boldsymbol{\alpha} = (\alpha_1, \alpha_2, \alpha_3), \alpha_i > 0 \forall i$, are the *hyperparameters* assessed by the biologist, with $B(\alpha_1, \alpha_2, \alpha_3) = \Gamma(\alpha_1)\Gamma(\alpha_2)\Gamma(\alpha_3)(\Gamma(\alpha))^{-1}$ and $\alpha = \sum_i \alpha_i$.

Now we suppose that condition *(c1)* is not verified, i.e. we observe in the population numerous consanguineous matings (*inbreeding*), while condition *(c2)* is still reasonable.

In this case, the biologist has elements to support the conjecture that the population has evolved towards a particular disequilibrium model introduced first by Bernstein in 1930. To this regard, see Emery (1976) and Lindley (1988).

According to *(c1)*, the probability that the second allele is *A[a]*, when also the first is A[a], is given by $\Pr_{HW}\{A|A\}=\Pr\{A\}=t\left[\Pr_{HW}\{a|a\}=\Pr\{a\}=1-t\right]$. By contrast, according to the Bernstein model, we have now $\Pr_{HW}\{A|A\}=u\left[\Pr\{a|a\}=v\right]$, where the vector *(u,v)* belongs to the unit square $Q=(0,1)\times(0,1)$. In words, *u[v]* represents the probability that the second allele is identical to the first, when the first is *A[a]*.

It follows that the frequencies of the genotypes *AA*, *Aa* and *aa* are now

$$\begin{cases} y_1=\Pr\{A\}\Pr\{A|A\}=tu, \\ y_2=\Pr\{A\}\Pr\{a|A\}+\Pr\{a\}\Pr\{A|a\}=t(1-u)+(1-t)(1-v), \\ y_2=\Pr\{a\}\Pr\{a|a\}=(1-t)v. \end{cases}$$

According to *(c2)*, the proportion of the allele *A* is constant in the population

$$\Pr\{A\}=tu+\frac{1}{2}\left[t(1-u)+(1-t)(1-v)\right]=t$$

from which we easily obtain

$$t=\frac{1-v}{2-u-v}.$$

In this way, the vector $\mathbf{y}=(y_1,y_2,y_3)$ can be expressed as a function of *(u,v), i.e.*,

$$\left\{y_1=\frac{u(1-v)}{2-u-v}, y_2=2\frac{(1-u)(1-v)}{2-u-v}, y_3=\frac{(1-u)v}{2-u-v}\right\} \tag{3}$$

Since the Jacobian associated with the transformation (3) is given by $|J|=2(1-u)(1-v)(2-u-v)^{-3}$, instead of prior (2) we have the prior *p.d.f.*

$$(U,V) \sim \mathcal{D}_b(u,v|\alpha) =$$

$$= \frac{2^{\alpha_2}}{B(\alpha_1,\alpha_2,\alpha_3)} \frac{u^{\alpha_1-1}(1-u)^{\alpha_2+\alpha_3-1} v^{\alpha_3-1}(1-v)^{\alpha_1+\alpha_2-1}}{(2-u-u)^{\alpha}} 1_Q(u,v). \tag{4}$$

We note that, in this new context, the *H-We* corresponds to the case that $\Pr_{HW}\{A|A\} = u = \Pr_{HW}\{A|a\} = 1-v$. In other words, the *H-We* is equivalent to the fact that the vector *(u,v)* belongs to the line $\rho \subset \mathcal{Q}$, given by equation $v = 1-u$, or in parametric form

$$\rho : \{u = t, v = 1-t, t \in (0,1)\}. \tag{5}$$

Although (3) determines the transformation $\mathcal{Y} \Leftrightarrow \mathcal{Q}$ (and consequently the transformation, $\gamma \Leftrightarrow \rho$), we stress the fact that (3) represents more than a mere change of variables. As we shall comment more in detail in the conclusions of our work, we point out that working with the vector *(u,v)*, in place of (y_1,y_2,y_3), suggests that any shifting away from the *H-We* appears in the form described by the Bernstein disequilibrium model.

Our analysis of the *H-We* assumes that a random sample is taken from the population. Let *n* independent trials be made and let $\mathbf{n} = (n_1, n_2, n_3)$ be a vector whose components $n_i \in \mathbb{N}_{\{0\}} \forall_i$ and $n = \sum_i n_i$,denote the numbers of trials resulting *AA*, *Aa* and *aa*. The probability distribution of data is given by the multinomial law

$$(N_1 N_2) | \mathbf{y} \sim \mathcal{M}(n_1 n_2 | \mathbf{y}, n) = \binom{n}{n_1, n_2, n_3} y_1^{n_1} y_2^{n_2} (1-y_1-y_2)^{n_3}$$

Given the prior (2) and **n** it is easy to obtain the posterior *p.d.f.* of the genotypic proportions $(Y_1,Y_2)|\mathbf{n} \sim \mathcal{D}(y_1, y_2 | \alpha')$, where $\alpha_i' = \alpha_i + n_i, \forall i$. In a similar way, if we assume the Bernstein model, from (4) we deduce the posterior *p.d.f.* $(U,V)|\mathbf{n} \sim \mathcal{D}_b(u,v|\alpha')$.

Example 1

Suppose that the expert elicits $\alpha_1 = 2, \alpha_2 = 5.6, \alpha_3 = 4.4$ and that the frequencies $n_1 = 2$, $n_2 = 11$, $n_3 = 9$ are observed. Figure 1.a [1.b] shows the curve γ [the line ρ] and the equal *p.d.f.* contours of the prior density $\mathcal{D}(y_1, y_2 \mid \alpha)$ on $\mathcal{Y}$ $\left[\mathcal{D}_b(u,v|\alpha) \text{ on } \mathcal{Q}\right]$. Figure 1.c [1.d] shows the curve γ[the line ρ] and the equal density contours of the posterior *p.d.f.* $\mathcal{D}(y_1, y_2 \mid \alpha')$ on $\mathcal{Y}$ $\left[\mathcal{D}_b(u,v|\alpha') \text{ on } \mathcal{Q}\right]$ for the same α_i's. The circumstance that γ $[\rho]$ intersects the equal density contours of $\mathcal{D}(y_1, y_2|\alpha')$ on $\mathcal{Y}\left[\mathcal{D}_b(u,v|\alpha') \text{ on } \mathcal{Q}\right]$ on having higher density is an evidence which supports the *H-We*.

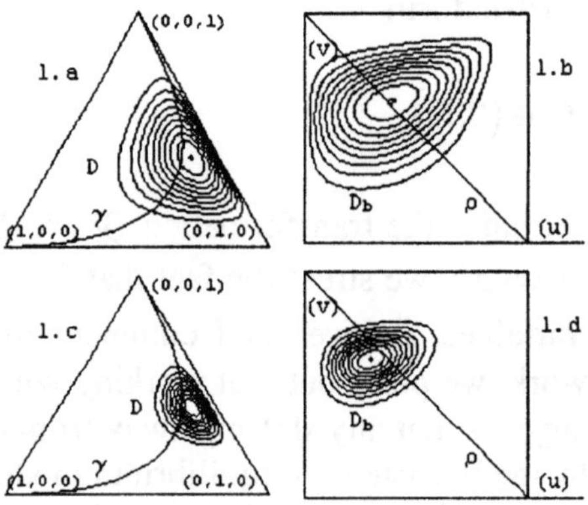

Figure 1. Equal density contours of the prior and posterior densities of (y_1, y_2, y_3) and (u,v) of, respectively in the simplex $\mathcal{Y}$ and in the simplex $\mathcal{Q}$.

The aim of the test is to establish whether this hypothesis is to be accepted or not. The following subsections will consider problems *(i)* e *(ii)* separately.

2.1 Problem (*i*): the Hardy-Weinberg equilibrium test

As we explained above, we assume that π_0, the prior (2) and the experimental result $\mathbf{n}$ are available for the analysis. Then we can compute the posterior probability of the null hypothesis H_0

$$\Pr\{H_0|\mathbf{n}\} = \left\{1 + \frac{1-\pi_0}{\pi_0}\frac{1}{B_{0,1}(\mathbf{n})}\right\}^{-1}, \tag{6}$$

where

$$B_{0,1}(\mathbf{n}) = \frac{m_{H_0}(\mathbf{n})}{m_{H_1}(\mathbf{n})}$$

is the Bayes factor of H_0 *versus* H_1 and $m_{H_j}(\mathbf{n})$ denotes the predictive of **n** given $H_j, j = 0,1$. The computation of $m_{H_1}(\mathbf{n})$, aside from numerical difficulties, is simple

$$m_{H_1}(\mathbf{n}) = \int_{\mathcal{Y}^*} \mathcal{D}(y_1, y_2 | \alpha) \mathcal{M}(n_1, n_2 | \mathbf{y}, n) \mathrm{d}y_1 \mathrm{d}y_2 =$$
$$= \binom{n}{n_1, n_2, n_3} \frac{B(\alpha_1 + n_1, \alpha_2 + n_2, \alpha_3 + n_3)}{B(\alpha_1, \alpha_2, \alpha_3)}.$$

By contrast, since H_0 corresponds to the measure zero set γ in $\mathcal{Y}$, the *B-Kp* arises and therefore the computation of the predictive $m_{H_o}(\mathbf{n})$ depends on the parametrization of the sample model. See Bertolino and Ratto (2002).

Using formulas (1) and (13), in Appendix, we easily compute the line Jacobian $|J_\gamma|(t) = 2^{2/3}\sqrt{3t^2 - 3t + 1}$. It follows now from (12) of the Appendix that

$$m_{H_0}(\mathbf{n}) = \frac{\int_0^1 \mathcal{M}(n_1, n_2 | \mathbf{y}(t), n) \mathcal{D}(y_1(t), y_2(t) | \alpha) | J_\gamma | (t) \mathrm{d}t}{\int_0^1 \mathcal{D}(y_1(t), y_2(t) | \alpha) | J_\gamma | (t) \mathrm{d}t} = \binom{n}{n_1, n_2, n_3} 2^{n_2} \frac{I_\gamma(\mathbf{n})}{I_\gamma(\mathbf{0})}.$$

where $I_\gamma(\mathbf{n}) = \int_0^1 t^{2(\alpha_1 + n_1) + \alpha_2 + n_2 - 3} (1-t)^{\alpha_2 + n_2 + 2(\alpha_3 + n_3) - 3} \sqrt{3t^2 - 3t + 1} \mathrm{d}t$. Thus the Bayes factor is

$$B_{0,1}(\mathbf{n}) = \frac{2^{n_2} B(\alpha_1, \alpha_2, \alpha_3)}{B(\alpha_l + n_1, \alpha_2 + n_2, \alpha_3 + n_3)} \frac{I_\gamma(\mathbf{n})}{I_\gamma(\mathbf{0})}.$$

Suppose now that we adopt the Bernstein disequilibrium model described above. In this context, the Bayes factor becomes

$$B_{0,1}^b(\mathbf{n}) = \frac{m_{H_0}^b(\mathbf{n})}{m_{H_1}(\mathbf{n})},$$

where $m^b_{H_0}(\mathbf{n})$ is now computed using (4). Since the line Jacobian is $|J_\rho|(t)=1$ and the equation of ρ is 2-u-v=1, we have

$$m^b_{H_0}(\mathbf{n})=\binom{n}{n_1,n_2,n_3}2^{n_2}\frac{\int_0^1 t^{2(\alpha_1+n_1)+\alpha_2+n_2-2}(1-t)^{\alpha_2+n_2+2(\alpha_3+n_3)-2}\,dt}{\int_0^1 t^{2\alpha_1+\alpha_2-2}(1-t)^{\alpha_2+2\alpha_3-2}\,dt}=$$

$$=\binom{n}{n_1,n_2,n_3}2^{n_2}\frac{B(2(\alpha_1+n_1)+\alpha_2+n_2-1,\alpha_2+n_2+2(\alpha_3+n_3)-1)}{B(2\alpha_1+\alpha_2-1,\alpha_2+2\alpha_3-1)}.$$

It follows that

$$B^b_{0,1}(\mathbf{n})=2^{n_2}\frac{B(\alpha_1,\alpha_2,\alpha_3)B(2(\alpha_1+n_1)+\alpha_2+n_2-1,\alpha_2+n_2+2(\alpha_3+n_3)-1)}{B(\alpha_1+n_1,\alpha_2+n_2,\alpha_3+n_3)B(2\alpha_1+\alpha_2-1,\alpha_2+2\alpha_3-1)}.$$

Thus we conclude (not without surprise) that, despite the same prior information concerning the experiment and the sample model, the choice of two different parametrizations has lead us to obtain two Bayes factors which do not imply univocal inferential conclusions. (Some precautions to avoid such ambiguities will be indicated in the final Section.) For the moment, we propose to measure such discrepancies by introducing an index of paradoxality, ϕ_{BK} say, given by the difference of the weights of evidence corresponding to two parametrizations, i.e.,

$$\phi_{BK}=\log B_{0,1}(data)-\log B^b_{0,1}(data)=W_{0,1}(data)-W^b_{0,1}(data),$$

where *BK* of course reminds the reader of the underlying *B-Kp*. In our specific instance, we have

$$\phi_{BK}=\log m_{H_0}(\mathbf{n})-\log m^b_{H_0}(\mathbf{n})=$$

$$=\log\frac{I_\gamma(\mathbf{n})}{I_\gamma(\mathbf{0})}-\log\frac{B(2(\alpha_1+n_1)+\alpha_2+n_2-1,\alpha_2+n_2+2(\alpha_3+n_3)-1)}{B(2\alpha_1+\alpha_2-1,\alpha_2+2\alpha_3-1)}.$$

Example 2

In order to show the trends of the weights of evidence in connection with different choices of the hyperparameters in (2) we assume, in Figures 2.a, 2.b and 2.c, $\alpha_1=2,\alpha_2=5.6$ and $\alpha_3=4.4$. In Figures 2.d, 2.e and 2.f,

$\alpha_1 = \alpha_2 = \alpha_3 = 4$. For the sake of convenience the vector $\mathbf{n}$ is given in the form $\mathbf{n} = n\boldsymbol{\nu}$, with $\boldsymbol{\nu} = (\nu_1, \nu_2, \nu_3)$ fixed and n variable.

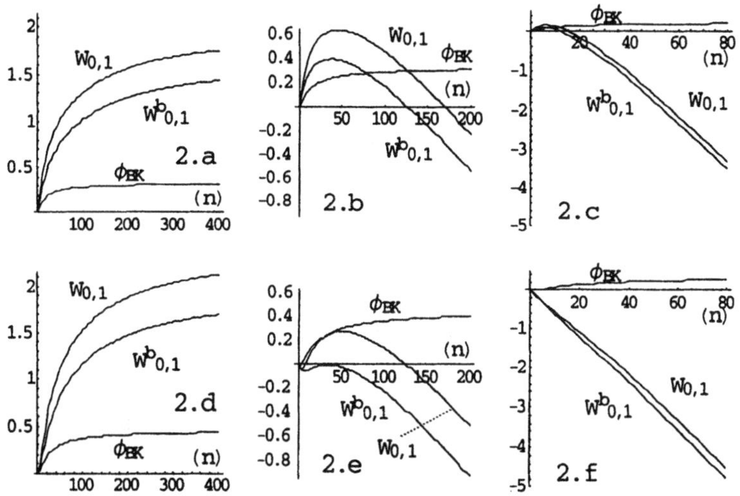

Figure 2. Weights of evidence $W_{0,1}(\mathbf{n})$ and $W_{0,1}^{b}(\mathbf{n})$ for two different elicitations and three sample proportions, with n increasing.

In Figures 2.a and 2.d we assume ν_1 = 0.07, ν_2 = 0.36, ν_3 = 0.57, $n = \{0,400,(40)\}$. The weights of evidence $W_{0,1}(\mathbf{n})$ and $W_{0,1}^{b}(\mathbf{n})$ increase with n, indicating the validity of H_0, though in different ways. In Figures 2.b and 2.e we assume ν_1 = 0.09, ν_2 = 0.32, ν_3 = 0.59, $n = \{0,200,(20)\}$; $W_{0,1}(\mathbf{n})$ and $W_{0,1}^{b}(\mathbf{n})$ and so in favour of H_0, for $n \le 100 \div 140$, and are negative so supporting H_1, for large n. In Figures 2.c and 2.f ν_1 = 0.15, ν_2 = 0.25, ν_3 = 0.60, $n = \{0,80,(10)\}$. The weights of evidence show a departure from *H-We* even for small values of n.

In all cases the index ϕ_{BK} is positive and grows slowly as n increases. For n = 400, ϕ_{BK} = 0.32 case 2.a and ϕ_{BK} = 0.43 case 2.d; for n = 200 ϕ_{BK} = 0.31 case 2.b and ϕ_{BK} = 0.41 case 2.b; for n = 80 , ϕ_{BK} = 0.19 case 2.c and ϕ_{BK} = 0.27 case 2.e.

To summarize our conclusions, in Table 1 we reported the posterior probabilities π_1 and π_1^b computed, according to (6), by means of Bayes factors $B_{0,1}(\mathbf{n})$ and $B_{0,1}^{b}(\mathbf{n})$ respectively. The prior π_0 is assumed to be equal to $\frac{1}{2}$. For brevity, only cases 2.a, 2.b and 2.c are considered (and for some values of n only), the other being similar.

Table 1. Posterior probabilities of H_0 for some values of *n*. The case where H_0 is to be rejected are in Italic.

case	(a)	(b)			(c)		
n	400	50	200	400	60	90	120
π_1	0.853	0.578	0.443	0.127	0.104	*0.020*	*0.003*
π_1^b	0.624	0.366	0.187	*0.040*	*0.037*	*0.007*	*0.001*

The choice of the prior distribution has a moderate influence on the resulting inference.

For brevity we did not present examples in which $W_{0,1}^b > W_{0,1}$ or in which $|\phi_{BK}|$ is greater than 1. Because of the *B-Kp*, the weights of evidence obtained by using two different parametrizations can differ substantially, as shown by the previous examples. The index ϕ_{BK} is very useful in such analysis.

Therefore, we conclude that the inferential implications of the *B-Kp* need a case by case evaluation.

2.2 Problem (*ii*): Allelic proportions distribution

Assuming the *H-We*, a biologist must be able to produce distributions and estimates regarding the allelic proportions. Since that implies the computation of a *p.d.f.* conditioned to a measure zero subset, once again the *B-Kp* again arises.

Following the Appendix (see also Theorem 1 and the Example 5 in Bertolino and Ratto, 2002), and assuming to work with (y_1, y_2, y_3), the posterior *p.d.f.* conditioned to $\mathbf{y} \in \gamma$ of the allelic proportion *t* is given by

$$T|\mathbf{n} \sim g_{HW}(t|\mathbf{n}) = \frac{\mathcal{D}(y_1(t), y_2(t)|\alpha')|J_\gamma|(t)}{\int_0^1 \mathcal{D}(y_1(t), y_2(t)|\alpha'|J_\gamma|(t)\mathrm{d}t)} \mathbf{1}_{(0,1)}(t) \propto$$

$$\propto t^{2\alpha_1'+\alpha_2'-3}(1-t)^{+\alpha_2'+2\alpha_3'-3}\sqrt{3t^2-3t+1}\;\mathbf{1}_{(0,1)}(t). \tag{7}$$

Recalling that $|J_\rho|(t)=1$, in an analogous fashion we obtain the posterior *p.d.f.* of *t* (conditioned to $(u,v,)\in\rho$)

$$T\,|\,\mathbf{n} \sim h_{HW}(t\,|\,\mathbf{n}) = \frac{\mathcal{D}_b(t,1-t\,|\,\alpha')}{\int_0^1 \mathcal{D}_t(t,1-t\,|\,\alpha')\mathrm{d}t}\mathbf{1}_{(0,1)}(t) \propto$$
$$\propto t^{2\alpha_1'+\alpha_2'-2}(1-t)^{+\alpha_2'+2\alpha_3'-2}\,\mathbf{1}_{(0,1)}(t). \tag{8}$$

To measure the distance between $g_{HW}(t\,|\,\mathbf{n})$ and $h_{HW}(\mathrm{t}\,|\,\mathbf{n})|\,\mathrm{d}t$ we use the scaled L_1-norm

$$d_1(g_{HW}, h_{HW}) = \frac{1}{2}\int_0^1 |\, g_{HW}(t\,|\,\mathbf{n}) - h_{HW}(t\,|\,\mathbf{n})|\,\mathrm{d}t\,, \tag{9}$$

which belongs to the interval [0,1]. Observe that while the *H-We* test requires that the (2) be a proper prior, for the calculation of $g_{HW}(t\,|\,\mathbf{n})$, (2) may be improper. The same is true for $h_{HW}(t\,|\,\mathbf{n})$.

If no experiment is available, we can calculate (7) and (8) provided that the hyperparameters α_i assessed by the biologist have "some consistence". Let $g_{HW}(t)$ and $h_{HW}(t)$ be the corresponding prior conditional (to the *H-We*) densities of the allele A.

Example 3

In Figure 3.a we reproduce the prior densities $g_{HW}(t)$ and $h_{HW}(t)$ when $\alpha_1 = 2, \alpha_2 = 5.6, \alpha_3 = 4.4$ in this case we have $d_1(g_{HW}, h_{HW}) = 0.095$. In Figure 3.b we find the corresponding posterior densities $g_{HW}(t\,|\,\mathbf{n})$ and $h_{HW}(t\,|\,\mathbf{n})$ with $n_1 = 2, n_2 = 11, n_3 = 9$. Now $d_1(g_{HW}, h_{HW}) = 0.063$.

We note that, as n increases, $g_{HW}(t\,|\,\mathbf{n})$ and $h_{HW}(t\,|\,\mathbf{n})$ tend to coincide and their distance approaches to zero. Therefore we conclude that, in this context, the *B-Kp* has an influence which is moderate when n is small and negligible for large n.

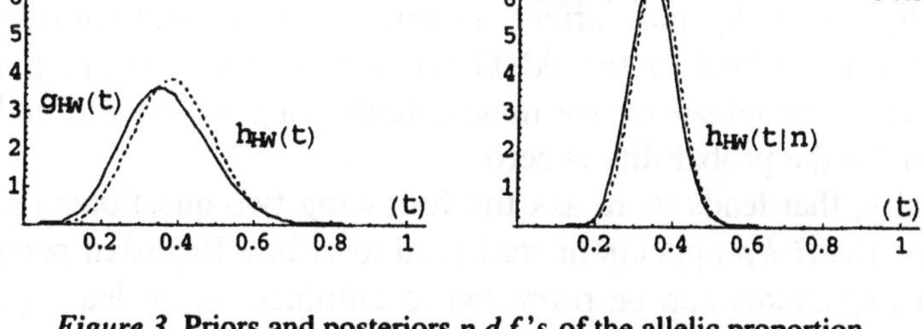

Figure 3. Priors and posteriors *p.d.f.*'s of the allelic proportion.

2.3 Some criticism

As shown through the above examples, the *B-Kp* can have remarkable effects in the Bayes factors computation, while its influence concerning the determination of the distribution of the allelic proportions is less appreciable.

A detailed statistical analysis of other (well-known to biologists) disequilibrium models is far beyond our scopes, though certainly it deserves future attention of Bayesian people.

By way of example, we briefly describe the following interesting context. Consider a homogenous population subdivided in small communities geographically far from each other, but all having numerous consanguineous matings (inbreeding) and similar fertility coefficients and, consequently, identical propensities to form homozygotes *AA* and *aa,u* and *v* respectively. (In this case condition *(c2)* of Section 2 becomes equivalent to test the hypothesis $H_0 : \Pr\{A \mid A\} = \Pr\{a \mid a\}$.)

Another worth mentioning instance concerns the case of populations which include distinct and (not necessarily) closed racial groups having rather dissimilar fertility coefficients. In this case, condition (c2) fails to hold and we encounter a disequilibrium model where the proportion of the allele *A* is modified. Other cases are possible, and all can be tackled (with the necessary modifications!) by means of the methods presented in this work.

However, our main aim was to stress the presence of the *B-Kp* in the study of the *H-We*, and to propose an evaluation of its consequences.

In this order of ideas, the next Section will explain that the *B-Kp* appears in usual statistical problems much more often than what generally people think. We shall end our work by proposing some precaution measures which may help to investigate or, at least, evaluate the ambiguities caused by the paradox.

3. GENERALIZATION AND PRECAUTIONS

We have shown that the *B-Kp* has relevant effects on the study of the *H-We*. Actually, the *B-Kp* may affect several other classical statistical tests, such as the Student test or the ANOVA, for instance. More generally, the *B-Kp* is present whenever we must calculate a *p.d.f.* conditionally to an event for which the probability is zero.

Essentially, that leads us to ask the following two questions: *(q1)* under which forms the *B-Kp* appears in statistical tests in a Bayesian perspective? *(q2)* which expedients can be proposed to eliminate or, at least, put under control the ambiguity generated by the paradox?

To answer question *(q1)*, we only assume, as it is common in experimental sciences, that it is necessary to carry out some parametric statistical test on the basis of a certain set of data z from a given sample model $f(z|\theta), \theta \in \Theta$, when some *p.d.f.* $g(\theta)$ has been elicited by an expert of the problem.

The system of hypotheses under consideration $\{H_0, H_1\}$ determines a partition of subsets $\{\Theta_j, j=0,1\}$ of Θ. In most applications Θ_0 and Θ_1 are common geometric *loci*, such as points, straight lines, planes or other simple curves and surfaces. When both Θ_0 and Θ_1 are *not* measure zero subsets, the computation of the Bayes factor of H_0 *versus* H_1 does not give rise to serious problems, aside from numerical difficulties, of course. Indeed, setting the prior in the form $\pi_0 g_0(\theta)\mathbf{1}_{\Theta_0}(\theta)+(1-\pi_0)g_1(\theta)\mathbf{1}_{\Theta_1}(\theta)$, where $g_j(\theta)$ is the *p.d.f.* of θ under the subset $\Theta_j, j=0,1$, and $\pi_0=\int_{\Theta_0} g(\theta)\mathrm{d}\theta$ denotes the prior probability of H_0, we can compute the Bayes factor

$$B_{0,1}(z)=\frac{m_{H_0}(z)}{m_{H_1}(z)},$$

where $m_{H_j}(z)=\int_{\Theta_j} f(z|\theta)g_j(\theta)\mathrm{d}\theta$ is the predictive of z given H_j, $j=0,1$.

When Θ_0 is a point, the calculation of $m_{H_0}(z)$ is also simple. By contrast, if Θ_0 is a curve or a surface (even a straight line or a plane!) in a higher dimensional ambient space Θ, then in the computation of $m_{H_0}(z)$ the *B-Kp* arises.

Without loss of generality, let us illustrate an elementary case to account for this.

Let $\theta=(\alpha,\beta)\in\mathbb{R}\times\mathbb{R}^+$ and let $\{H_0:\alpha=0, H_1:\alpha\neq 0, \forall\beta>0\}$ the hypotheses to be tested. (In this case, since Θ_0 is a measure zero subset, the expert assigns to H_0 the prior probability π_0). We have $m_{H_1}(z)=\int_{\Theta} f(z|\theta)g(\theta)\mathrm{d}\theta$ and $m_{H_0}(z)=\int_0^{+\infty} f(z|0,\beta)g_0(\beta|0)\mathrm{d}\beta$ where

$$g_0(\beta|\alpha)=\frac{g(\alpha,\beta)}{\int_0^{+\infty} g(\alpha,\beta)\mathrm{d}\beta}$$

is the *p.d.f.* of β given α.

Next, let us assume the following reparametrization $\phi=\alpha\beta$ and $\zeta=\beta$, whose Jacobian $|J| = \zeta^{-1}$. Now, our hypotheses become $\{H_0:\phi=0,\ H_1:\phi\neq 0, \forall\zeta>0\}$. While $m_{H_1}(z)$ is independent of the parametrization, we cannot say the same for $m_{H_0}(z)$.

Now, we have $m^d_{H_0}(z)=\int_0^{+\infty} f(z\,|\,0,\zeta)h_0(\zeta\,|\,0)\mathrm{d}\zeta$ where

$$h_0(\zeta\,|\,\phi)=\frac{g(\phi/\zeta,\zeta)\zeta^{-1}}{\int_0^{+\infty} g(\phi/\zeta,\zeta)\zeta^{-1}\mathrm{d}\zeta}$$

is the *p.d.f.* of ζ given ϕ.

It is immediate to observe that, in general, $m^d_{H_0}(z)\neq m_{H_0}(z)$, a surprising fact which leads us to conclude that the Bayes factor, together with all its inferential implications, does depend on the choice of the model parametrization!

Because of this problem, we consider as rather illusive the idea, frequent in the literature, of introducing a nuisance parameter to be eliminated afterwards, by means of some marginalization techniques. The difficulty does not lie in the choice of the nuisance parameter, but rather in the nonuniqueness of the inferential conclusions.

In this order of ideas, it is possible to answer question *(q2)*, at least in the sense of proposing some common sense precautions: *(i)* when possible, avoid using measure zero hypotheses; for instance, in the example above, $H_0:\alpha\in[-\varepsilon,+\varepsilon]$ is preferable with respect to $H_0:\alpha=0$; *(ii)* if there is no way to by-pass a measure zero hypothesis, then the experimenter should be able to produce some justification in favour of the parametrization that he has adopted; *(iii)* if an uncertainty remains between choosing a certain parametrization or another, then the different inferential implications should be pointed out, possibly, by introducing an appropriate *criterion* to evaluate this discrepancy.

Of course, precaution *(i)* may be difficult to apply because in many practical instances the complexity of the problem makes an accurate estimation of ε impossible.

However, even if one is ready to give up any routinist aptitude, in the case of the *H-We* precaution turns out to be of little help. Indeed, no convenient criterion can indicate a specific neighborhood $\mathcal{Y}_0$ of γ in $\mathcal{Y}$.

Therefore, it becomes necessary to produce some justification in favour of the parametrization which is adopted. Otherwise, the alternative is to make a comparison between the different inferential conclusions deriving from reasonable parametrizations, possibly by means of the index of paradoxality ϕ_{BK}.

APPENDIX

Let $\{\mathcal{X}, \mathcal{A}, \mathcal{P}\}$ be a probability space. For simplicity, we assume that the sample space $\mathcal{X}$ is an open set in $\mathbb{R}^n$, the σ-algebra $\mathcal{A}$ is the Borel field, and $\mathcal{P}$ is expressed by means of an absolutely continuous density $\varphi : \mathcal{X} \to [0, +\infty)$, i.e.,

$$\mathcal{P}(E) = \int_E \varphi(\mathbf{x})d\mathbf{x}, \forall E \in \mathcal{A}.$$

Next, assume that random variable $\mathbf{X}$ belongs to a measurable subset $\Lambda \subset \mathcal{X}$, so that Λ is our new sample space. Given the event $B \in \mathcal{A}$ such that $B \subset \Lambda$, the conditional probability of B given Λ is

$$\mathcal{P}_\Lambda(B) = \frac{\mathcal{P}(B)}{\mathcal{P}(\Lambda)}, \text{ provided that } \mathcal{P}(\Lambda) > 0. \tag{10}$$

In the important case that Λ is an *m*-dimensional $(m < n)$ submanifold of $\mathcal{X}$ (in particular, in the present work, Λ will be a curve in a 2- or 3-dimensional ambient space), we have $\mathcal{P}(\Lambda = 0)$. Therefore (10) must be replaced by a well specified procedure of the type

$$\mathcal{P}_\Lambda(B) = \lim_{\varepsilon \to 0} \frac{\mathcal{P}(B_\varepsilon)}{\mathcal{P}(\Lambda_\varepsilon)}, \tag{11}$$

where B_ε and Λ_ε are suitable n-dimensional neighborhoods of B and Λ, respectively, which restrict to B and Λ as $\varepsilon \to 0$.

The shape of these neighborhoods is not univocally defined: different choices may lead to different results in (11), and this ambiguity is the so-called Borel-Kolmogorov paradox. In Bertolino and Ratto (2002), a systematic method is developed to establish a geometrically significant limit procedure of the type (11), where the involved neighborhoods are bounded by suitable parallel submanifolds.

In this way, we obtained a general definition of $\mathcal{P}_\Lambda(B)$, which was adopted in this article as well. Therefore we have

$$\mathcal{P}_\Lambda(B) = \frac{\int_B \varphi_\Lambda(\mathbf{x}) d\ell_\Lambda}{\int_\varphi \varphi_\Lambda(\mathbf{x}) d\ell_\Lambda}, \tag{12}$$

where $d\ell_\Lambda$ is the line element on Λ. Thus assuming for the curve Λ the parametric representation, $\Lambda:\{\mathbf{x}(t)\}=\{x_1(t),x_2(t),x_3(t)\}$, the line element $d\ell_\Lambda$ is simply given by the arc length

$$d\ell_\Lambda = |J_\Lambda|(t)dt = \sqrt{\left(\frac{\partial x_1(t)}{\partial t}\right)^2+\left(\frac{\partial x_2(t)}{\partial t}\right)^2+\left(\frac{\partial x_3(t)}{\partial t}\right)^2}\,dt\,.$$

In the present work, we shall only be concerned with the case that Λ is the curve γ, given by (1), or the line ρ, given by (5).

It is easy to compute their line Jacobians

$$|J_\gamma|(t)=2^{3/2}\sqrt{3t^2-3t+1} \tag{13}$$

and $|J_\rho|(t)=\sqrt{2}$, respectively.

REFERENCES

BERNARDO, J. M. AND SMITH, A. F. M. (1994), Bayesian Theory, J.Wiley, Chichester.

BERTOLINO, F. AND RATTO, A. (2002), A note on conditional probability in a geometric context, (*preprint*).

DEGROOT, M. H. (1986), Probability and Statistics, Addison-Wesley, Reading, Mass.

EMERY, A. E. H. (1976), Methodology in Medical Genetics, Churchill, Livingstone, Edimburgh.

LINDLEY, D. V. (1988), Statistical inference concerning Hardy-Weinberg equilibrium, in *Bayesian Statistics 3*, eds. J. M. Bernardo, M. H. De Groot, D. V. Lindley and A. F. M. Smith, Oxford University Press, 307-325, (with discussion).

PEREIRA, C. A. DE B. AND ROGATKO, A. (1984), The Hardy-Weinberg equilibrium under a Bayesian perspective, *Brazilian J.Genetics 7*, 689-707.

Chapter 4

IDENTIFYING A BAYESIAN NETWORK FOR THE PROBLEM "HOSPITAL AND FAMILIES: THE ANALYSIS OF PATIENT SATISFACTION WITH THEIR STAY IN HOSPITAL".

A. Brogini*, M. Bolzan and D. Slanzi
University of Padova, Department of Statistics, Padova, Italy

1. THE PROBLEM: GENERALISATION AND CONTEXT

In the evolution of the epidemiological profile of present day communities, the phenomena of "chronicity" and "disability" are more and more important. These phenomena find a natural place for their manifestation and for the research of their solution in the family context. The health of some members, in a family context, proves to be an experience which affects the whole family unit and the more the condition of the individual is one of suffering, the greater the hardship the family finds itself having to face. We can therefore talk of "family hardship" as the adverse condition, perceived by the family in various ways, which directly (e.g. due to the sudden onset of critical events) and/or indirectly (due to structural conditions of the family or the context of family life) prevents the carrying out of the functions necessary for the optimal achievement of expected objectives such as a better quality of life (Bolzan, M., 2002; Pless, I. B., 1984). However, an initial definition of family hardship stands on the three-dimensional level of: i) main family functions; ii) resources the family have at their disposal for the reaching of their own objectives; iii) the system of institutions and services in which the policies and interventions on health and care operate. On this level all the exchanges of relationships – between

* For correspondence: brogini@stat.unipd.it

people united by a history of behaviours and by a dominant culture in which the social unity is linked to other social unities – commonly known as the "social network", are activated.

The system of interdependence present in the concept of social network can be divided into formal and informal. The first relates to relations with public services, services provided by the public operator and by services available and purchasable on the market. Such services, in particular in the medical field (including preventive, rehabilitative, therapeutic), are available and offered according to proven criteria of professionalism. The functions carried out by the service are organised and destined for use when an objective need exists which, in order to be satisfied, requires the availability of competence, ability and professionalism which the individual, holder of the need, does not possess. The contribution that these formal networks of care offer (in Italy the National Social-Health Service), is gauged according to the express request of the single patient. Thus the family condition, which is however involved in making access to the service possible for the family member, is not considered. Often the family feels that a very efficient service is available but that access to it is demanding because of binding limits linked to the daily running of a family. A partial answer to such a need is authoritatively represented by the system of informal networks of care between and within the family, voluntary groups and associations and private social organisations. The informal system, which represents the relationships between relatives, friends, voluntary associations and groups of mutual help, involves goods and services which the individual or the family can or must draw upon out with market logic (Cioni, E. 1997; Donati, P., 1991; Facchini, C., 1997). The essential elements for classifying such help are the contemporaneous absence of profit and cohabitation.

The present work is part of a wider project of work and study intended to research and describe variables, indicators, and their relationships associated with the experience of families which, together or through one of their members, live through exceptional experiences, such as for example hospitalisation, or much more commonly and on a more daily level, access to the most elementary social and health services. In particular the level of satisfaction perceived from hospital use with regard to care received will be explored and described. Naturally such events take on different characteristics depending on the demographic, epidemiological, social and economic typology of the family involved. The database used in the work project is the one obtained in the sample surveys which ISTAT (Central Institute of Statistics) organised in Italy on health conditions and the use made of social and health services by Italian families. Since 1980 ISTAT has organised and carried out these surveys through families in order to learn about health conditions, use of social and health services, and some habits or lifestyles including some risk factors (smoking, alcohol, etc.). These surveys had at most a three-year time limit and are characterised by the fact that they were carried out over the whole national territory, each time involving more than 23000 families and over 93000 people (Eurostat, 1999; Istat, 1994b; Istat, 2000a; Istat, 2000b). For the present analysis the data were selected from the Multipurpose Survey on Families carried out by ISTAT in 1998 called "Families, social subjects and infancy conditions". Among the variables which arose (concerning single members and the family as a whole) there is also information concerning the structural characteristics of the family, the level of accessibility to some important social and health services, the level of satisfaction with the services (in particular hospital services), and to a lesser extent the network of interfamily relationships (help received and given). These surveys, which observe important modalities and conditions of social and health care, are of particular importance both for scientific purposes and for the government of the system of services in Italy. In fact health care takes the form of a system of relationships (which can be demanding for the resources involved) between operators, services and care given, in which the users who have access to them are identified for their particular conditions of need and dependence. In such a context the user often finds himself in conditions of particular, dramatic weakness, with a family background often unprepared for the experience of the event of the relative. For this reason relationships with the environment, the services and the personnel seem to be articulated, complex and difficult to classify (Ware, J. E., 1978; Ware, J. E., 1981; Ware, J. E., Hays, R.D., 1988). On the other hand, in health, just as in other services, interest in the judgement of quality based on the user/patient's perception has grown. Donabedian states that "the satisfaction of the patient can be considered one of the results of the care, even the element of well-being in itself" (Donabedian, A., 1980; Donabedian, A., 1988) and that information about the patient's satisfaction may be considered essential for the evaluation, planned and managed by the health systems, of services (Bolzan, M., 2001; Øvretveit, J., 1992; Ross, C. K., Steward, C. A., Sinacore, J. M., 1983). It therefore seems clear that the measurement of quality in the field of health care cannot be set aside from the observation of the patient's satisfaction with the services received. In this field of research hospital care is among the areas of greatest interest, both for the commitment of resources which it involves in terms of personnel and services, and for the typologies of relationships between user and service.

Gathering data and measuring the satisfaction of the patient with services received, is however advised i) to better understand the growing sensitivity of users; ii) for an ever more widespread awareness of the decisive elements and to operate in competitive conditions in offering health care; iii) to have at one's disposal an adequate informative base necessary in the management of available resources and evaluation of interventions; iv) to measure the satisfaction of the user as an index of performance, i.e. as an indicator of quality.

Although in Italy and in these ISTAT surveys we are still far from the consolidation of a procedure for the evaluation of "patient satisfaction", the need to design valid, reliable, standardised measurements of satisfaction which measure specific welfare aspects is, however, more and more noticeable. Here we remember one of the first approaches for the evaluation and improvement of services: *total quality management* (T.Q.M), supported mainly by Deming (1982), which met with a vast and articulated development, documented by an interesting amount of publications as well as normative provisions recently approved in Italy. The Italian legislative provisions allow for the description of several guidelines which should shape the whole activity of the national health system, both at a local and central level, where it clearly emerges that evaluation of quality must become a constant component and therefore an ordinary component of the modalities of management of the National Health Service. The first rules are those of the legislative decree n. 502 of 1992. Article 2, in defining regional competences, establishes that "...activities of a technical, promotional and supporting nature with regard to Local Health Units and Hospitals, including the control of management and the evaluation of the quality of health care" are the concern of the regions. Article 8, among the directive criteria and principles of the act of policy and coordination concerning minimum requirements for the practice of health activities, inserts the prevision with "the obligation to check the quality of the services provided". Article 12, which regulates the distribution of the national health fund, in fixing the criteria for the distribution of the funds in stock accounts, identifies instruments for evaluating efficiency and among these quality and quantity indicators of health care are highlighted.

The legislative dispositions on the matter of the Public Services Card (19/5/95) and the URP – Public Relations Office (Presidency of Council of Ministers Law 11/10/94), highlighted "the importance not only of safeguarding the users' rights (transparency, participation, information), but also of the attribution to the users of a power to directly check the quality of services". It seems clear, therefore, that patient satisfaction should not concern only the more strictly professional and specialised dimensions of hospital care (medical and nursing) for which the patient is often not in the condition to express an opinion in a pertinent manner. Vice versa, the logistic conditions of the service deserve particular attention, including those represented by hygienic services and the food offered in the hospitalisation ward. Article 14 of the earlier legislative decree provides for indicators of the quality of services and care given relative to the personalisation and humanisation of the care, the right to be informed, accommodation services, as well as the state of activities of disease prevention. Here too it is prescribed that the Ministry of Health defines the contents and modalities of use, in order to guarantee the constant adjustment of structures and health care to the needs of citizens. It is dutiful to guarantee them those conditions which, although not comparable to family conditions, are at least sustainable with what the patient is used to in his own home. In this evaluation merciless comparisons will certainly be easy to make, conditioned not only by the global state of necessity (acute, chronic, level of autonomy, etc.) which is also homogeneous among patients in the same structure, but also by foreseeable personal, social, psychological, family and prejudicial factors. Moreover, again the Services Card indicates the duty to "evaluate the quality of services, not only through inspections and reports on the reaching of the quality standards", but also through the "sending of forms and questionnaires to the user, sample interviews with the users even after the provision of the service and public meetings with the participation of users by area or by unit providing the service" as an instrument to put the fundamental principles into effect. Finally the Italian National Health Plan for the three-year period 1998-2000 had as its priority objective "the guarantee of adequate levels of quality in health care", based on a "national programme for quality". In the three-year period it was necessary to "introduce mechanisms directed towards making the development of the activity of evaluation and promotion of quality of care from health operators binding and widespread... increase the forms of social evaluation of the services, valorizing the contribution of the user and of the organizations which represent them", favour recognition as an integral part of the tasks of the national health service, of the participation in the activity of evaluation and promotion of the quality of the health care provided by health system. The problem described looks like a complex system, which we informally define as one which is made up of a large number of various sub-elements which interact. From a pragmatic point of view, trying to understand the whole behavior is not a trivial matter. If we apply this perspective, the implication is that the process of analysis should be the process of identifying and understanding the aspects of the social-health system and their interactions; the objective should be to obtain a representation which is good enough across all relevant aspects of the problem and easy to interpret. We will use the Bayesian network (B for short) as our method of analysis. It is a powerful tool for knowledge representation and inference for problems in conditions of uncertainty. Given a set of observations in a certain domain, it permits a credible reasoning to the complex model system. The B offers a strategy for summarizing our current state of knowledge, subjecting it to a critical empirical evaluation. We will use B for its ability to reason about the events (relations between events) and to model the environment accurately, offering a useful formalism for representation of (in)dependency structures in a multivariate domain. In the paper we concentrate on the Bayesian approach where our interest is turned to the construction of the topology of the network (learning) directed towards the complex system. Operationally the problem is to infer the most probable (MAP) model from a complete database in the context of Bayesian Networks.

2. BAYESIAN NETWORK

In this section we introduce notations and describe the Bayesian network. We denote random variables by an upper case letter like "X", a set of random variables by a bold-face capital letter like "**X**"; the states, that represent all possible situations of the corresponding random variable or sub-set of random variables, by the same letter in lower-case with an apex letter like "x^k" or "$\mathbf{x}^k$" and we leave the set of each variable implicit. The Bayesian network is constructed starting with a graphical model, where each node corresponds to a variable in the domain of the system and each edge (direct link or arrow) between nodes is used to describe the direct influence among the set of the random variables of interest. The edge pointing from a variable represents the direct stochastic dependence of Y on X, so that Y is called the parent of X and X is called the child of Y and we use **Pa**(X) to denote the set of parent nodes of X and so on for each variable. We also use the same upper case letter to refer to both the variable and the corresponding node. We consider a domain **U** of n variables $X_1, \ldots, X_n$, and throughout this discussion, we limit our attention to discrete variables with a finite number of states.

Formally a Bayesian network consists of the following elements:

- A set of variables and a set of edges between variables.
- Each variable contains a finite set of exhaustive and mutually exclusive states.
- The variables, coupled with the edge, construct a direct acyclic graph, G=(V,A), G for short, where V is a finite set of nodes and A is a finite set of directed edges between the nodes.
  The graph is acyclic if there is no direct path, we suppose $X_1 \rightarrow X_2 \rightarrow \ldots \rightarrow X_n$, such that $X_1 = X_n$.
- Each variable X_i with parents **Pa**(X_i), has a conditional probability distribution $P(X_i|Pa(X_i))$ associated with it, and can be represented as a table (CPT).
  If the variable X_i has no parent, the conditional probability distribution is replaced by the unconditional probability, $P(X_i)$, which must be defined.

This probability can arise from data previously observed or can be the subjective assessment elicited by a domain expert.

The Bayesian network satisfies interesting properties such as:

➢ **D-separation**

It is a graphical criterion which constitutes the semantics for the Bayesian network and intuitively represents the idea of the impossibility of passage of information between the nodes of the network. Thus we call evidence on a variable a statement of the certainties of its states, i.e. we have assigned to it a value and this value is called instantiation. We instantiate a set of variables by assigning a value to each variable in the set. Let X_i, X_i', X_i'' be different nodes (or subset of nodes) in G, and X_i'' is instantiated. If X_i and X_i' are d-separated in G by X_i'', the changes in the certainty of X_i have no impact on the certainty of X_i'. X_i and X_i' are conditionally independent given X_i''. $P(X_i|X_i'',X_i')=P(X_i|X_i'')$ or equivalently $P(X_i,X_i'|X_i'')=P(X_i|X_i'')P(X_i'|X_i'')$. The block by evidence is reflected in the assumptions

➢ **Conditional independence**

Each node X_i is conditionally independent of all its non descendents in G given its parents $Pa(X_i)$ in G. We use the term descendent of a node X_i, for all nodes that can be reached from X_i through a directed path which is following the directionality of the edge. In particular, it is implied that a variable X_i is conditionally independent of all other network variables, given its Markov blanket ([29]), that is roughly speaking the set consisting of X_i's parents, its children and the other parents of its children.

➢ **Chain rule**

Let B be a Bayesian network over U, then the joint probability distribution over U is the product of all conditional probability distributions specified in B

$$P(U)=\prod_i P(X_i\,|\,\mathbf{Pa}(X_i))$$

A Bayesian network has two components:

- **qualitative**, a structure G, which captures the dependencies between the variables of the system
- **quantitative**, a local probability set, i.e. the set of conditional probability distributions of each variable given each combination of states of its parents. It looks for a more compact representation of the underlying distribution, making calculations easier.

Specifically, a Bayesian network will be denoted by $B=(G,P:\Theta_G)=(G,\Theta_G)$ where Θ_G is the set of parameters which quantifies the network, encoding local probability distributions. The set of parameters Θ_G contains a single parameter $\theta_{i,j,k}$ for each node X_i, for each state k of X_i and for each state parent j, that is $\theta_{i,j,k} = P(X_i = x_i^k \mid \mathbf{Pa}(X_i) = \mathbf{pa}_i^j)$. Let r_i denote the number of states of the variable X_i and q_i denote the number of states of the set $\mathbf{Pa}(X_i)$. We use $\Theta_{i,jG}$ to denote the set of parameters characterising the distributions $P(X_i \mid \mathbf{Pa}(X_i) = \mathbf{pa}_i^j)$, i.e. for every i, j, $\boldsymbol{\theta}_{i,j}=(\theta_{i,j,k})_{k=1,\ldots,ri}$, and Θ_{iG} to denote the set of parameters characterizing all conditional distributions $P(X_i|\mathbf{Pa}(X_i)=\mathbf{pa}_i)$, i.e. for every i, $\boldsymbol{\theta}_i=(\boldsymbol{\theta}_{i,j})_{j=1,\ldots,qi}$.

3. BAYESIAN LEARNING BAYESIAN NETWORK FROM DATA.

The Bayesian network originally developed as a knowledge representation formalism with a human expert. Construction of a Bayesian network with a domain expert is difficult and a time consuming task. As a result experts have problems making the relations between variables explicit, which hinders the construction of network structures and even if the human experts are good enough at judging qualitative relations, they are not usually so good at quantizing these relations. During the late 1980s people realized that the statistical foundation of Bayesian networks make it possible to learn from data rather than from an expert. By exploiting information contained in databases and using computational techniques, an automatically constructed Bayesian network is obtained, which gives insight into the dependences of the variables in the domain and can be applied in the automated discovery of dependency relationships, turning Bayesian networks into a powerful tool for the analysis of data. However the information about the real problem from the expert will be incorporated during the analysis.

Learning about Bayesian networks means to learn about:

- The conditional probability distributions: the parameter of B
- The graphical model of dependencies: structure of B

3.1 Basic assumptions

In order to learn about Bayesian networks from data, a database is used. We will introduce the concept of database and we will give some notational conventions.

A database D over **U** is a multi-set of configurations of **U**. A configuration of **U** in D is referred to as an "instance", that is to say we observe the state for each variable in **U**.

For D we make the assumptions that:

- The set of variables in the domain is agreed upon by the involved expert
- The variables are discrete

- There are no instances in D in which the variables have unspecified values
- All instances are independent of each other, given the model

We will write:

- N to denote the cardinality of the database D, D=[$\mathbf{u}_1,\ldots,\mathbf{u}_N$], where every $\mathbf{u}_m$, m=1,...,N, is an n-ple $(x_1^{k1},\ldots,x_n^{kn})$
- N_{ijk} to denote the number of instances in D where $X_i=x_i^k$ and $\mathbf{Pa}(X_i)=\mathbf{pa}_i^j$, $j_i(u)=j$ and $k_i(u)=k$
- $N_{ij} = \sum_{k=1}^{r_i} N_{ijk}$, to denote the number of instances in D where $\mathbf{Pa}(X_i)=\mathbf{pa}_i^j$

D is complete, with reference to the model, if for every i,j, $N_{ij}\neq 0$

3.2 Bayesian approach for learning Bayesian network

The Bayesian approach is a well founded method for selecting statistical models given a dataset. It is a formal mechanism which, by the application of Bayes' theorem, allows us to incorporate the prior distribution, reflecting a prior knowledge, and the likelihood function, reflecting the sample information, to form a posterior distribution: a process of learning from experience. In our context, the statistical model is a Bayesian network, where we are uncertain about the probabilities and we are also uncertain about the structure which encodes them. The basic idea of this approach is to use the posterior probability distribution which we will gain later, having subdivided the problem into learning parameters and learning structure. In the Bayesian interpretation, the probability will always depend on the information I, currently available, so we will have to write the probability for every event as $P(\cdot|I)$. Hereafter I is omitted for short.

3.2.1 Learning parameters

Our problem consists of $\mathbf{U}=\{X_1,\ldots,X_n\}$ and a fully observed data set D=[$\mathbf{u}_1,\ldots,\mathbf{u}_N$] which is a random sample from an unknown multivariate probability distribution P for **U**. We assume that this distribution is encoded by $B=(G,\Theta_G)$, where G denotes the hypothesis that the database is generated from a fixed network structure G.

Given G, our task is to estimate, from D, the conditional probabilities quantifying the dependencies in G. The essential aspect of the Bayesian approach is to regard Θ_G as a random variable whose prior distribution represents the observer's belief about the conditional probabilities before data are seen.

Bayesian learning parameters means to update the prior belief on the basis of evidence, so we compute the posterior distribution for Θ_G, using Bayes' theorem

$$p(\theta_G \mid D) = \frac{p(\theta_G)p(D \mid \theta_G)}{p(D)}$$

where $p(D) = \int p(\theta_G)p(D \mid \theta_G)d\theta_G$ is called marginal likelihood.

We assume the following assumptions (Heckerman, D., Geiger, D., Chickering, D. 1995) for which these computations can be done efficiently and in a closed form with a complete database

- **Multinomial sample**

The likelihood term $p(\mathbf{u}|\theta_G)$ is factorised as follows

$$p(\mathbf{u} \mid \theta_G) = \prod_{i=1}^{n} P(X_i = x_i \mid \mathbf{Pa}(X_i) = \mathbf{pa}_i, \boldsymbol{\theta}_i)$$

where each local likelihood is a collection of multinomial distributions, one distribution for each configuration of $\mathbf{Pa}(X_i)$, that is

$$p(\mathbf{u} \mid \theta_G) = \prod_{i=1}^{n} P(X_i = x_i^{k_i(u)} \mid \mathbf{Pa}(X_i) = \mathbf{pa}_i^{j_i(u)}, \boldsymbol{\theta}_i) = \prod_{i=1}^{n} \theta_{ijk} > 0,$$

$$\sum_{k=1}^{r_i} \theta_{ijk} = 1; \; k_i(u)=k, \; j_i(u)j$$

where $\boldsymbol{\theta}_i=((\theta_{ijk})_{k=2,\ldots,ri})_{j=1,\ldots,qi}$ are the parameters.

For convenience we consider the parameter $\boldsymbol{\theta}_{ij}=((\theta_{ijk})_{k=2,\ldots,ri}$ for all i, j, associated to the conditional distribution $P(X_i|\mathbf{Pa}(X_i)=\mathbf{pa}_i^j)$.

We present one short argument on the multinomial sample, with reference to a single variable.

Given a discrete variable X with r states, let us consider a finite sequence of outcomes $\mathbf{x}_1,\ldots,\mathbf{x}_N$ of this variable, D for $\mathbf{U}=\{X\}$. This sequence is said to be exchangeable if the sequence obtained by interchanging any two outcomes has the same probability as the original sequence, i.e. a judgement of complete symmetry among the outcomes under considerations. Given exchangeability, De Finetti (1937) showed that a parameter vector $\boldsymbol{\theta}=(\theta_1,\ldots\theta_k)$, $\theta_k>0$, k=1,…,r and $\sum_{k=1}^{r}\theta_k = 1$ exists such that $\boldsymbol{\theta}$ renders the individual outcome in the sequence conditionally independent, so the probability of obtaining any outcome of X in the state k is θ_k; θ_k can be thought of as the limiting relative frequency, the long run fraction of outcomes where $X=\mathbf{x}^k$. An exchangeable sequence is a random sample known as a (r-1)-dimensional multinomial sample with parameters $\boldsymbol{\theta}$ (Good, I., (1965), Heckerman, D., (1998)).

➢ **Parameter independence**

An assumption which leads to local computation is that the parameters $\boldsymbol{\theta}_{ij}$ and $\boldsymbol{\theta}_{i'j'}$ associated to different variables X_i and X_i' are independent for $i \neq i'$ (global independence) and the parameters $\boldsymbol{\theta}_{ij}$ and $\boldsymbol{\theta}_{ij'}$, associated to the distribution of X_i, given different configurations $\mathbf{pa}_i^j$ and $\mathbf{pa}_i^{j'}$ ($j \neq j'$) are independent (local independence) (Spiegelhalter, D. J., Lauritzen, S. L., 1990). So the joint prior density factorises in to the product

$$p(\theta_G) = \prod_{i=1}^{n} \prod_{j=i}^{q_i} p(\boldsymbol{\theta}_{ij})$$

and given D the parameters remain independent and can be updated independently

$$p(\theta_G \mid D) = \prod_{i=1}^{n} \prod_{j=i}^{q_i} p(\boldsymbol{\theta}_{ij} \mid D)$$

➢ **Prior Dirichlet**

Each variable Θ_{ij} has a Dirichlet distribution as a prior (Bernardo, J. M., Smith, A. F. M. 1994), because it turns out that most of the interesting calculations can be done in a closed form. The Dirichlet prior which is the conjugate distribution for multinomial sampling, allows us to have the posterior distribution in the same form as the prior distribution. A Dirichlet distribution over Θ_{ij} is defined via a set of hyperparameters ($\alpha_{ij1}=N'_{ij1},\ldots,\alpha_{ijk}=N'_{ijk}$) and we use the notation $\Theta_{ij}\sim Dir(\alpha_{ij1},\ldots,\alpha_{ijk})$. In this case the prior density of Θ_{ij} is (up to a proportionality constant)

$$p(\boldsymbol{\theta}_{ij}) \propto \prod_{k=1}^{r_i} \theta_{ijk}^{\alpha_{ijk}-1}, \quad \alpha_{ijk}>0$$

The prior hyperparameters α_{ijk} encode the observer's prior belief and can be regarded as frequencies of imaginary datasets needed to formulate the prior distribution. As a matter of fact the marginal probability of

$(X_i=x_i^k|\mathbf{Pa}(X_i)=\mathbf{pa}_i^j)$ is α_{ijk}/α_{ij} where $\alpha_{ij}=\sum_{k=1}^{r_i}\alpha_{ijk}$ is the prior precision on θ_{ij} and $\alpha_i=\sum_{j=1}^{q_i}\alpha_{ij}$ is the size of the imaginary dataset which reflects how much confidence we actually have. The situation of initial ignorance can be represented by assuming $\alpha_{ijk}=\alpha/(r_i q_i)$, for all i, j, k so the prior probability of $(X_i=x_i^k|\mathbf{Pa}(X_i)=\mathbf{pa}_i^j)=1/r_i$ (Ramoni, M., Sebastiani, P., 1999). The choice of appropriate values can most easily be carried out with a computer-based elicitation tool. The posterior distribution over Θ_{ij}~$Dir(\alpha_{ij1}+N_{ij1},\ldots,\alpha_{ijk}+N_{ijk})$ and the posterior density of Θ_{ij} is (up to a proportionality constant)

$$p(\boldsymbol{\theta}_{ij}\mid D)\propto\prod_{k=1}^{r_i}\theta_{ijk}^{\alpha_{ijk}+N_{ijk}-1}$$

We examine the consequences of the assumptions

- The likelihood function $L(\theta_G)=p(D|\theta_G)$ is

$$L(\theta_G)=\prod_i\prod_j\prod_k\theta_{ijk}{}^{N_{ijk}}$$

The likelihood decomposes according to the structure of the network.

The N_{ijk} counts are sufficient statistics that summarise the relevant information for the likelihood from the data.

- The posterior density over Θ_G is

$$p(\theta_G\mid D)\propto\prod_i\prod_j\prod_k\theta_{ijk}{}^{\alpha_{ijk}+N_{ijk}-1}$$

If the parameters are non related, they can be estimated independently of each other and the standard Bayesian estimate of θ_{ijk} is the posterior expectation that is

$$\hat{\theta}_{ijk}=\frac{\alpha_{ijk}+N_{ijk}}{\alpha_{ij}+N_{ij}},\ \alpha_{ij}=\sum_{k=1}^{r_i}\alpha_{ijk},\ N_{ij}=\sum_{k=1}^{r_i}N_{ijk}$$

and can be implemented by accumulating sufficient statistics.

- The marginal likelihood is obtained

$$p(D) = \prod_{i=1}^{n} \prod_{j=1}^{q_i} \frac{\Gamma(\alpha_{ij})}{\Gamma(\alpha_{ij} + N_{ij})} \prod_{k=1}^{r_i} \frac{\Gamma(\alpha_{ijk} + N_{ijk})}{\Gamma(\alpha_{ijk})}$$

where $\Gamma(\cdot)$ is the Gamma function and can be efficiently computed.

3.2.2 Learning Structure

In the previous section we considered the situation in which we are uncertain about probabilities but certain about the network structure. Now we suppose that we are also uncertain about the structure which encodes them. The problem of the learning structure Bayesian network can be stated as follows: given a fully observed database $D=(\mathbf{u}_1,\ldots,\mathbf{u}_n)$ of instances of $U=\{X_1,\ldots,X_n\}$ our task is to select $G \in \mathbf{G}$, where $\mathbf{G}$ is a family of graphical models over U and to estimate the parameters.

This problem is useful when there is a large database available and we would like to interpret the data.

In addition to providing a model, the structure also gives the expert some indications of what variables are correlated.

Adopting the Bayesian approach, let G be a discrete random variable with an assigned prior distribution. Also we assume that every $G \in \mathbf{G}$ can be represented by the parameters Θ_G and it is possible to define a probability distribution over Θ_G. The sample information is used to compute posterior distributions for each G and Θ_G via Bayes' theorem:

$$p(G \mid D) = \frac{p(G,D)}{p(D)} = cp(G,D)$$

$$\begin{aligned} p(G \mid D) &= \int p(G,\theta_G, D) d\theta_G \\ &= \int p(D \mid G,\theta_G) p(\theta_G \mid G) p(G) d\theta_G \\ &= p(G) \int p(D \mid G,\theta_G) p(\theta_G \mid G) d\theta_G \\ &= p(G) p(D \mid G) \end{aligned}$$

where $p(D|G,\Theta_G)$ is simply the probability of the data given a specific network structure.

- **Prior distribution over G**

  The prior distribution over G is uniform.

The prior distribution over structures is usually considered the less important of the two components, a simple prior distribution is often chosen for pragmatic reasons and the most common choice is uniform distribution (Heckerman, D., 1998); alternative prior distributions can be founded in (Buntine, W. 1991; Heckerman, D., Meek, C., Cooper, G., 1997; Madigan, D., Garvin, J., Raftery, A., 1995). We note that every G uses the same complete database and has equal probability prior distribution, so

$$p(G|D) \propto p(D|G) \text{ for every } G \in \mathbf{G}$$

We will restrict ourselves to the assumptions of the previous section, thus we only need the marginal likelihood which we gained before.

3.2.3 Model selection and search

In learning network structures, several networks are generated and compared to decide which one is the best structure, given the database. For the purpose of comparing structures a quality measure is used: the better the network fits the data, the higher the quality.

In order to construct network structures a learning algorithm is employed which selects network structures that are likely to be of high quality from the space of all possible structures. It also searches for a network structure with the highest quality, which may be seen as the solution to an optimisation problem.

A Bayesian network algorithm requires the following components to be determined:

1. Scoring function
2. Search procedure

Each component will be discussed separately

➢ **Scoring function**

We refer to a quality measure of how likely a graphical model is for the database. In our problem we assume as scoring function, the Bayesian score (**BD score**), that is the relative posterior probability of a network structure, given the data. This posterior probability, by the assumptions, is proportional to marginal likelihood

$$\mathbf{Score_{BD}}(G|D)=p(D|G)$$

Without loss of generality we can use its natural logarithm and the marginal likelihood is decomposable precisely in the sum of the marginal log likelihood of each dependency in the graphical model.

Now the goal is to find the network structure with the highest posterior probability which is called a maximum a posteriori, **MAP** model.

- **Search procedure**

The search procedure involves the definition of two elements: the search space, that is operators which take on a structure and modify it to produce another and a search algorithm which does the optimisation search. A search space is defined when the states in the space are possible structures and operators denote the adjacency of structures. The typical operators in the search space are add edge, delete edge, reverse edge. The search starts with a candidate network, which may be the empty one (or one that an expert has provided as a starting point) and by applying the operators, the high scoring network is searched in the space.

The space of a Bayesian network is a combinatorial space, consisting of a super-exponential number of structures. As the number of variables increases, the evaluation of all graphical models becomes intractable. Therefore it needs smaller domains or those in which additional constraints (Heckerman, D., Meek, C., Cooper, G., 1997) restrict the space. However heuristic methods have to be used to limit the search space to a sub-set of models.

A heuristic search usually limits its attention to the subset of network structures that are consistent with a partial ordering "<" among the variables, that is if $X_i < X_j$, $i \neq j$, X_i can never be a parent of X_j.

The most commonly used algorithm for an optimisation search was originally proposed by Cooper and Hersokovitz (1992), i.e. the **K2** algorithm, which is a Greedy Hill-Climbing algorithm. The **K2** algorithm works on a predefined ordering on the set of variables creating a list upon which the Greedy search is performed. The rank of each variable defines the set of variables which will be tested as possible parents - the higher the order of a variable, the higher the number of variables to be tested. The use of the **K2** algorithm starts with the highest rank variable and the calculation of the score of the model which has no edge towards the variable from the others on the list. The next step is to calculate the score of the models with a single edge to this variable from the others on the list. If none of these dependences has a higher score than the model without edges, the latter is taken as the most probable model and the next variable on the list is evaluated. If at least one of these models has a higher score than the model without edges directed towards the variable, the corresponding edge is accepted and the search continues, trying to add two edges towards the variable and so on until the score no longer increases. Once the evaluation of a variable has ended, the algorithm removes it and substitutes it with the second variable on the original list and repeats the same search. The fact that the database is complete, or rather that no entry has an unknown value in the database, is a key characteristic making the induction of Bayesian networks computationally feasible.

A Hill-Climbing algorithm may produce inconveniencies such as Local Maximums where all the changes of a single edge reduce the score, and Plateaux where some changes on a edge leave the score unaltered. To avoid these problems some expedients such as Tabu-Search, Random Restarts and Simulated Annealing are adopted.

Search algorithms have had various proposals, but in general the performance differences are not so evident, and the **K2** works in the same way when a good ordering is available. However, some experimental research has shown that the Greedy search method is efficient. In addition, carrying out the Greedy search in a space where **Markov equivalent models** are present, i.e. network structures that represent the same set of conditional independence assertions for the domain problem (Heckerman, D., Meek, C., Cooper, G., 1997; Pearl, J, Verma, T., 1990) are represented by a single model, there has been an improvement in performance.

4. MATERIAL AND ITS APPLICATIONS

4.1 The database

The statistical unit is the family. To build the database only families with at least two members were considered. The analysis to be carried out concerns the condition of patients in particular; for this reason the choice has been made to analyze the answers to the questionnaire of the family member who has had at least one period of hospitalization. Should two or more persons in this condition be present in a family, one of them is chosen at random. Some variables do however refer directly to the family or head of the family. We then give a short presentation of the analyzed variables, specifying for each of these all possible states and the person considered to be the reference. By construction the variables are all observable and the database does not show missing cases.

***Titolo di studio* - Qualification**: "1=research doctorate or post-degree specialisation"; "2=degree", "3=university diploma", "4=secondary school diploma (4-5 years)", "5=secondary school diploma (2-3 years)", "6=junior secondary school-leaving certificate", "7= elementary school-leaving certificate", "8=no qualification (can read and write)", "9=no qualification (cannot read and/or write)". The head of the family is considered the reference person.

Condizione professionale **- Professional situation**: "1=employed", "2=in search of new job", "3= in search of first job", "4=on military call up or civilian alternative", "5=housewife", "6=student", "7=unfit", "8=retired", "9=other condition". The head of the family is considered the reference person.

Tipo di nucleo **- Type of family unit**: "0=no unit", "1=couple with children", "2= couple without children", "3=single parent father", "4=single parent mother". Referring directly to the family.

Tipologia familiare **- Family typology**: this variable was constructed with the help of the expert in such a way as to present 6 possible states (in the gathering of data it gave a total of 41 possible states): "1=family without unit", "2= couple with children", "3= couple without children", "4=male single parent", "5=female single parent", "6=families with two units". Referring directly to the family.

Parentela **- Relationship**: "1=head of family", "2=spouse", "3=cohabitant", "4=parent of head of family", "5=parent of head of family's spouse", "6=child of head of family", "7=child born of previous marriage", "8=child's spouse", "9=child's cohabitant", "10=grandchild", "11=nephew/niece", "12=brother/sister", "13= brother/sister of head of family's spouse", "14=spouse of brother/sister of head of family", "15=cohabitant of brother/sister of head of family", "16=other relative of head of family", "17=person linked by friendship". The patient is considered the reference person.

Ripartizione zona geografica **- Geographic area distribution**: "1= Northwest Italy", "2= Northeast Italy", "3= Central Italy", "4=Southern Italy", "5=Italian Islands". Referring directly to the family.

Fonte reddito principale **- Main source of income**: "1=from subordinate employment", "2=from self-employment", "3=pension", "4=various benefits and allowances", "5=property", "6=support from family" The head of the family is the reference person.

Assicurazione salute **- Health insurance**: "1=No", "2=Yes". State 2 is present in the variable if at least one family member possesses health insurance.

Assicurazione vita **- Life insurance**: "3=no", "4=yes". State 4 is present in the variable if at least one family member possesses life insurance..

Componenti famiglia **- Number of family members**: adopts the state corresponding to the number of family members, therefore the possible states number from 1 to 12.

Età discretizzata **- Age**: this variable was constructed with the help of the expert in such a way as to present 4 possible states: "1=[0,14]", "2=[15,35]", "3=[36,65]", "4=[65+]". The subdivision into these states was made in accordance with the significance which this variable can adopt within the analysis. The patient is considered the reference person.

Sesso **- Sex**: "1=male", "2=female". The patient is considered the reference person.

Malattie croniche **- Chronic illnesses**: "1=yes", "2=no". The variable adopts state 1 if at least one family member has one of the following chronic illnesses:

- Diabetes
- Arterial hypertension
- Myocardium infarct
- Angina pectoris or other heart diseases
- Chronic bronchitis, emphysema, respiratory insufficiency
- Bronchial asthma
- Allergic illnesses
- Tumour
- Gastric and duodenal ulcer
- Liver and biliary calculosis
- Hepatic cirrhosis
- Renal calculosis
- Arthrosis, arthritis
- Osteoporosis
- Nervous illnesses

Media gg ricovero1 **- Average number of days in hospital**: "1=[0,4]", "2=[5,7]", "3=[8,14]", "4=[15,30]", "5=[30+]". This variable was initially constructed by finding the average number of days in hospital of the hospitalised person, or rather by dividing the number of days in hospital over the previous three months by the number of hospitalisations over the previous three months. This was then discreeted with the help of the expert in such a way as to present 5 possible states, in accordance with their significance for the purposes of the analysis.

Assistenza medica **- Degree of satisfaction with hospitalisation for medical care**: "1=very", "2=quite", "3=not very", "4=not at all" "5=don't know". The patient is considered the reference person.

Assistenza inferm **- Degree of satisfaction with hospitalisation for nursing care**: "1=very", "2=quite", "3=not very", "4=not at all" "5=don't know". The patient is considered the reference person.

Vitto **- Degree of satisfaction with hospitalisation for food**: "1=very", "2=quite", "3=not very", "4=not at all" "5=don't know". The patient is considered the reference person.

Servizi igienici **- Degree of satisfaction with hospitalisation for hygienic services**: "1=very", "2=quite", "3=not very", "4=not at all" "5=don't know". The patient is considered the reference person.

***Farmacia* - Difficulties met by family in reaching pharmacy services**: "1=no difficulties", "2=some difficulties", "3=many difficulties", "4=don't know". Referring directly to the family.
***Pronto soccorso* - Difficulties met by family in reaching emergency services**: "1=no difficulties", "2=some difficulties", "3=many difficulties", "4=don't know". Referring directly to the family.
***Collaboratore domestico* - Private domestic help in the family**: "1=no", "2=yes". Referring directly to the family.
***Assistenza anziani disabile* - Private care for elderly or disabled in the family**: "1=no", "2=yes". Referring directly to the family.

The database thus constructed gives 2269 records.

4.2 Network structure

The "Main Source of Income" variable, present in the database as suggested by the expert, is not initially considered in the analysis.

The remaining variables have been divided into three subgroups:

- **Context variables**: these are the general variables of the social-demographic characteristics of the statistical units; in this group only the variables "Age", "Sex", "Relationship", "Qualification", "Professional situation", "Type of family unit", "Family typology", "Number of family members", "Geographic area distribution" have been considered.
- **Intermediate variables**: these are concomitant variables which interact with the context variables to condition the target variables: "Chronic illnesses", "Health insurance", "Life insurance", "Private domestic help in the family", "Private care for elderly or disabled in the family", "Average number of days in hospital", "Difficulties met by family in reaching pharmacy services", "Difficulties met by family in reaching emergency services".
- **Target variables**: these are the variables we wish to investigate: "Degree of satisfaction with hospitalisation for medical care", "Degree of satisfaction with hospitalisation for nursing care", "Degree of satisfaction with hospitalisation for food", "Degree of satisfaction with hospitalisation for hygienic services".

The first step was to find the ordering of the variables which leads to a network with a higher score. In order to do so, all possible networks were built, each time modifying the order of the variables and evaluating the marginal likelihood function of each network created, starting with the context variables and keeping the others fixed. Having found the most efficient order within each subgroup, the best order for the construction of the network is the following:

- age

- sex
- geographic area distribution
- professional situation
- qualification
- type of family unit
- relationship
- family typology
- number of family members
- chronic illnesses
- life insurance
- health insurance
- private domestic help in the family
- private care for elderly or disabled in the family
- average number of days in hospital
- difficulties met by family in reaching pharmacy services
- difficulties met by family in reaching emergency services
- degree of satisfaction with hospitalisation for nursing care
- degree of satisfaction with hospitalisation for medical care
- degree of satisfaction with hospitalisation for hygienic services
- degree of satisfaction with hospitalisation for food

The software used in the analysis is Bayesware Discoverer (BD). It is based on all the assumptions specified in sections 3.2.1, 3.2.2, 3.2.3. Moreover, it uses marginal likelihood as its scoring function and the **K2** algorithm as its research method. For further information see the internet site www.bayesware.com.

An initial network has been defined through the automatic generation supplied by BD software. Since this provided three blocks of variables connected within a block but free from the variables of the other blocks, it was necessary to globally research which relations were best capable of linking together the blocks of variables. Preliminary tests of independence among variables were used to do this, calculated with the R software (Chi Square, Kendall, Spearman Tests).

The "Main Source of Income" variable was evaluated separately, following the expert's suggestion, because some of the answers to the questionnaire were not reliable. The variable is introduced after a preliminary cleaning of the data, thus the database has been reduced to a number of records equal to 2197. In order to decide where to insert it, a network was created for every possible position in the ordering, evaluating the respective marginal likelihood function assumed by the network. The "Main Source of Income" variable is inserted into the context variables group and is placed immediately after "Geographic Area Distribution". After consultation with the expert several variables were eliminated from the network because they were considered superfluous for the analysis – "Type of family unit" because it gives similar information to "Family typology", "difficulties met by family in reaching pharmacy services" and "difficulties met by family in reaching emergency services" because they are marginal and do not influence the other variables.

5. BAYESIAN NETWORK FOR THE PROBLEM "HOSPITAL AND FAMILIES: THE ANALYSIS OF PATIENT SATISFACTION WITH HOSPITAL RECOVERY"

The graphic model we produced is shown in figure 1. We show that its general structure can be subdivided into three sub-graphs or "clusters" of nodes which are highlighted in the figure by a dotted line aimed at simplifying the reading and interpretation of the network.

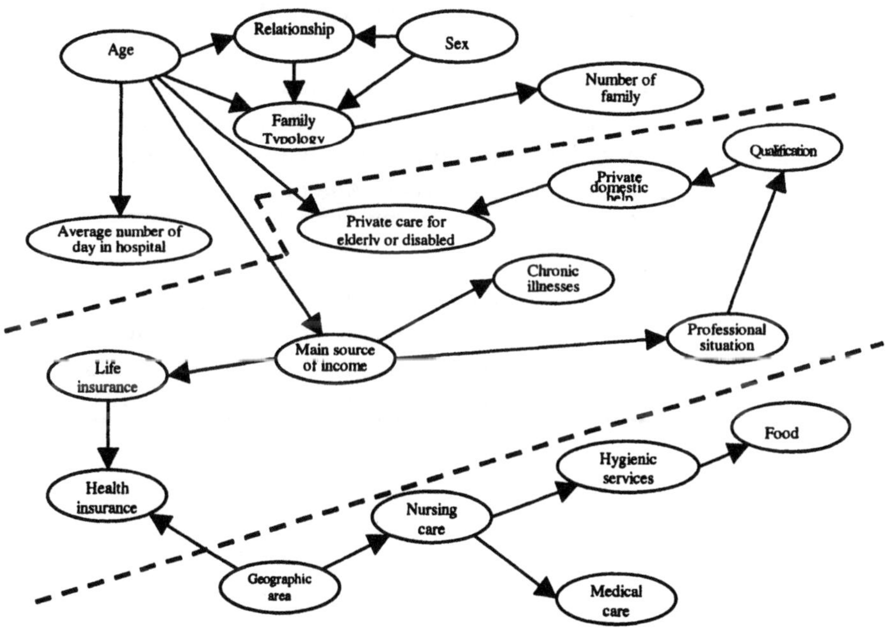

Figure 1. Bayesian network structure. The dotted lines separate the three sub-graphs described in the text.

These three areas aggregate around three variables of differing but important nature and can be thought of as the centres of the three sub-graphs, arranged in an approximately chronological and causal sequence.

The first variable has a demographic nature - the age of the hospitalised family member. The next is a social and economic variable such as the source of income of the head of family. Finally there is a variable of strategic importance in Italy, whose relevance is documented and confirmed by many other studies in this area of research (Bolzan, M., Frigo, A. C., Fabbris, M. L., Rausa, G. 1998). It is represented by the geographic subdivision of residence of the patient (even if there is, to a certain extent, hospital mobility in Italy, from hospitals in the south to those in the north).

After defining the structure of the network, the next step consists in determining the joint probability distribution on the whole structure, or rather in specifying a table of conditional probability (CPT) for each node – a table of conditioned probability of the states of that node, given every combination of states of its parent nodes.

From an operational and interpretative point of view, it is useful to ask the expert to simplify the number of CPTs based on his knowledge and experience with reference to the sub-graphs characterized in figure 1, which we shall examine later.

5.1 Bayesian Network: structure and parameters

- At the top of the network we have a cluster of nodes representing general variables of the social-demographic characteristics associated with the statistical unit (family of hospitalized patient), with nodes for the various sources of evidence relating directly to the Age of patient.

Average no. of days in hospital	1	2	3	4	5
Age					
1	0,657	0,197	0,107	0,039	0
2	0,496	0,288	0,143	0,066	0,007
3	0,381	0,226	0,241	0,136	0,016
4	0,262	0,198	0,303	0,207	0,03

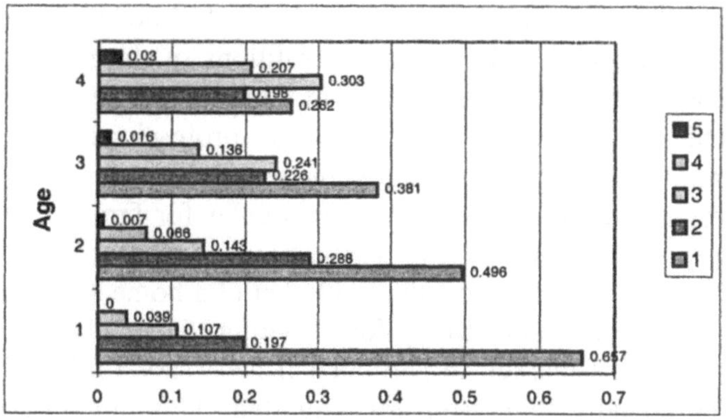

Moreover it seems clear that age also defines the role within the family, in that if older, it is reasonable to assume he or she is the head of the family.

Relationship	1	2	3	4	5	6	7	8
Age								
1	0,000	0,000	0,000	0,000	0,000	0,983	0,017	0,000
2	0,133	0,286	0,019	0,000	0,000	0,546	0,009	0,007
3	0,538	0,393	0,013	0,011	0,001	0,034	0,002	0,009
4	0,565	0,270	0,012	0,087	0,042	0,023	0,000	0,000

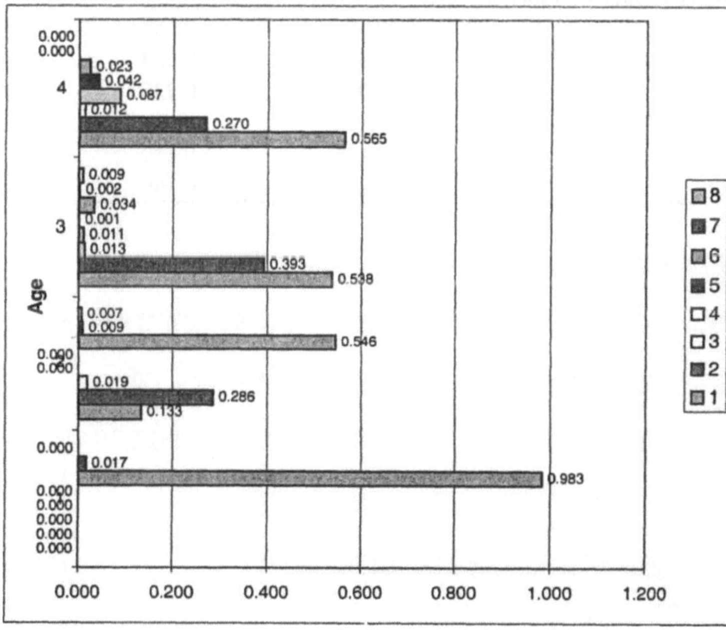

➤ In the intermediate part of the network there is a cluster representing variables associated to the social and economic life conditions of the family. All the nodes branch off from the central node "Source of Main Income". The social and economic conditions of the family, explained mainly by the typology of source of family income, which is itself associated to the head of family's professional position and qualifications, is interesting to know the resources available to the family in confronting the needs of care, in particular for families with elderly patients, justified also by the seriousness of an extended period of hospitalisation. This care together with that of a home help, more widely used by families, are not easily found within the family. They must be looked for on the market, in particular if necessary abilities in a family with a chronically ill person are requested. This circumstance merits attention in this analysis because it highlights the relationship between source of income of the head of family and presence of a chronically ill person. The elevated probability of being chronically ill (according to a list of large and varying groups of illnesses) is normal in families with elderly or hospitalised persons (in this case conditions may reasonably coincide), or where a source of income no longer from work (pension or insurance) is declared.

Chronic illnesses	0	1
Main source of income		
1	0,345	0,655
2	0,371	0,629
3	0,075	0,925
4	0,194	0,806
5	0,111	0,889
6	0,231	0,769

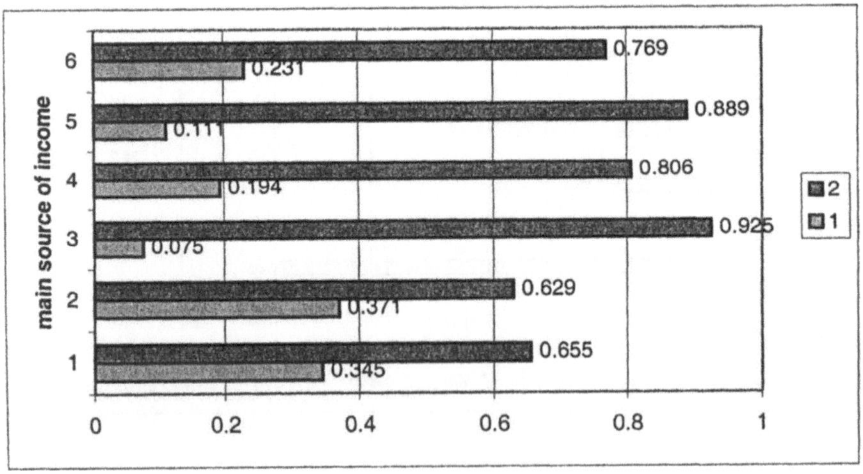

The role of the central node here is essential. This help, therefore, is precious just as much as it is burdensome for the family, particularly where an increased need of care is present, such as in the case of hospitalization of a family member.

- At the bottom of the network, the geographic area of residence in Italy expresses an important dimension of the level of quality of life and in particular of quality of hospital care offered in the national territory. The different distribution, among the country's large geographic areas, of those who have taken out health or life insurance, are indicative of different life conditions and availability of resources of the populations resident in the various regions of Italy.

Health insurance	1	2
Geographic area		
1	0,675	0,325
2	0,607	0,393
3	0,721	0,279
4	0,851	0,149
5	0,830	0,170

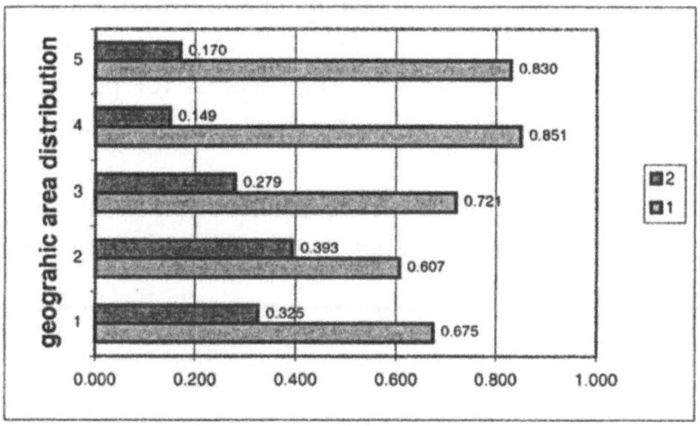

Health insurance	1	2
Source of income		
1	0,697	0,303
2	0,483	0,517
3	0,841	0,159
4	0,871	0,129
5	0,889	0,111
6	0,865	0,135

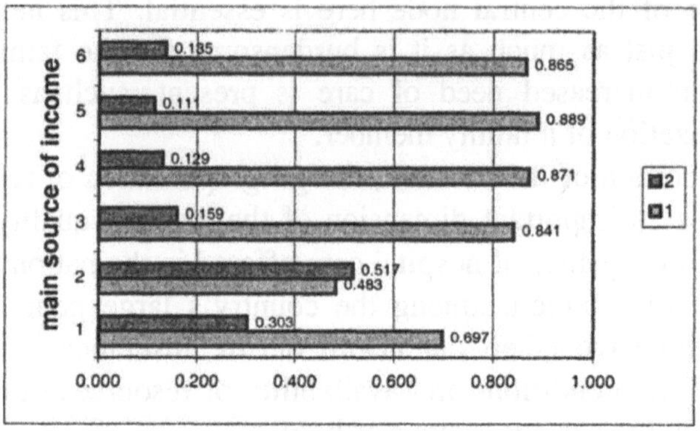

Naturally such resources, reasonably made available by the family in the circumstances of hospitalization, represent further help which is useful in confronting a critical event. Confirming what has emerged from other studies (Bolzan, M., Frigo, A. C., Fabbris, M. L., Rausa, G. 1998; Bolzan, M. 2001; Bolzan, M.2002), the satisfaction expressed by patients with regard to hospital care according to the four typologies of services (here information on other services present in hospital care and of equal interest was not gathered, such as all the service activated at the time of hospitalization and those concerning the request for personal information), expresses varying satisfaction on the part of patients in the country's hospitals.

In the north there is a high level of satisfaction with services and care received, while the trend reverses heading south and to the islands.

Nursing care	1	2	3	4	5
Geo. area distribution					
1	0,45	0,436	0,075	0,035	0,002
2	0,502	0,406	0,068	0,017	0,007
3	0,282	0,603	0,083	0,022	0,01
4	0,188	0,612	0,152	0,042	0,005
5	0,242	0,536	0,157	0,062	0,003

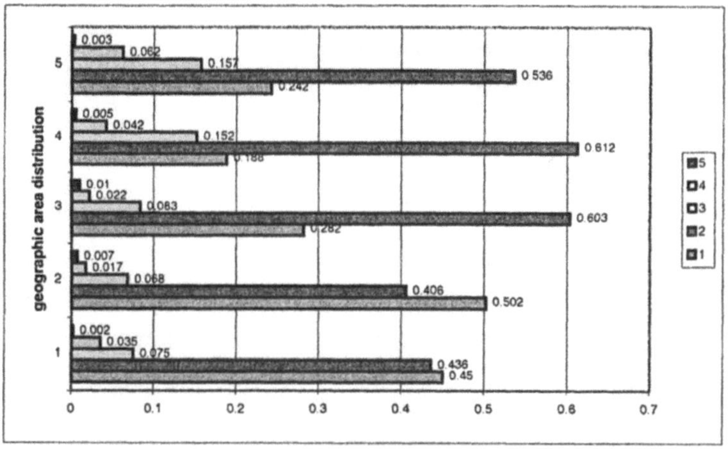

Nursing care seems to represent an important node in perceiving the quality of hospital care received during hospitalization. This is further confirmed by other studies and is understandable given that the nurse, for how the hospital care service is organized in Italy, has a very intense, frequent and personal relationship with the patient (Bolzan, M. 2001).

In fact the nurse carries out a function of mediator between the doctor and the patient, plus he or she coordinates all health services, including specialist services, all day long. In this sub-graph, the latter characteristic highlights itself well from the distinct relationship which this care has with medical care and clearly with the other two residential services (food and hygienic services).

Medical care	1	2	3	4	5
Nursing care					
1	0,874	0,108	0,013	0,006	0
2	0,076	0,852	0,053	0,018	0
3	0,071	0,537	0,342	0,046	0,004
4	0,104	0,156	0,245	0,494	0
5	0,167	0,25	0	0	0,583

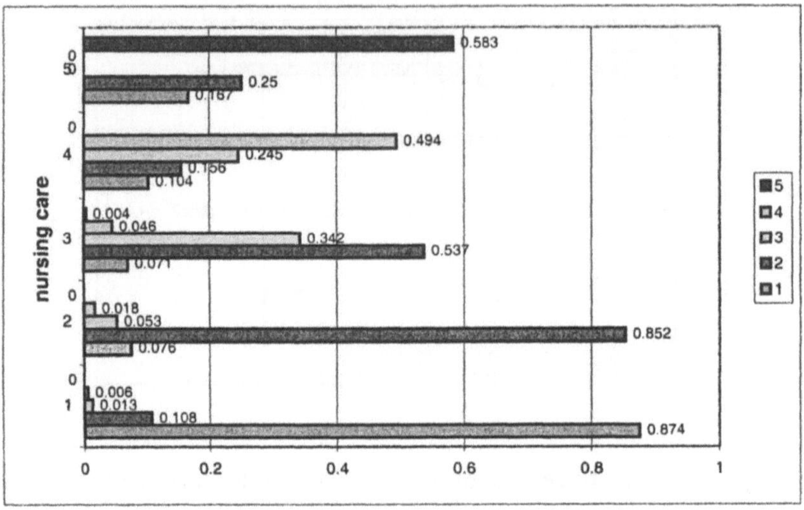

6. CONCLUSIONS

The application of the Bayesian network carried out on data gathered during the ISTAT National Survey on Family in 1998, concerning satisfaction with hospital services of about 2200 patients (all those within the sample families who declared they had been hospitalised during the three months prior to the interview), is part of a wider research intended to analyse the relationship between families and systems of services (primarily social and health). The database contains information on over 23000 families interviewed and represents an original and wide basis of statistical analysis. The matter under study is particularly relevant in Italy where the family has undergone remarkable, radical changes. There has been a significant change in family structure and dynamics, producing a greater number of singles, couples without children, and elderly family units (alone or couples). Along with other social and economic factors, this has consequently led to a gradual disappearance of the nets of care within and between families, which characterised the Italian social tissue until the 1960s and which represented one of the resources of the system of care (Bragatta, G., Arcaleni, E, 2000; Donati, P., 1991; Facchini, C., 1997; Saraceno, C., 1998). Parallel to these demographic phenomena there has been a remarkable strengthening and spread of services for citizens (social, health and care) across the territory. This development has, on the one hand, strengthened the efficiency of the system of services (increasing the production of services offered) and, on the other, has been unable to adequately respond to and resolve the real needs and problems of users (increase in efficacy). Analysis of the satisfaction of patients in hospital thus presents one of the main activities in governing health services. This work is intended to focus attention on the role the family plays or at least how the family enters and activates itself in a moment of particular difficulty and commitment, both in terms of emotions and resources, such as when a family member is in hospital. The results obtained with this initial application find substantial and interesting confirmation with what was obtained in other ways and with other statistical methods of analysis (Bolzan, M., Frigo, A. C., Fabbris, M. L., Rausa, G., 1998; Bolzan, M., 2001; Bolzan, M., 2002). Certainly they introduce interesting new elements, particularly concerning methodological properties and the typology of the relationships between variables (and the possibility of graphically representing them – not to be neglected when results must also be presented to non statisticians such as those responsible for governing public health and programming services).

The social and demographic characteristics of the patient (age, role within the family, professional situation) interact among themselves and highlight the relations and family typologies of patients in Italy. Together with these relationships and variables the (economic and caring) resources of the family intervene, considerably contributing to the understanding of the phenomena in question. The territorial dimension, and therefore organisational dimension, of the hospital service in Italy is inserted in the framework of family/services relationships. The difference in level of satisfaction expressed by the patient appears to be significantly different in different areas of the country. In addition, the territorial component appears to be indicative, not only of the different perceived level of quality, which may be the real expression of a qualitatively inferior service in the south with respect to the north, but also of the different social and economic conditions of the family. Reasonably, the bitterness of not having the resources at their disposal which would have perhaps guaranteed better care is added to the dissatisfaction expressed concerning care services received during hospitalisation. The application of the Bayesian network has at this point made it possible to appreciate some results which, with other applications, would have been of dubious interpretation. The reference is on the side of the ISTAT database, particularly with regard to the relationship between social and economic variables and territorial variables of the family of the patient. The ISTAT survey is the most important carried out on a national level and is certainly the widest but the chapter concerning the use of services contains some gaps which this application has in part permitted us to overcome. The territorial reference is connected to the residence of the patient's family and not to the hospital where the patient is treated (migration from south to north of patients for hospital care has become quite consistent in Italy). Thus interpretation of the relationship between residence and hospital satisfaction is not immediate. Vice versa, application of the Bayesian network has highlighted and permitted us to appreciate the relationship between geographic area and caring resources of the family (life and health insurance). In particular the presence in the south of the country (more than in the north) of a lower level of satisfaction and availability of family resources expresses a validation of the informative contribution summarised by the territorial dimension, on the perceived quality of care.

Finally, the relationship between the various types of services and care, and the centrality of the role of nursing care, highlight the complexity of the hospital system in Italy and express the importance of investing not only in so-called fixed resources (installations and structures and greater specialist personnel) but also in the humanisation and personalisation of health care based on people and not on use.

ACKNOWLEDGEMENTS

Thanks go to Roberto Boggiani for the computational support given to this work.

REFERENCES

BERNARDO, J. M., SMITH, A. F. M. (1994), Bayesian Theory, Wiley and Sons, New York.

BINDA, W. (1994), La famiglia come risorsa nella salute e nella malattia. In L'arco di Giano, rivista di medical humanities, 5, Angeli, Mi.

BOLZAN, M., FRIGO, A. C., FABBRIS, M. L., RAUSA, G. (1998), Qualità espressa dai pazienti sui servizi igienici ospedalieri in Italia. In *L'Igiene Moderna*, 109:681-690.

BOLZAN, M. (2001), Nuove misure del disagio familiare e di accesso ai servizi socio-sanitari per condizione di salute. In *LA SALUTE IN FAMIGLIA. Per un sistema statistico Informativo in grado di valutare la salute nella famiglia,* Atti del Convegno (a cura di M. Bolzan), Padova 6 Aprile: 113-126.

BOLZAN, M.(2002), Le famiglie valutano l'accessibilità ai servizi socio-sanitari. Risultati di un'analisi in Italia e nel Triveneto, *Argomenti 4*:101-118.

BUNTINE, W. (1991), Theory refinement on Bayesian networks. In Proceedings of Seventh Conference on Uncertainty in Artificial Intelligence, Los Angeles, CA. Morgan Kaufmann.

BRAGATTA, G., ARCALENI, E, (2000) La tipologia familiare per nuclei e per generazioni. In *SIS, Atti dalla XL Riunione Scientifica,* Firenze 26-28 Aprile 2000.

CHICKERING, D. (1996), Learning equivalence classes of Bayesian network structures. In Proceedings of Twelth Conference on Uncertainty in Artificial Intelligence, Portland, OR. Morgan Kaufmann.

CIONI, E. (1997), Il sistema di parentela. In Lo stato delle famiglie in Italia, Barbagli M., Saraceno C. (a cura di), il Mulino, Bologna.

COOPER, G., HERSKOVITS, E. (1992), A Bayesian method for the induction of probabilistic networks from data, *Machine learning*, *9*:309-347.

DE FINETTI, B. (1937), La prévision : ses lois logiques, ses sources subjectives. In *Ann. Inst. H. Poincaré*, 7:1-68 (trad. In (1964) Studies in Subjective Probability. Kyburg, H. E., Smokler, H. E., Wiley, New York)
DEMING, W. E., (1982), Out of the crisis, Cambridge Univ. Press.
DONABEDIAN, A., (1980), Explorations in quality assessment and monitoring. In The definition of quality and approaches to its assessment, Vol.1, Ann Arbor, Michigan, University of Michigan
DONABEDIAN, A., (1988), The quality of care. How can it be assessed?, Jama
DONATI, P., (1991), Famiglia, servizi e reti informali in Italia. In La famiglia nella società relazionale: nuove reti e nuove regole, Ed. F. Angeli, Milano .
EUROSTAT, (1999), European Community Household Panel: selected indicators from the 1995 wave, Eurostat, Luxemburg.
GOOD, I., (1965), The Estimation of Probability, MIT Press, Cambridge MA.
FACCHINI, C., (1997), Gli anziani e la solidarietà tra le generazioni. In Lo stato delle famiglie in Italia, Barbagli, M., Saraceno, C., (a cura di), il Mulino, Bologna.
HECKERMAN, D., GEIGER, D., CHICKERING, D. (1995), Learning Bayesian Networks: The combination of knowledge and statistical data, *Machine Learning, 20*:197-243.
HECKERMAN, D., MEEK, C., COOPER, G., (1997), A Bayesian Approach to Causal Discovery. Technical report, *Technical report MSR-TR-97-05*, Microsoft Research.
HECKERMAN, D., (1995), A Bayesian Approach to learning Causal Networks. Technical report, *Technical report MSR-TR-95-04*, Microsoft Research.
HECKERMAN, D., (1998), A tutorial on learning with Bayesian networks. In M.I. Jordan (ed): Learning in Graphical models, Dordrecht, Netherlands, Kluwer.
JENSEN, F. V., (1996), An Introduction to Bayesian Networks, London, UK: University College London Press.
ISTAT (1994b), Condizioni di salute e ricorso ai servizi sanitari. *Collana indagine multiscopo sulle famiglie. 10*, Roma.
ISTAT (2000a), Rapporto annuale. La situazione del Paese nel 1999. Istat, Roma
ISTAT (2000b), Le strutture familiari. Indagine Multiscopo sulle famiglie "Famiglie, soggetti sociali e condizioni dell'infanzia". 1998, Istat, Roma.
MADIGAN, D., GARVIN, J., RAFTERY, A., (1995), Eliciting prior information to enhance the predictive performance of Bayesian graphical models. *Communications in Statistics: Theory and Methods, 24*:2271-2292.
ØVRETVEIT, J., (1992), Health service quality. Blackwell Scientific Pubblication.
PEARL, J., (1988), Probabilistic Reasoning in Intelligent System: Networks of Plausible Inference, Morgan Kaufmann, San Mateo, CA.
PEARL, J, VERMA, T., (1990), Equivalence and synthesis of causal models. In Proceedings of Sixth Conference on Uncertainty in Artificial Intelligence. Boston, MA, Morgan Kaufmann
PLESS, I. B., (1984), The family as a resource unit in health care: changing patterns. In *Soc. Sci. Med. 19*, 4:385-389.
ROSS, C. K., STEWARD, C. A., SINACORE, J. M., (1983), The importance of patient preference in the measurement of the health care satisfaction, In *Medical care*, 31-12
RAMONI, M., SEBASTIANI, P., (1999), Bayesian Methods for Intelligent Data Analysis. In M. Berthold and D.J. Hand (eds): Intelligent Data Analysis : An Introduction, Springer, New York, NY.
SARACENO, C., (1998), Mutamenti della famiglia e politiche sociali in Italia, Il Mulino, Bologna.
SPIEGELHALTER, D. J., LAURITZEN, S. L., (1990), Sequential updating of Conditional Probabilities on Directed Graphical Structures, In Network, 20: 579-605

SPIRTES, P., MEEK, C., (1995), Learning Bayesian networks with discrete variables from data. In Proceedings of First International Conference on Knowledge and Data Mining. Montreal, QU, Morgan Kaufmann.

WARE, J. E., (1978), A taxonomy of patient satisfaction . In *Health and Medical Care Service Review, 1*:2-15

WARE, J. E., (1981), How to survey patient satisfaction. In *Drug International and Clinical Pharmacy, 15*:892-899.

WARE, J. E., HAYS, R. D., (1988), Methods for measuring patient satisfaction with specific medical encounters, In *Medical care*, 26-4.

Chapter 5

RELIABILITY OF GIST DIAGNOSIS BASED ON PARTIAL INFORMATION

A. Capotorti[1*] and S.F. Leite[2]

Dipartimento di Matematica e Informatica, Università degli Studi di Perugia, Italy[1]; Istituto di Anatomia e Istologia Patologica, Divisione di ricerca sul cancro, Università degli Studi di Perugia, Italy[2].

1. INTRODUCTION

In several medical diagnostic procedures there is the absence for a "golden standard" to follow, especially when new advances in the understanding of the biology are done or new techniques are discovered. In such situations, different opinions appear in scientific literature and they are based on disparate case studies, each one with its peculiarity and heterogeneity of data. Due to these discrepancies, it is reasonable the physician tries to "replicate" such evaluations to have a better (scientifically based) idea of which diagnostic procedure to adopt. But there are situations where new sophisticated techniques are required and, either they are so expensive that only few selected trials can be performed, or they are at such initial stage that it is hard to fully trust on them. Moreover, the physician could have the opportunity to make only a "retrospective" study and usually reliability and accuracy of such data are not very high.

A "prototype" of such situation is, for example, the diagnosis of gastrointestinal stromal tumors (GISTs), where only recently a new and reliable phenotypic marker (the KIT protein CD117) for these neoplasm has been introduced. It's a common behavior that few other area of surgical pathology has caused as much confusion and controversy as GISTs. In the past, because of a lack of effective therapeutic options, GISTs were a neglected area and they have been regarded as very rare, while a more

* For correspondence: capot@dipmat.unipg.it

accurate GIST diagnosis is nowadays even more important because a new targeted therapy is available. In fact, because this new interest on them, official estimates of GISTs annual incidence of clinically detected new cases have been continuously revised, till the point that now GISTs represent the majority of mesenchimal tumors of the gastrointestinal tract (except esophagus).

There is no doubt about the confirmatory relevance of KIT immunopositivity for histologically suspected GISTs, on the contrary there is not jet precise or reliable information about its specificity and about the actual incidence of GISTs among intrabdominal mesenchymal lesions. Hence the need to "cross" the results of personal pathologist's case studies and the controversial results on the subject reported in the recent literature. This has induced us to focus on the problem of the whole diagnostic procedure based on such premise.

Usual (either classical or Bayesian) statistical analysis for diagnostic features crucially depend on or try to propose well specified statistical models to adopt in the different situations, but in the context we are "moving in", a preliminary step is required: an explicit quantitative and/or qualitative evaluation of the probabilistic bounds induced by the partial and heterogeneous available information on the main quantities (e.g. sensitivity, specificity, positive predictive value, negative predictive value, etc.) usually adopted to manage the problem at hand. Such bounds will be obtained in a fully "model-free" framework, using only relevant conditional probabilistic assessments, and they should represent a sound background for any further prior and/or likelihood model selection procedure.

To perform such basic analysis, we will profit of the methodological tools offered to us by the simple requirement to stay in a coherent setting. Coherence has its roots on the opera of de Finetti (1970) and it has been nowadays refreshed and widely developed, reaching considerable results, both for theoretical and practical issues (main ideas and results can be found on the two major latest books of Lad, 1996 and of Coletti and Scozzafava, 2002). Our methodological choice has been induced by the peculiarity of such approach to deal with arbitrary domains (i.e. not necessarily well-structured) and to require a minimal information effort. In particular, we will use the more general framework of a "mixture" of precise, imprecise (lower-upper) and qualitative conditional probabilities assessments.

Anyway, before to pass to the analytical part, in the next Section 2 there will be a detailed illustration of GISTs' features, focusing on the more debated themes and on the more uncertain aspects of their diagnosis. In Section 3 we will "embed" the available information inside a framework suitable to perform a quantitative evaluation and, apart from numerical considerations on the diagnostic procedure, it will been shown how coherence obliges a revision of some ambiguous results in the personal case study. Finally, in Section 4 we will show how results modify by introducing reasonable qualitative requirements.

2. GIST FEATURES AND DIAGNOSIS PROCEDURE

2.1 Tumor description and historical overview

The stromal gastrointestinal tumors are the most common mesenchimal neoplasm of the digestive system. They occur often in the stomach and in the small intestine as a mass of the inner/outer gastrointestinal wall. Such tumors represent an heterogeneous group of neoplasms with different morphological aspects (spindle cell and epithelioid types) and biological behavior depending on their anatomical site.

For many years GISTs were classified as smooth-muscle neoplasms (leiomyoma, leiomyosarcoma and leiomyoblastoma). In subsequent studies the ultrastructural evaluation has been applied and it has shown absence or only weak presence of smooth-muscle differentiation. In the early 1980s, with the introduction of the immunohistochemistry, Mazur and Clark described a group of gastric mesenchimal neoplasms without the immunophenotipic aspects of the smooth-muscle differentiation, associated with the expression of the neural antigen S-100 protein. For this group of neoplasms the same authors introduced the term "stromal tumor". However, at that time there was still a lack of knowledge about the line of differentiation (histogenesis), since there was not a selective tumor marker. In the 1990s many authors had described consistent immunopositivity for the marker CD34 for the GISTs. This aspect was not confirmed by others that, furthermore, have shown similar immunopositivity in different types of tumors.

Only recently the new KIT protein (CD117 antigen) has been identified by immunohistochemistry in GIST's cells. This protein, together with mutations of the gene KIT, clarified the GIST histogenesis. In fact, the unique compatible cell of the gastrointestinal tract that expresses the KIT protein is the interstitial cell of Cajal, considered nowadays the original cell of stromal tumors.

The most recent works confirm a significant immunopositivity for the KIT protein in the GISTs, both of spindle cell and epithelioid type, which arises in each anatomical site and with either malignant or benign behavior.

Moreover, an accurate detection of the KIT protein in the context of the GIST diagnosis has became fundamental since there is now a new and successful mode of therapy, which is based on the inactivation of the KIT molecule.

2.2 Diagnostic process

The GIST diagnostic approach begins with a conventional histopathological evaluation with the optical microscope. The purpose is to recognize the morphological aspects of the neoplastic cells. In fact, the finding of a neoplastic proliferation formed by fascicles of spindle cells, without significant atypia and/or nests of epithelioid cells, is highly suspected to belong to the GISTs group. Other elements to evaluate are the presence of necrosis and the mitotic rate.

According to few authors, an experienced pathologist should be able to conclude the diagnosis at this stage. However this is a debatable point because it is a current opinion that the immunophenotype is necessary to recognize the mesenchimal lesions of the gastrointestinal tract. In fact, there is a "consensus" approach (see for example Fletcher et al., 2002) that prescribes to submit to immunohistochemistry a tumor sample of cases suspected to be GISTs. The usual immunohistochemical schema consists of the KIT protein, the CD34, the muscle (smooth-muscle Actin and Desmin) and neural (S-100 protein) markers. The last three markers are employed to exclude the belonging to the smooth-muscle tumors previously described and to the Schwannomas.

Note that ultrastructural evaluation by electronic microscope is not usually performed in the GISt diagnosis routine, since the immunohistochemical technique permits for the moment accurate results.

Purpose of this paper is to evaluate the relevance of the immunohistochemical part of the diagnosis quantifying the reliability of the first stage based only on the histopathological evaluation. For this, literature expectations have been crossed with the personal research described in the next subsection.

2.3 A personal case report

We have re-examined all neoplasms suspected to belong to the GIST group that have been occurred at the *Istituto di Anatomia e Istologia Patologica - Divisione di ricerca sul cancro* - Università degli Studi di Perugia – Italy, during the period January 1998 – September 2002. In this period, 47 mesenchimal neoplasm have been diagnosed, among those 24 (41,4 %) were suspected to be GISTs. At a first stage, all the 24 cases have been reviewed with respect to their morphology (cell type, mitotic rate and necrosis). Subsequently, it was possible to obtain immunohistochemical profiles only for 13 of them. We adopted for them the "micro-array tissue" methodology, which consists of embedding tumoral samples of different patients in the same paraffin block, together with a known positive control case. Results obtained with such method are summarized in Table 1 where each single marker response has been classified by one label of the scale *negative* (-), *focal positivity* (+/-) and *diffuse positivity* (+), according to the expression intensity. Anyway, for the diagnosis purposes, single cases have been discriminated between those negative (-) from all the others, thought to be positive.

Table 1. Immunohistocehmical results for specific markers obtained on 13 cases among the 24 suspected to be GISTs

Case n°	CD117	CD34	DESMIN	ACTIN	S100
3	+	+	-	.	-
6	-	+	+	-	-
7	+	+	-	-	+/-
10	+	+	-	+	-
11	-	+	-	+	-
15	+	-	-	+	-
16	+/-	-	+	+	-
18	+	+	-	+	-
19	+	-	-	+/-	+
20	+	-	-	-	+/-
21	+/-	-	.	+	-
22	+	+	-	+	-
23	+	-	+	+	-

Note that we had two missing data, precisely the Actin answer for case n. 3 and the Desmin answer for case n. 21.

Moreover, the S-100 focal positivity (+/-) for the two cases n. 7 and 20 was actually very uncertain, so that also negativity (-) was thought to be a possible right answer.

3. EVALUATION OF THE DIAGNOSTIC CRITERIA

3.1 Quantities' specification

From the available "mass" of information about GISTs we must now isolate the relevant quantities, with their interconnections, that can be used to perform an analytical study. For this, in the sequel we will introduce binary random variables (events), each one describing the presence of a particular feature of intrabdominal mesenchymal lesions and they will be referable to any individual case.

Since we will deal with events, in the sequel we will use the usual "logical" style notation to describe combined statements. In particular, | will be used to express conditioning, the negation operator will be denoted by the symbol $\neg$, the conjunction operator $\wedge$ will be sometimes omitted to do not make the notation too heavy, while the disjunction $\vee$ and the implication $\subseteq$ will be always maintained.

First of all we can distinguish between cases diagnosed on histological basis to belong to the GIST group and those really being GIST and for this we introduce two events DIAGNOSIS and GIST, respectively. Hence the former event summarizes the satisfaction of all the preliminary features to suspect a lesion to be a GIST, while the last one represents the crucial discriminant feature among the tumors we are considering.

Apart from these two events, which are comprehensive of several details, we introduce one event for each immunopositivity at a specific marker of the immunohistochemical schema adopted for the GIST differential diagnosis as they are summarized in Table 2.

Table 2. List of the events involved in the procedure with their description

Events	Description
DIANOSIS	Tumor is histologically suspected to be a GIST
GIST	tumor is really a GIST
CD117	KIT protein expression
CD34	hematopoietic progenitor cell antigen expression
SMA	smooth-muscle actin expression
DESM	desmin expression
S100	S-100 protein expression

Of course several other events could be introduced, but either they are implicitly embedded in the first two or they have been judged irrelevant for our goal.

3.2 Logical relations

One of the main component for an assessment that wants to describe a complex domain is the explicit expression of possible restrictions (usually named logical relations) among the quantities involved. In fact, thanks to them it is possible formalize situations where some configurations (combinations) of events are impossible or there are some material relationships (like implications, identities, exhaustiveness, etc.). This has an influence also on the operational side because the logical relations can reduce the number of possible scenarios to consider and hence the number of "degree of freedom" involved in the computation (for a more detailed exposition refer to Lad, 1996, chapt. 2 and to Coletti and Scozzafava, 2002, chapt. 2).

About the quantities introduced in the previous Subsection, there aren't particular restrictions for combinations, apart from the widespread conviction of the full specificity of the KIT for GISTs. This imply to consider KIT positive tumors as subset of the GIST group.

Hence, with the notation already introduced, we will deal with the single constraint

$$\mathrm{CD117} \subseteq \mathrm{GIST} \tag{1}$$

Note that in several qualified papers (see for example Miettinen et al., 1999-2001, or Fletcher et al., 2002) such strong relation between KIT immunopositivity and GIST is so overestimated (or better, misunderstood) to the point of proposing to restrict the GISTs to the group of intrabdominal mesenchymal lesions showing CD117 positivity, completely neglecting the possibility of observing false-negative cases. Moreover, the term "specificity" that they adopt should not be confused with the specificity of the CD117 immunopositivity test that should formally defined as the conditional probability

$$P(\neg\mathrm{CD117}|\neg\mathrm{GIST}) \tag{2}$$

while the peculiarity of the KIT expression for GISTs can be probabilistically represented by

$$P(\mathrm{GIST}|\mathrm{CD117}) = 1 \tag{3}$$

as it obviously derives from (1).

3.3 Information matching

We can pass now to deal with the numerical expression of the information the pathologist can rely on. As already described in the previous sections, we have to join two different source of information, the personal case study reported in subsection 2.3. and literature reports and reviews. Before to perform any inference step we have to check the consistency (coherence) of these two. Coherence requirement can be explained as the need of having at least a conditional probability distribution (a model) agreeing simultaneously with all the knowledge we have, if such model does not exist any further consideration would be based on inconsistent premises. This is realizable by introducing the available information as constraints a conditional distribution must fulfill and searching for their satisfiability. It will be operationally obtained by searching the solvability of particular sequences of linear systems where the unknowns will represent probabilities that can be adopted for the different combinations of events (usually named atoms and representing all the possible detailed scenarios), while the equations will represent the constraints we mentioned before expressed trough usual probabilistic properties (non negativity, additivity, chain rule, etc.). Moreover, since the literature source will give us vague bounds for expected frequencies, we will deal also with weaker constraints expressed by inequalities and hence we will actually search the existence of a *class* of conditional distributions whose closed envelop will agree with the bounds we impose (i.e. we will check the coherence of the assessments with a lower-upper conditional probability model).

More precisely, denoting by A_r a generic atom obtained by a possible combination of the events (i.e. a full conjunction of events or negations) and by x_r its associated possible probability, for each conditional event $E|H$ with an assigned conditional probability $P(E|H)$ (e.g. one of the frequencies obtained in the personal case study) we will have a constraint of the form

$$\sum_{A_r \subseteq EH} x_r = P(E|H) \sum_{A_r \subseteq H} x_r \qquad (4)$$

(where EH stays for the logical conjunction $E \wedge H$), while for each conditional event $F|K$ with assessed probabilities bounds $[P_l(F|K), P_u(F|K)]$ (e.g. declared expected frequencies for particular situations) we will have two constraints of the form

$$\begin{aligned} \sum_{A_r \subseteq FK} x_r &\geq P_l(F|K) \sum_{A_r \subseteq K} x_r \\ \sum_{A_r \subseteq FK} x_r &\leq P_u(F|K) \sum_{A_r \subseteq K} x_r \end{aligned} \qquad (5)$$

Denoting by bold lower-case letters the characteristic vectors of the events (i.e. those vectors associated to each event and whose components are 1 or 0 depending if the corresponding atom implies or not the event) and by $\mathbf{x}^T$ the transpose row vector with components x_r, the previous constraints can be easily rewritten in the more compact form

$$(\text{eh} - \text{P(E|H) h})\cdot\text{xT} = 0 \qquad (4')$$

and

$$(\mathbf{fk} - P_l(F|K)\,\mathbf{k})\cdot\mathbf{x}^T \geq 0$$
$$(\mathbf{fk} - P_u(F|K)\,\mathbf{k})\cdot\mathbf{x}^T \leq 0 \qquad (5')$$

respectively, where · denotes the usual row-column product.

How these constraints are operationally handled and why a set of sequences of linear systems is needed are out of the scope of this paper because it would take us away from the description of the GIST diagnosis procedure. Anyway, we can just mention that the methodological features rely on the theoretical work started in Coletti (1993) and later developed till the full formulation reported in Coletti and Scozzafava (2002) (see in particular chapt. 15 and 16), with technical details about the computational part presented in Capotorti et al. (2002-2003). The most relevant ideas are the linearity of probabilities and the peculiarity of conditional assessment to be separable in different "zero layers" where the usual representation by unconditional probabilities ratios can hold, with all the properties and computational advantages that derive from this.

Let us turn to the practical application we are dealing with. We start by accepting the first "reading" of the two ambiguous cases with S100 = (+/-) (see subsection 2.3) as positive and we can summarize the results of the personal case study by the conditional probability assessment reported in Table 3. Such evaluation can be thought as the pathologist's "knowledge base" and it represent our first source of information.

Table 3. Pathologist's knowledge based on the personal case study reported in subsect. 2.3

Statements	**Cond. Probabilities** (estimated by obs. freq.)
DIAGNOSIS	24/47
CD117 CD34 ¬DESM ¬S100 | DIAGNOSIS	4/13
¬SMA ¬CD117 CD34 DESM ¬S100 | DIAGNOSIS	1/13
¬SMA CD117 CD34 ¬DESM S100 | DIAGNOSIS	1/13
SMA ¬CD117 CD34 ¬DESM ¬S100 | DIAGNOSIS	1/13
SMA CD117 ¬CD34 ¬S100 | DIAGNOSIS	3/13
SMA CD117 ¬CD34 ¬DESM S100 | DIAGNOSIS	1/13
¬SMA CD117 ¬CD34 ¬DESM S100 | DIAGNOSIS	1/13

Note that the conditional statement reported represent the different cases observations and that whenever there was some missing data (like SMA or DESM responses for cases number 3 and 21, respectively) we have just considered them unknown and hence such cases are described by combinations of less features. Hence, we neither neglect nor try to estimate them as in other approach is usually done, but we profit of all the available information, even if it is not fully detailed.

As already stressed, this knowledge base is referred to cases suspected to be GISTs on histological basis and we have to cross them with expected immunohistochemical behaviors obtained by joining different literature results (Miettinen et al., 1999-2001, Fletcher et al., 2002) where usually only CD117 positive cases are considered. The last can be thought as an overall accepted rule base representing our second source of information which is summarized in the following table:

Table 4. Rule base for expected immunohistochemical behaviors

Statements	Frequencies' bounds
CD34 | CD117	60% - 70%
SMA | CD117	30% - 40%
S100 | CD117	Around 10%
DESM | CD117	1%- 2%

Note that the statements reported are conditioned to the single event CD117 since from our logical imposition (1) it coincides with the conjunction CD117∧GIST. Obviously, whenever the frequencies will be used as estimates of conditional probabilities, the percentages are transformed in numbers between 0 and 1. Moreover, the vague bounds for S100 | CD117 will be translated in the interval 9.5% - 10.49%, due to the rounding usually adopted in medical reports (hence also all the other values will be input by their closest values of a second decimal number approximation).

While the two source of information are separately consistent, putting together the knowledge and the rule base it turns out[1] that they are incoherent. It means that it is impossible to have a probabilistic model agreeing with all such requirements. This is technically expressed by the not existence of an array **x** of values satisfying constraints like (4′) and (5′).

Analyzing the two evaluations we have found that the incoherence is due to the discrepancy between the expected percentage, among those CD117 positive, of S100 positive cases and those implied by the observed cases. In fact, performing an inference based only on the knowledge base of Table 3, we obtain that the coherent interval for S100|CD117 should be 13% - 70% while we are trying to force it to be around 10%. On the contrary, all the other bounds of the rule base Table 4 are consistent (i.e. included) in the coherent extensions of the knowledge base Table 3.

We consider the extension computations as inference steps because they represent the only consistent probabilistic conclusions one can obtain for a different statement starting from some initial evaluation (in our previous case the new statement is the conditional event S100|CD117 while the starting evaluation is represented by Table 3). Such coherent extensions are computed by linear optimization techniques with the starting evaluation as constraints. Even at a first glance it seems strange that the optimization can be linear (usually with conditional events fractional tolls are considered), this is an other of the important results obtainable operating with simple coherent tools (once again for a detailed explanation refer to Coletti and Scozzafava, 2002, chapt. 16).

Going back to the incoherence detected before, since the rule base is considered more reliable then the personal case study, and since there were two cases where the S100 positivity was judged uncertain, we revise the knowledge base assigning a negative S100 reading for the two ambiguous cases (the other revision of considering unknown the result of the two doubtful cases is possible, but our choice will lead to better results). With such revision on the knowledge base the two source of information result jointly consistent so that we can use them to perform a sound inference for the statements measuring the reliability of the diagnostic procedure. The whole knowledge-plus-rule base is shown in Table 5 where everything has been reported trough conditional probabilities assessments. Note moreover that we have added bounds for the sensitivity CD117|GIST of the KIT marker. In fact, even in literature we do not have detailed reports on the expected percentage of false negatives, in Fletcher et al. (2002) we found some hint about the causes of exceptions at the KIT immunopositivity, so that the range of 95% - 99% of true positives (expressed by $0.95 \leq P(CD117|GIST) \leq 0.99$) sounds reasonable.

Table 5. Whole coherent knowledge-plus-rule base system (expressed trough a conditional probability assessment)

P(DIAGNOSIS) = 24/47
P(CD117 CD34 ¬DESM ¬S100 | DIAGNOSIS) = 5/13
P(¬SMA ¬CD117 CD34 DESM ¬S100 | DIAGNOSIS) = 1/13
P(SMA ¬CD117 CD34 ¬DESM ¬S100 | DIAGNOSIS) = 1/13
P(SMA CD117 ¬CD34 ¬S100 | DIAGNOSIS) = 4/13
P(SMA CD117 ¬CD34 ¬DESM S100 | DIAGNOSIS) = 1/13
P(¬SMA CD117 ¬CD34 ¬DESM ¬S100 | DIAGNOSIS) = 1/13
0.095≤ P(S100 | CD117) ≤ 0.1049
0.595≤ P(CD34 | CD117) ≤ 0.7049
0.295≤ P(SMA | CD117) ≤ 0.4049
0.005≤ P(DESM | CD117) ≤ 0.0249
0.95≤ P(CD117 | GIST) ≤ 0.99

3.4 Reliability evaluation

Taking the assessment of Table 5 as a consistent inference basis, we can compute how it will bounds some index usually adopted to measure the "goodness" of a diagnostic "device" (either it being a clinical test or a physician personal decision). Practically speaking, we will compute how our available information constraints the values attainable by some relevant conditional probabilities. As already stated in subsection 3.3, these inferences will be performed by linear programming techniques, profiting from all the potentiality of having embedded our evaluation in a coherent setting. With extreme synthesis, we can say that an inference on a conditional statement $S|C$ reduces to a sequence of linear programming problems of the form

minimize/maximize $\mathbf{sc}\cdot\mathbf{x}^T$

$$\text{subject to}\quad \begin{aligned} &\mathbf{E}\cdot\mathbf{x}^T = \mathbf{0}\\ &\mathbf{L}\cdot\mathbf{x}^T \geq \mathbf{0}\\ &\mathbf{U}\cdot\mathbf{x}^T \leq \mathbf{0}\\ &\mathbf{c}\cdot\mathbf{x}^T = 1\\ &x_r \text{ nonnegative}\end{aligned}$$

where **E**, **L** and **U** are the matrices whose rows express the constraints of Table 5 expressed as in (4′) and (5′), respectively, while the $\mathbf{c}\cdot\mathbf{x}^T = 1$ constraint is a kind of normalization that allow the program to be linear instead of fractional. We will need "sequences" of such linear optimizations both because constraints deriving from conditional event having null conditioning must be treated separately, and because the inequalities constraints of type (5′) must be cyclically (i.e. one each time) forced to be equalities (to be sure about the existence of a class of conditional distributions whose closed envelope fulfill all the constraints). Once again the interested reader should refer to the relevant literature on the subject, in particular the technical details reported in Capotorti et al. (2002-2003).

Applying such procedure with $S|C$ being alternatively the sensitivity DIAGNOSIS|GIST, the specificity ¬DIAGNOSIS|¬GIST, the positive predictive value GIST|DIAGNOSIS and the negative predictive value ¬GIST|¬DIAGNOSIS we finally have[2] a numerical quantification of the reliability of the diagnostic procedure histologically based (as synthesized in the event DIAGNOSIS). Results are reported in the following table and are expressed in percentage frequencies for an easier interpretation:

Table 6. Evaluation of the common indexes to measure the diagnostic reliability

Indexes	Description	Frequencies bounds
DIAGNOSIS | GIST	Sensitivity	47% - 76%
¬DIAGNOSIS | ¬GIST	Specificity	0% - 88%
GIST | DIAGNOSIS	Positive predictive value	85% - 94%
¬GIST | ¬DIAGNOSIS	Negative predictive value	0% - 69%

4. RESULTS' IMPROVEMENT

As stated in the introduction, the bounds computed in the previous Section 3 represent a first quantification of the goodness of the diagnostic procedure. On them now it should be possible to set particular statistical models, specifying priors and likelihood distribution families, estimating parameters and so on. But, if we want to limit ourselves to use the partial information we have, such results should anyway suffice to judge the soundness of the criteria adopted to suspect a lesion to belong to the GISTs' family.

For this, the last to indexes are particularly meaningful, and the upper bounds of 94% and 69% attained for the positive and negative predictive values, respectively, show a quite good reliability of the procedure. On the other hand, apart from the positive predictive value, the bounds result so large (i.e. the interval are so wide) that they suggest a too weak "influence" of the constraint considered. At this point it is reasonable to analyze more deeply the framework we have built and ask if there is some further consideration to take into account. Qualitative statements, i.e. comparisons between conditional probabilities not stated at the beginning, could be particularly important.

For example, it sounds reasonable for the pathologist that his/her diagnostic procedure, being anyway scientifically based, behaves properly, i.e. in percentage the right diagnosis should exceed the wrong one. This can be probabilistically translated by adding to our assessment a constraint such as

$$P(\text{DIAGNOSIS}|\text{GIST}) \geq P(\text{DIAGNOSIS}|\neg\text{GIST}) \qquad (6)$$

Note that we don't have direct information on the conditional probabilities here involved (actually they are the targets of our inference) and that they are, usually, not uniquely determined by the other constraints we have. Hence, when (6) is added to the constraints of the linear optimizations procedure, it becomes quadratic because it will be introduced as

$$x \cdot [(\text{diagnosis gist})^T \cdot \neg\text{gist} - (\text{diagnosis } \neg\text{gist})^T \cdot \text{gist}] \cdot x^T \geq 0 \qquad (6')$$

This makes impossible the use of common linear programming techniques (like the simplex algorithm) and introduces the need of more sophisticated optimization procedures, like for example the primal-dual log-barrier algorithm. Anyway numerical computations[3] performed with such further quadratic constraint have shown negligible improvements on the already stated bounds.

Anyway, further qualitative considerations are possible. Note, for example, that coherence of the knowledge-plus-rule base is possible thanks to particular "a priori" values of GIST's incidence. In fact, if we perform inference on the unconditional statement GIST with the starting assessment expressed in Table 5 we obtain

$$0.59 \leq P(\text{GIST}) \leq 0.97 \qquad (7)$$

that is consistent with the common behavior that GISTs represent the majority of mesenchimal tumors of the gastrointestinal tract. Anyway, such bounds are extremely weak and hence it is reasonable to limit them. Looking carefully at the class of conditional probabilities consistent with the starting assessment, we can observe that there is some of them that is compatible with a GIST incidence of about 81%. If we then take as good such restriction, we can include it in the rule base and re-compute the bounds of the relevant indexes, obtaining.

Table 7. Bounds for reliability's indexes computed with GIST incidence limitation

Indexes	Description	Frequencies bounds
DIAGNOSIS | GIST	Sensitivity	53% - 59%
¬DIAGNOSIS | ¬GIST	Specificity	58% - 80%
GIST | DIAGNOSIS	Positive predictive value	85% - 93%
¬GIST | ¬DIAGNOSIS	Negative predictive value	22% - 32%

Since the bounds now are narrower, these results are much more informative. They confirm a good positive predictive performance of the diagnostic procedure, while they express a really bad reliability in the case of a negative diagnosis, suggesting a more careful inspection whenever the lesion is suspected to be something different from a GIST.

Of course these last conclusions depend on the last limitation we impose to the "a priori" GIST incidence, slightly different results could be obtained with different assumptions but we do not report them because they would be just numerical considerations.

5. CONCLUSIONS

In this paper we have shown how a diagnostic procedure can be quantitatively evaluated even when the available information contains several uncertain aspects. All the specific considerations we have stated about the practical application to the GIST diagnosis can be easily generalized to any similar decisional procedure. In fact, thanks to a genuinely probabilistic reasoning we have shown that it is possible to deal with situations where the information is partial (i.e. not fully detailed) and originated by different (and sometimes apparently contradicting) sources.

In such situations the check of consistency is a compulsory step to perform, and we have shown that it could lead to a revision of some consideration. Moreover, once coherence is assured, it is also possible to perform a preliminary inference on relevant statements, so that subsequent more or less sophisticated statistical models can be built in the light of such results. Otherwise, introducing further qualitative judgements it is possible to obtain considerable conclusions remaining inside an original "model-free" framework.

Of course, such extreme general approach can lead to not definite answers, in such cases a skilful reading of the results is needed (especially when answers are interval based and not uniquely determined) or we must search for more constraining considerations or assumptions.

NOTES

[*] All our computations has been performed with the specific CHK Interface software developed by the PAID (Partial Information and Decision) Italian Research Group.

[2] For these particular computations, the number of unknowns is 40 and binding together the matrices **E**, **L**, **U** and the vector **c** it leads to a 18×40 matrix.

[3] For such computations we used the Maple software with its specific *Nonlinear Programming* package.

REFERENCES

CAPOTORTI, A. AND VANTAGGI, B. (2002): Locally strong coherence in inference processes, *Annals of Mathematics and Artificial Intelligence, 35*: 125-149.

CAPOTORTI, A., GALLI L., AND VANTAGGI *B.*,(2003): How to use locally strong coherence in inferential processes based on lower-upper probabilities, *Soft Computing*,. 7(5): 280-287.

COLETTI, G. (1993): Numerical and qualitative judgements in probabilistic expert systems, in: Proc. Of the International Workshop on Probabilistic Methods in Expert Systems (Ed. R.Scozzafava), SIS, Roma, 37-55.

COLETTI, G. AND SCOZZAFAVA, R. (2002). Probabilistic Logic in a Coherent Setting, Kluwer Acad. Pub., Dordrecht.

DE FINETTI, B. (1970). Teoria della Probabilità, Einaudi, Torino, – Engl. Transl. (1974) Theory of Probability, Vol. 1 and 2, Wiley, Chichester.

FLETCHER, C. D. M., BERMAN, J. J., CORLESS C. *et al.* (2002): Diagnosis of gastrointestinal stromal tumors: a consensus approach, *Human Pathology, 33(5)*, 459-464.

LAD, F. (1996). Operational Subjective Statistical Methods: a mathematical, philosophical, and historical introduction, Wiley, New York.

MIETTINEN, M., SARLOMO-RIKALA, M. AND LASOTA, J. (1999): Gastrointestinal stromal tumors: recent advances in understanding of their biology, *Human Pathology, 30(10):* 1213-1219.

MIETTINEN, M. AND LASOTA, J. (2001): Gastrointestinal stromal tumors : definition, clinical, histological, immunohistochemical, and molecular genetic features and differential diagnosis. *Virchows Arch 438*: 1-12.

Chapter 6

COMPARING TWO GROUPS OR TREATMENTS-A BAYESIAN APPROACH

J. Deely*

Department of Statistics, Purdue University, West Lafayette Indiana, USA.

1. INTRODUCTION

The purpose of this paper is to illustrate the value of a Bayesian approach in practical problems involving two groups (treatments) which are to be compared. Using practical criteria for comparisons, the advantage of the Bayesian approach will be demonstrated in two situations. Problem I will deal with cholesterol data from two groups of people and it is the aim of the experiment to say which group has the higher cholesterol levels. Problem II will compare two treatments in a clinical trial situation at an interim before the trial is completed. This situation is referred to as ***interim analysis*** because only part of the data in the planned trial has been collected. At this interim stage it is desirable to decide whether to stop the experiment now or to continue until the end.

Both of these problems lend themselves to a Bayesian analysis. That is, there is a likelihood function that describes the data's relationship to some quantity (or quantities) of interest labeled a parameter. This parameter of interest will then be given a prior distribution, which will depend on the type of prior information available in any given situation. Then using Bayes theorem the posterior distribution of the parameter of interest can be computed. It is to be noted that this posterior distribution is always conditional upon the data that has been observed. It does not suppose that imaginable data sets have occurred and that probabilities of imagined data

* For correspondence: jdeely@stat.purdue.edu

have been computed for various values of this parameter. These statements will be illustrated specifically in the two problems discussed in this paper.

In Problem I, we first of all introduce a published data set concerning a study of the cholesterol levels in black American men and black American women. The frequentist analysis of that data is discussed and the aspects to be addressed by a Bayesian analysis are mentioned. In Section 2.2 we develop the formulas and notation for the Bayesian analysis. We also introduce the main quantity of interest to be used for comparisons. In Section 2.3, various Bayesian approaches are introduced and computations displayed. A concluding discussion is given in Section 2.4.

In Problem II, we discuss the situation surrounding interim analysis and why it is important. In Section 3.2, we develop the particular Bayesian approach to be implemented and in Section 3.3, we perform computations that describe the value of the Bayesian approach. A concluding discussion is given in Section 3.4.

Since both Problems will implement the Bayesian approach, we state here a general overview of that paradigm.

Firstly there is some operationally defined quantity (or quantities) of interest whose value is unknown to us. We will label this unknown quantity θ for notational convenience noting that it has a practical and operationally defined meaning. There is a likelihood function, denoted by $f(x|\theta)$, which links the data x to be observed to this quantity θ.There is a prior distribution describing our uncertainty about the quantity θ, denoted by $\pi(\theta)$.

Using Bayes Theorem we then compute the posterior distribution, denoted by $\pi(\theta|x)$, which is given by

$$\pi(\theta|x) = \frac{f(x|\theta)\pi(\theta)}{f(x)}$$

where

$$f(x) = \int f(x|\theta)\pi(\theta)d\theta.$$

The posterior describes our uncertainty about the quantity of interest θ after the data x has been observed. This highlights the very basic difference between the frequentist and the Bayesian approaches. Frequentists condition on some value or values of the unknown quantity θ and then using the likelihood function compute probabilities for values of the data. The Bayesian approach conditions on the observed data at hand and by way of the posterior distribution computes probabilities for values of the unknown quantity θ. This latter approach uses Bayes Theorem to modify our original uncertainty expressed in the prior distribution to a posterior description of our uncertainty now that some data has been observed. These general concepts will be made specific in the following discussion of each of the two Problems of interest.

2. PROBLEM I CHOLESTEROL LEVELS

2.1 Introduction

In the paper Ford *et al* (1988) cholesterol data is reported on 119 black American men and 130 black American women. A summary of the data concerning just the cholesterol values is contained in Figure 1. The aim of the research is to ascertain the extent to which black American men and women differ in their cholesterol levels. It is to be noted that high levels of total cholesterol (TC) are thought to be hazardous while high levels of high density lipoprotein (HDL) can offer protection against coronary artery disease.

	Total cholesterol (mg/dl)		
	men	women	P-value
mean	209.5	215.6	0.322
stdev	50.6	47.4	
n	119	130	
sterr	4.64	4.16	
	HDL cholesterol (mg/dl)		
mean	55.2	59.2	0.0621
stdev	16.5	17.2	
sterr	1.51	1.51	

Figure 1.

In analyzing this data the authors state in their results that "Only the difference in HDL cholesterol was of borderline statistical significance....." and "total cholesterol was also higher in women, but the difference was not significant".

In making these statements the authors allude to the P- values concerning this data and as is quite often the practice in a frequentist approach, the lower the P-value the more strength is given to rejecting the null hypothesis. In fact, some practitioners interpret (quite wrongly) the P-value as the probability of rejecting a true hypothesis and thus, think of one minus the P-value as the probability that the alternative hypothesis is true.

In the Bayesian paradigm these ad hoc interpretations are corrected with probability statements that are properly derived and are totally coherent. The quantity that is so important in the Bayesian approach is the posterior distribution since it allows computation of important other quantities of interest. For this data the computation of the posterior probability that one group has a mean cholesterol level larger than the other group is the important quantity of interest. It can easily be computed and more particularly, the posterior probability that one group mean is larger than the other group mean by any specified amount can also be computed. It is this latter computation that highlights the advantage of the Bayesian approach. This will be illustrated more specifically in Section 2.3.

2.2 Mathematical Model

Firstly we point out that we will set up the model for cholesterol levels without distinguishing between TC and HDL. However in the analysis we will treat each of these separately using the same notation.

Let θ_1 and θ_2 denote respectively the true unknown mean levels of cholesterol in the population of women and men being studied. In this example we could imagine in the first instance that the population being studied is the Chicago area population of black American men and women. This is reasonable since the sample was taken from Cook County hospital in Chicago. Inference to a larger population may be possible provided a case is made for similarities in the populations.

Let X_1 and X_2 denote respectively the cholesterol levels in an individual woman and man from the population. We will use the notation that $N(m,v^2)$ indicates a normal distribution with mean 'm' and variance 'v^2'. In this paper we ill assume that the likelihood function is normal, namely that

$$f\left(x_i \mid \theta_i\right) = N\left(\theta_i, \sigma_i^2\right) \; for \; i = 1, 2.$$

To describe our uncertainty about θ_1 and θ_2, we will use a normal prior distribution and write

$$\pi\left(\theta_i\right) = N\left(\beta, \tau^2\right) \; for \; i = 1, 2.$$

It will be the case that various Bayesian approaches are described via their treatment of β and τ^2. These ideas will be discussed later.

Data has been collected in the form of a sample of n_1 women and n_2 men and we can compute the means from these samples which we will denote by $\overline{X}_1$ and $\overline{X}_2$ respectively. Then the likelihood function for $\overline{X}_i$ is given by

$$f\left(\bar{x}_i \mid \theta_i\right) = N\left(\theta_i, \sigma_i^2 / n_i\right) \; for \; i = 1,2.$$

We will be interested in the quantity $w=\theta_1-\theta_2$ since this quantity can be used to describe the differences between cholesterol levels from the two groups. Thus the prior distribution of w is $N(0,2\tau^2)$ and the distribution of $Y=\bar{X}_1-\bar{X}_2$ conditional on w is $N(w,\sigma^2)$ where $\sigma^2=\frac{\sigma_1^2}{n_1}+\frac{\sigma_2^2}{n_2}$. In the data set analyzed here in the sample size is large enough so that we can take σ^2 as known. In particular we will be interested in the posterior distribution of w which will be used to describe the extent of the cholesterol differences between the women and men. This distribution conditional on β and τ^2 is given by

$$\pi\left(w \mid y\right) = \frac{f\left(y \mid w\right)\pi\left(w\right)}{f\left(y\right)}$$

$$= N\left(\frac{2\tau^2 y}{2\tau^2+\sigma^2}, \frac{2\tau^2\sigma^2}{2\tau^2+\sigma^2}\right).$$

2.3 Some different Bayesian models

1. Naïve Noninformative

In this approach it is assumed that the prior is 'flat' and unbounded which corresponds to letting τ^2 go to infinity in the prior distribution for w. Even though this is an improper prior, the posterior is proper and is $N(y,\sigma^2)$. This approach is often taken because it corresponds to some frequentist methods. For example, a frequentist C% confidence interval on w is given by ($y-Z_C\sigma$, $y+Z_C\sigma$) in which Z_C is the standard normal value with (1+C)/2 probability below it. But using the posterior above, it can be seen that

$$P\left(y - Z_C\sigma \le w \le y + Z_c\sigma\right) = C$$

which is the same as the frequentist interval. It is to be noted however that entirely different interpretations are given in the two approaches.

For the cholesterol data we are interested in computing $P(w \geq b \mid y)$ as a function of 'b' where 'b' is a specified amount which is of interest to the practitioner. For the posterior above this function is given by

$$P\left(w \geq b \middle| y\right) = \Phi\left(\frac{y - b}{\sigma}\right)$$

and is shown in the Figure below.

b	TC	HDL
0	0.917	0.996
1	0.877	0.977
2	0.824	0.909
3	0.759	0.748
4	0.683	0.500
5	0.599	0.252
6	0.509	0.091
7	0.419	0.023
8	0.333	0.004
9	0.255	0.000
10	0.188	0.000
11	0.133	0.000
12	0.090	0.000
13	0.058	0.000
14	0.036	0.000
15	0.022	0.000

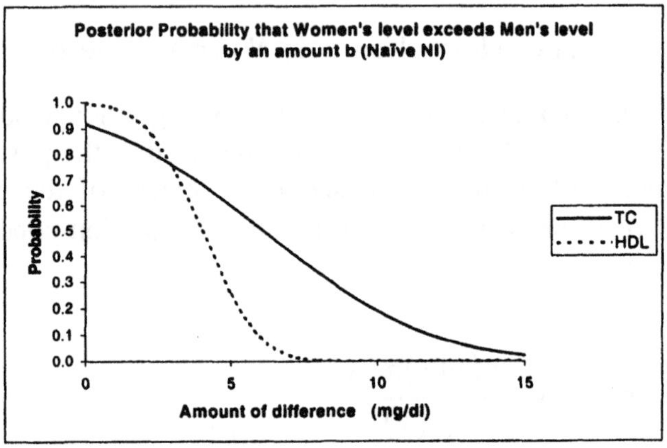

Figure 2.

This graph enables the practitioner to decide whether there is a clinically significant difference between the cholesterol levels of the two groups. In this case we note that there is a 0.9 probability that the mean HDL level for women is larger than that of the men by an amount of 2 mg/dl. But this probability drops to 0.25 for a difference of 5 mg/dl. (i.e. about a 10% shift from the mean level of 50 mg/dl). Thus there is very little chance that these two groups are different by any amount that is clinically significant.

Similarly, looking at the values for TC there is a very small chance (probability of 0.188) that the women's mean level exceeds that of the men by 10 or more. This is about a 5% shift from a mean level of 200 mg/dl. So again we can see that the two groups are very unlikely to be different by an amount that is clinically significant.

The point about this approach is that the frequentist problem of having a statistically significant result which may not be clinically significant disappears and is replaced with a more practical statistical analysis.

2. Naïve Informative

In this approach information about the unknown quantities is elicited to obtain an informative prior distribution. Using the general form of the posterior distribution for w, it is clear that we need elicit information about τ^2 only. More particularly we only need to assess the relative size of τ^2 to σ^2 since that will provide enough information to give values to the posterior mean and variance thus enabling calculations using the posterior. To do this elicitation, we can think about the variability of the unknown quantity w relative to the variability in the data. We will consider two examples herein. Suppose firstly that we assess the variability of w to be about the same as σ^2, which is the variability in the difference of the two sample means. Then the posterior mean is $\frac{2\tau^2 y}{2\tau^2+\sigma^2}=0.5y$ and the posterior variance is $\frac{2\tau^2\sigma^2}{2\tau^2+\sigma^2}=0.5\sigma^2$. For TC we take $\frac{\sigma_1^2}{n_1}=\frac{\sigma_2^2}{n_2}=(4.4)^2=19.4$ thus giving σ^2=38.8. For HDL we take $\frac{\sigma_1^2}{n_1}=\frac{\sigma_2^2}{n_2}=(1.5)^2=2.25$ thus giving σ^2=4.5

For Example 2 we imagine the variability of w to be 2 σ^2. The Table below summarizes the calculations.

Table 1.

		Posterior mean	Posterior variance
$2\tau^2=\sigma^2$	TC	3	19.4
	HDL	2	2.25
$\tau^2=\sigma^2$	TC	4	25.9
	HDL	2.67	3

With these values we can now calculate the same posterior probability that we used in (1) above. In this case it is given by

$$P(w \geq b \mid y) = \Phi\left(\frac{m-b}{v}\right)$$

where m is the posterior mean and v is the posterior standard deviation. The Figure below displays the calculations for a range of 'b' values.

	Example 1		Example 2	
b	TC	HDL	TC	HDL
0	0.756	0.909	0.788	0.938
1	0.679	0.748	0.727	0.832
2	0.594	0.500	0.658	0.650
3	0.505	0.252	0.583	0.424
4	0.415	0.091	0.505	0.221
5	0.329	0.023	0.427	0.089
6	0.251	0.004	0.352	0.027
7	0.185	0.000	0.282	0.006
8	0.130	0.000	0.219	0.001
9	0.088	0.000	0.166	0.000
10	0.057	0.000	0.121	0.000
11	0.035	0.000	0.086	0.000
12	0.021	0.000	0.059	0.000
13	0.012	0.000	0.039	0.000
14	0.006	0.000	0.025	0.000
15	0.003	0.000	0.016	0.000

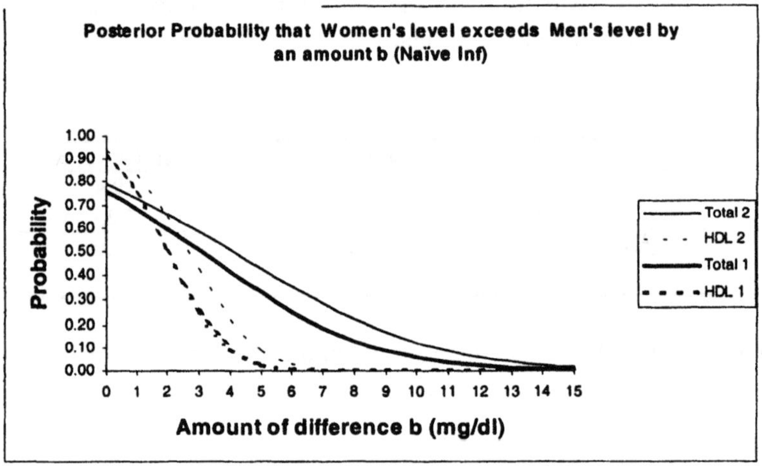

Figure 3.

This graph is similar to the one obtained in the Naïve noninformative case and has the same interpretation. There is not a large difference between the two informative examples. It is also to be noted that the probabilities have been lowered in this informative case which is to be expected. For example, the posterior probability that the women's TC level exceeded the men's level by five mg/dl was 0.599 in the naïve noninformative case and this probability was lowered to 0.427 for Example 2 in the Table. Again this approach substantiates the basic idea that there is very little chance that these two groups are different by any amount that is clinically significant.

3. Hierarchical Bayesian (Exchangeable) informative (HBI)

In this approach we exploit the concept that knowledge of one of the θ_i 's may help decide the value of the other, i.e. θ_1 and θ_2 are not independent. In fact in some situations it is possible to assert that θ_1 and θ_2 are exchangeable.

The interested reader is referred to de Finetti. This assumption implies that the prior on θ_1, θ_2 is a mixture. In this paper we will assume that it is a mixture of normal distributions and that the mixing distribution is the joint distribution of the hyperparameters β and τ^2. This model can also be justified by starting as in previous sections with θ_1 and θ_2 having the same normal distribution, $N(\beta,\tau^2)$ but now assuming that we cannot give values to β and τ^2. To describe our uncertainty about β and τ^2, we use a probability distribution, called a hyperprior. Specifically, herein we will assume that our uncertainty about β and τ^2 can be described as the product of two distributions, i.e. β and τ^2 are independent. Our notation will be that the joint distribution on β and τ^2 can be written as $h(\beta,\tau^2)=h_1(\beta)h_2(\tau^2)$.

Thus the prior distribution on θ_1 and θ_2 is

$$\pi(\theta_1,\theta_2)=\int \pi(\theta_1,\theta_2|\beta,\tau^2)h_1(\beta)h_2(\tau^2)d\beta d\tau^2$$

where $\pi(\theta_1,\theta_2|\beta,\tau^2)$ is the product of the two normal distributions given in the Bayesian model in Section 2.2. It will be the case that we do not require the calculation of the prior in closed form to effectively do our posterior analysis. Using the notation $\underline{\theta}=(\theta_1,\theta_2)$ and $\underline{x}=(x_1,x_2)$, the posterior distribution of $\underline{\theta}$ can be written as

$$\pi(\underline{\theta}|\underline{x})=\int \pi(\underline{\theta}|\underline{x},\underline{\beta},\underline{\tau}^2)h_1(\beta|\underline{x})h_2(\tau^2|\underline{x})d\beta d\tau^2$$

where $\pi(\theta|x,\beta,\tau^2)$ is the posterior in the naïve case when values for β and τ^2 were given. The distributions $h_1(\beta|x)$ *and* $h_2(\tau^2|x)$ are the posterior distributions of the hyperparameters which will not be of interest in this paper but are necessary to carry out the calculations which are required. We are now in a position to calculate the quantity of interest as

$$P(w\geq b|\underline{x})=\int P(w\geq b|\underline{x},\underline{\beta},\underline{\tau}^2)h_1(\beta|\underline{x})h_2(\tau^2|\underline{x})d\beta d\tau^2$$

where $P(w\geq b|x,\beta,\tau^2)$ is the quantity that was computed in the naïve cases above. Thus it can be seen that the quantity of interest in the ***HBI*** model is the average value of the quantity of interest in the naïve case where the average is taken over the updated distributions of the unknown values β and τ^2. As noted then, the quantity $P(w\geq b|x,\beta,\tau^2)$ does not depend on β and thus we need an expression for only $h(\tau^2|x)$. To calculate this distribution, we must give the distributions $h_1(\beta)$ and $h_2(\tau^2)$ which describe our uncertainty about the values β and τ^2. Our uncertainty about β expresses the fact that we are uncertain about the ***mean*** value of the θ_i 's and our uncertainty about τ^2

expresses the fact that we are uncertain about how ***variable*** the θ_i 's are around their mean. Thus these distributions can be elicited in many cases. In the next section we consider the case in which elicitation is not feasible. In this section for purposes of illustration we consider the case in which $h_1(\beta)$ is taken as $N(\beta_0,A^2)$ with elicited values for β_0 and A^2 and $h_2(\tau^2)$ will be taken as a triangular distribution on an elicited interval. The elicitation we suggest here is just one possible scenario to illustrate the possibilities of the Bayesian model. The elicitation of the values for β_0 and A^2 can be obtained by asking the practitioner questions such as:

a) When you think about the *average value* of the θ_i 's, what is your best opinion regarding what that value is?
b) Can you give a range of that value ?

To elicit an interval for values of τ^2, we can ask questions such as:

a) Can you give a distance for which you are reasonably sure that the θ_i's are no father apart than this value?
b) Can you give a distance for which you are reasonably sure that the θ_i's are apart by at least this value?

Answering questions (a) and (b) with a distances d_u and d_l respectively and probabilities p_u and p_l respectively gives the equations

$$P\left(\left|\theta_1 - \theta_2\right| \le d_u\right) \ge p_u \text{ and } P\left(\left|\theta_1 - \theta_2\right| \ge d_l\right) \ge p_l.$$

From these equations we can obtain an upper and lower bound on τ^2.

We now give a possible set of answers to our elicitation questions above to obtain the values for β_0 ,A^2 and $h_2(\tau^2)$.

Table 2.

	Common Sterr	β_0	A^2	d_l	p_l	Lower bd on τ^2	d_u	p_u	Upper bd on τ^2
TC	4.5	210	25	1	0.8	8	20	0.95	50
HDL	1.5	55	4	0.5	0.8	2	5	0.95	3.1

Using these values we will compute $P(w \ge b \mid x)$ as we did in the previous sections.

To perform that computation we require an expression for $h(\tau^2 \mid x)$ which appears in the expression for of $P(w \ge b \mid x)$. This distribution is given by

$$h_2\left(\tau^2 \mid \underline{x}\right) = \frac{f\left(\underline{x} \mid \tau^2\right) h_2\left(\tau^2\right)}{\int f\left(\underline{x} \mid \tau^2\right) h_2\left(\tau^2\right) d\tau^2}$$

where

$$f\left(\underline{x}\middle|\tau^2\right)=\int f\left(\underline{x}\middle|\beta,\tau^2\right)h_1(\beta)d\beta$$

and

$$f\left(\underline{x}\middle|\beta,\tau^2\right)=\int f\left(\bar{x}_1,\bar{x}_2\middle|\theta_1,\theta_2\right)\pi\left(\theta_1,\theta_2\middle|\beta,\tau^2\right)d\theta_1 d\theta_2$$

$$=\prod_{i=1}^{2} N\left(\beta,\tau^2+\sigma_i^2/n_i\right).$$

In this paper as mentioned in the naïve case we will take $\sigma_1^2/n_1=\sigma_2^2/n_2=\lambda^2$, where λ^2 is given in the Table as the common standard error for each of TC and HDL. This assumption is not necessary in a general Bayesian model but is made here to keep the calculations simplified. Furthermore since the sample sizes are large and the standard errors are very close in our data, it is a reasonable assumption in this case.

This allows computation of

$$f\left(\underline{x}\mid\tau^2\right)=\left[2\pi\sqrt{\left(\lambda^2+\tau^2\right)\left(2A^2+\lambda^2+\tau^2\right)}\right]^{-1}\exp\left[-\frac{\left(\bar{x}_1-\bar{x}_2\right)^2}{8\left(\lambda^2+\tau^2\right)}\right]\cdot$$

$$\cdot\exp\left[-\frac{\left(0{,}5\left(\bar{x}_1-\bar{x}_2\right)-\beta_0\right)^2}{2A^2+\lambda^2+\tau^2}\right]$$

which is required to compute $h(\tau^2 \mid x)$.

We can now compute the quantity $P(w\geq b \mid x)$ and it is shown in the graph below.

b	TC	HDL
0	0.795	0.946
2	0.677	0.691
4	0.537	0.272
6	0.393	0.043
8	0.263	0.002
10	0.159	0.000

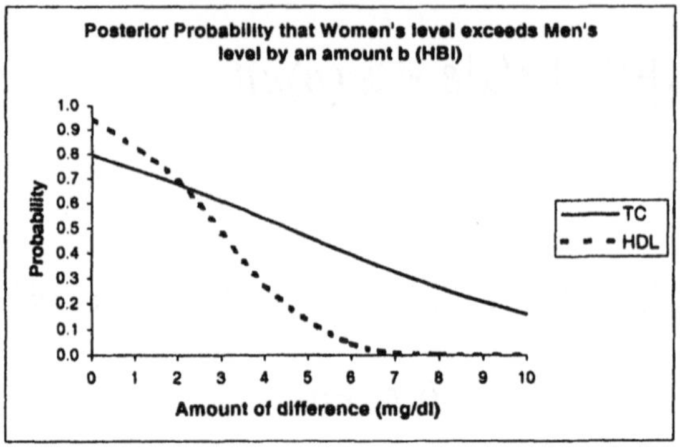

Figure 4.

This graph is again similar to those obtained previously and does not differ significantly from the naïve informative case. The fact that there is very little difference implies that the data itself is indicating just what the situation is.

4. Hierarchical Bayesian (Exchangeable) noninformative (HBN)

This approach uses the same model and notation as in the previous section but with the assumption that eliciting values for β and τ^2 is not feasible. Thus we use a noninformative model for these values. In particular the distributions $h_1(\beta)$ and $h_2(\tau^2)$ are taken as noninformative. For $h_1(\beta)$ this is accomplished by letting A^2 go to infinity. The usual noninformative choice for $h_2(\tau^2)$ would be $1/\tau^2$ but this does not yield a proper $h(\tau^2|\underline{x})$. However setting $h_2(\beta) = 1/(\lambda^2+\tau^2)$ does yield a proper. $h(\tau^2|\underline{x})$. With these choices we can now compute $P(w \geq b|x)$ and it is shown in the graph below.

b	TC	HDL
0	0.773	0.934
2	0.620	0.666
4	0.471	0.326
6	0.337	0.092
8	0.227	0.013
10	0.143	0.001

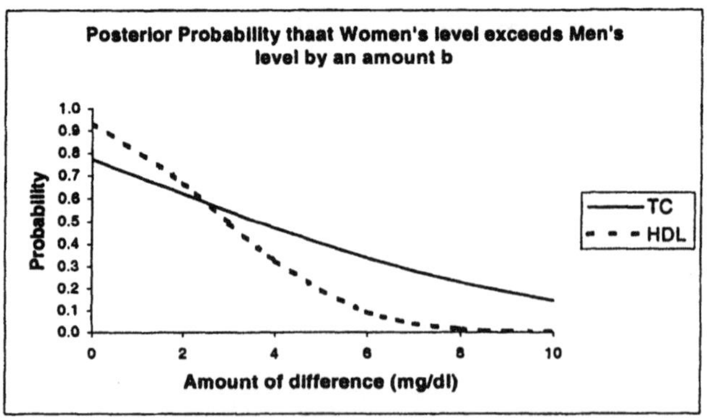

Figure 5.

This graph depicts the fourth and final method of analysis and differs very little from the naïve noninformative. Once again this similarity indicates that the data is quite overpowering in its information about the cholesterol differences in these two groups.

2.4 Discussion

What we have tried to show in these four Bayesian approaches to the cholesterol data is the fact that the posterior probability that cholesterol level of one group exceeds that of the group by some specified amount, is an ideal description of the situation. It is a quantitative method whereby practical clinically significant discriminations can be determined. There is no comparative frequentist analogue. Usually frequentist methods depends on confidence intervals and these are not generally definitive enough to make precise statements. The Bayesian approach offers a precise quantitative method of making this discrimination. We also have tried to show that there are different Bayesian approaches and when they all agree, this gives greater confidence in the conclusions.

It is the case that more complicated Bayesian analysis is available. The assumption that the variances are equal and known, is not necessary. In that case additional prior distributions are used. This merely provides a more complicated numerical solution, but with the advent of Markov Chain Monte Carlo "MCMC" methods, this type of approach is feasible. The cholesterol data analyzed in this paper, had good evidence for equal variances and taking them as known. There are situations in which this assumption is not valid, in which case, the analysis would be carried on in a different way.

3. PROBLEM II CLINICAL TRIALS AND INTERIM ANALYSIS

3.1 Introduction

In this section we consider a practical problem involved with clinical trials which will be used to illustrate the advantages of Bayesian methodology. Suppose a new treatment for a type of cancer is being proposed. The treatment labeled T is rather expensive and is to be compared with a standard treatment labeled S. The length of time until the next operation (or death) is the primary concern, but overall well-being can also be evaluated. A typical scenario might be that on the standard treatment it is expected that 20% of the patients would survive two years (say 650 days)after surgery. The purpose of the clinical trial is to establish whether T is sufficiently better than S based on a sample of 500 patients from each of S and T. For purposes of this talk we will take "sufficiently better" to mean "at least 10% larger".

This means that the end of the trial we will declare T better than S if the probability of surviving at least 650 days using T exceeds that for S by an amount 0.1; i.e.

$$P(X_T \geq 650) \geq P(X_S \geq 650) + 0.1$$

In this type of clinical trial it is becoming increasingly common and advisable that an ***interim*** analysis be performed before the trial is completed. In fact, there are situations in which there are several interim analyses performed. There are two general motivations for this type of interim analysis. One arises when a monitoring committee is in charge of overseeing the clinical trials. In this case, the monitoring committee has access to all of the data obtained up to that stage and would like to assess the viability of the new treatment. This committee has the power to stop the treatment if it is not as good as expected. In this way the monitoring committee can make sure that ethical procedures are being implemented for all of the patients.

The second motivation arises from the pharmaceutical company proposing the new treatment. The company clearly does not want to spend money on completing a trial that has very little chance of succeeding i.e. being proven to be better than the standard treatment. Of course they also have ethical concerns, but they are not in charge of the trials and hence cannot interpret them in the interim. However, it is being suggested that the data collected so far can be given to the pharmaceutical company without knowledge of which treatment the patients received. The statistical analysis in this case, is much more difficult than the first case above. In this paper we will restrict ourselves to the first situation.

The frequentist approach to this kind of problem has again been influenced by the use of P-values and of course, the concern is what does interim analysis do to the "α level"? In the Bayesian paradigm, two computations are the basis of decision-making. The first computation is similar to that used in Problem I, namely, the posterior probability that the new treatment is in fact better than the standard treatment by an amount agreed upon. However, in addition, it is then required at the interim analysis stage to predict what is likely to happen if the remaining patients are treated as indicated in the protocol. Since the survival times of these remaining patients are unobserved, we need to anticipate in some way what their values will be. In the Bayesian paradigm the predictive distribution can be used to solve this problem.

3.2 Mathematical Model

We will use the same basic Mathematical Model as used in Problem I noting that treatments T and S are identified with 'Women' and 'Men' respectively. In particular at a stage k we will have observed k survival times (uncensored) on each of T and S. The relevant distributions of the sample means and the prior for θ_T and θ_S are given by

$$\bar{x}_{k,T} \,|\theta_T \sim N\left(\theta_T, \frac{\sigma^2}{k}\right) \text{and } \bar{x}_{k,S} \,|\theta_S \sim N\left(\theta_S, \frac{\sigma^2}{k}\right)$$

$$\theta_T \text{ and } \theta_S \sim N\left(\beta, \tau^2\right) \text{so that } w = \theta_T - \theta_S \sim N\left(0, 2\tau^2\right).$$

We use the subscript 'k' on the sample means because it will be convenient to distinguish between the sample means at the interim and at the final stage. Also for simplicity we will assume that the variances of the two treatments are equal with a known common value.

The basic probability inequality we must satisfy in order to declare *T* better than *S* is

$$P\left(X_T \geq 650\right) \geq P\left(X_S \geq 650\right) + 0.1.$$

This will be satisfied if the difference between θ_T and θ_S is sufficiently large. Assuming that the range of values for θ_S will be between 600 and 700 days, it was determined numerically that sufficiently large means $\theta_T > \theta_S + 20$, i.e. $w = \theta_T - \theta_S > 20$.

The Bayesian approach is to compute the posterior probability of this event at the end of the trial and if that probability is sufficiently large, say larger than 0.95, we could confidently say that T is superior to S by the required amount. This computation is given by

$$P(\omega > 20 \,|\bar{y}_n, \beta, \tau^2) = \Phi\left(\frac{m - 20}{v}\right)$$

where $\bar{y}_n = \bar{x}_{n,T} - \bar{x}_{n,S}$ is the difference in the sample means, $m = \frac{\tau^2}{\left(\sigma^2/m\right) + \tau^2} \bar{y}_n$ is the posterior mean and $v^2 = \frac{2\sigma^2\tau^2}{\sigma^2 + n\tau^2}$ is the posterior variance.

3.3 Bayesian Interim Analysis

Interim analysis is required after observing k patients on each of S and T. We then want to predict what is likely to happen if the remaining n-k patients are treated as indicated in the protocol. The survival times of these remaining n-k patients are unobserved and we need to anticipate in some way what their values will be. The Bayesian predictive distribution is ideally suited for this computation.

In general terms the Bayesian ***predictive distribution*** of a future observation y given the data x is given by

$$f(y|x) = \int f(y|x,\theta)\pi(\theta|x)d\theta$$
$$= \int f(y|\theta)\pi(\theta|x)d\theta.$$

Thus it can be seen that the Bayesian predictive distribution is the average of the likelihood function where the average is taken with respect to the posterior distribution.

In our model discussed above we require the predictive distribution of the mean of the future n-k observations conditioned upon the data seen at stage k. This distribution is obtained as follows.

Firstly, we obtain the distributions relevant at interim stage k.

Let $w=\theta_T-\theta_S$ and $\overline{Y}_k = \overline{X}_{k,T} - \overline{X}_{k,S}$ then

$$f(\overline{y}_k|\omega) = N\left(\omega, \frac{2\sigma^2}{k}\right)$$

$$\pi(\omega|\overline{y}_k) = N\left(\frac{\tau^2}{\tau^2+\frac{\sigma^2}{k}}\overline{y}_k, \frac{\frac{2\sigma^2\tau^2}{k}}{\frac{\sigma^2}{k}+\tau^2}\right).$$

In a similar fashion to Problem I note that the posterior of w does not depend on β. Also we will be dealing with rather large values of k which has the effect of making σ^2/k much smaller than τ^2. Thus the posterior at stage k becomes

$$\pi(\omega|\overline{y}_k) = N\left(\overline{y}_k, \frac{2\sigma^2}{k}\right).$$

Next we can compute the predictive distribution of the mean of the remaining n-k observations as

$$f\left(\bar{y}_{n-k} \mid \bar{y}_k\right)=\int f\left(\bar{y}_{n-k} \mid \bar{y}_k, w\right)\pi\left(w \mid \bar{y}_k\right)dw$$
$$=N\left(\bar{y}_k, 2\sigma^2\left(\frac{1}{n-k}+\frac{1}{k}\right)\right).$$

Thus at interim stage k we desire an indication of whether or not T is sufficiently better than S to continue the trial. Computing the quantity $P(w\geq 20 \mid \bar{y}_k)$, we can assess whether or not T is sufficiently better than S. If it is , then there are still n-k observations to be taken and we would like to predict what would be the likely value of this probability then. In particular suppose at the end of the trial we would want $P(w\geq 20 \mid \bar{y}_n)\geq 0.95$ to be true in order to assert that T is sufficiently better than S. At the interim stage k, we compute this probability and suppose it is 0.97. What we want to know is how likely is it that this probability will be at least 0.95 if we complete the trial.

We thus need to make a 'prediction' of how likely the experiment will turn out as we would hope. The mathematical details follow.

We require

$$P\left(\omega \geq 20 \mid \bar{y}_n\right)=\Phi\left(\frac{\bar{y}_n-20}{\sqrt{\frac{2}{n}}\sigma}\right)\geq 0.95$$

and this will be true provided

$$\bar{y}_n \geq 20+1.645\sqrt{\frac{2}{n}}\sigma.$$

But how likely is it based on the data seen at the interim stage k that this result will be achieved? Using the Bayesian predictive distribution given above, we can compute the predictive distribution of $\bar{Y}_n=\frac{n-k}{n}\bar{Y}_{n-k}+\frac{k}{n}\bar{Y}_k$ as

$$f\left(\bar{y}_n \mid \bar{y}_k\right)=N\left(\bar{y}_k, 2\sigma^2\left(\frac{1}{k}-\frac{1}{n}\right)\right).$$

With this distribution we can compute how likely the required result is as

$$P\left(\bar{y}_n \geq 20 + 1.645\sqrt{\frac{2}{n}}\sigma \,\middle|\, \bar{y}_k\right) = \Phi\left(\frac{\bar{y}_k - 20 + 1.645\sqrt{2}\,\sigma/\sqrt{n}}{\sqrt{2}\sigma\sqrt{\frac{1}{k}-\frac{1}{n}}}\right).$$

Some values of this function for hypothetical sample values are given in the table below.

Table 3.

Table of Predictive Probabilities

values of sample mean at stage k=250 (top row) and for n-k future observations

n-k	25	26	27	28	29	30	31
1	0.000	0.000	0.114	0.990	1.000	1.000	1.000
5	0.000	0.020	0.326	0.874	0.997	1.000	1.000
10	0.006	0.083	0.404	0.815	0.979	0.999	1.000
50	0.174	0.348	0.562	0.759	0.895	0.964	0.991
100	0.305	0.464	0.628	0.772	0.878	0.943	0.977
200	0.436	0.569	0.695	0.801	0.881	0.935	0.968
250	0.582	0.684	0.775	0.848	0.904	0.942	0.968
1000	0.666	0.751	0.823	0.881	0.923	0.953	0.973
1300	0.691	0.772	0.838	0.891	0.930	0.957	0.975
2000	0.727	0.800	0.860	0.906	0.940	0.963	0.979
5000	0.782	0.843	0.892	0.929	0.955	0.973	0.984
Posterior Prob(w>20) at k	0.868	0.910	0.941	0.963	0.978	0.987	0.993

For example take the interim stage k=250 and suppose the sample mean for T is 30 days longer than the sample mean for S. Then $P(w \geq 20 \mid \bar{y}_k = 30) = 0.987$. That is, at this interim stage after observing 250 survival times on each treatment, we are 98.7% sure that the treatment T is better than the standard treatment S by the required amount. If there are 250 observations still to be taken, we are 94.2% sure that this posterior probability will be larger than 0.95 at the end of the trial.

3.4 Discussion

In Problem II we have tried to show that the Bayesian approach offers a much clearer interim analysis methodology. It is also much easier to interpret quantitatively than P-values. The fact that this approach can yield a Table of Predictive Probabilities gives the practitioner considerable information about the trial. For example, it can indicate how many more observations might be necessary to have a reasonable chance of obtaining the desired result. It can also indicate that there is such little chance of the desired result, that the trial should be stopped. It is not possible for a frequentist to give this type of information to the practitioner.

It should be noted that we have handled a very simple data set scenario. For example, we have assumed that the data was uncensored. In many cases, the observations are on censored data. Whereas this model is more complicated, it can still be analyzed using the Bayesian approach. Also as in Problem I, the assumption of equal variances is not necessary and was made simply for convenience. In many problems such an assumption may not be valid, in which case prior distributions would be obtained for the unknown and unequal variances. Application of MCMC techniques could then obrtain a Table of Predictive Probabilities as we have done here.

REFERENCES

FORD E., COOPER R., SIMMONS B., KATZ S., PATEL R., (1988), Sex differences in high density lipoprotein chpolesterol in urban blacks. *American Journal of Epidemiology, 127*, 753-761.

DE FINETTI,B,. (1974, 1975), Theory of Probability, Vols 1 and 2, Wiley.

Chapter 7

TWO EXPERIMENTAL SETTINGS IN CLINICAL TRIALS: PREDICTIVE CRITERIA FOR CHOOSING THE SAMPLE SIZE IN INTERVAL ESTIMATION

F. De Santis* and M. Perone Pacifico
Dipartimento di Statistica, Probabilità e Statistiche Applicate, Università di Roma "La Sapienza".

1. INTRODUCTION

Determination of the optimal sample size is a fundamental step in many statistical designs, especially relevant in biomedical studies and in all situations where data are difficult to collect.

As motivating examples, we consider two experimental settings in which sample size determination is the central issue.

In the first (see Example 2, Section 4), we are concerned with choosing the appropriate number of statistical units to consider in a clinical trial. In this setting researchers are interested in comparing the effects of two alternative therapies for the treatment of pelvic cancer. This problem can be formalized as a problem of estimation of a quantity that measures the difference in the "expected" effects of the two alternative cures. In the planning stage of the experiment, that involves persons affected by a serious pathology, it is of crucial importance to select both the overall size of the experiment and the number of individuals to assign to each treatment under comparison. Specifically, researchers are interested in planning the experiment so to be guaranteed, at a controllable level, to have an informative outcome, represented by a "short" interval estimate. In the same

* For correspondence: fulvio.desantis@uniroma1.it

context, it is also important to exploit information that is potentially available from previous studies on the same disease.

The second motivating experimental problem (see Example 4, section 6) is about estimating the effect on the expected lifetime of a group of patients of a drug for maintaining remission in acute leukemia. As in the previous setting, researchers are interested in planning the experiment so to be confident, at certain controllable levels, to observe an accurate estimate - represented by a set of possible values - of the quantity of interest. Also in this case we are interested in considering methods that allow researchers to model and to introduce in the analysis pre-experimental clinical knowledge on the phenomenon.

From a statistical point of view, both the above can be formalized as problems of optimal sample size determination in the context of interval estimation of a quantity of interest. We propose the use of Bayesian methods, that are particularly suitable not only for incorporation of pre-experimental information in the analysis, but also for dealing with unknown parameters of not direct inferential interest, such as, for instance, the variance of experimental observations.

While the two experimental settings considered pose essentially the same methodological issues, namely optimal sample size determination and modelling of historical data, they still present their own specificities. In particular, in the clinical trial experiment we also need to come up with an allocation rule to assign patients to the two treatments under control. We show that, under assumptions that do not seem too restrictive, closed-form expressions for the sample size determination problem can be given. The survival analysis example is characterized by the potential presence of censoring, that is of truncation in the observation time, that is shown to affect the optimal sample size. Furthermore, in this context, unlike the former, closed-form expressions for the formulas are not available, motivating the need for a numerical method, proposed in Section 5.

The literature regarding sample size choice and, more generally, optimal design is quite large, especially within the frequentist inferential framework. The most common frequentist criteria for sample size determination are related to power considerations when the statistical problem is testing and, in estimation problems, to either size of intervals or variance of estimators. Typically, standard frequentist criteria for sample size choice depend on one or more unknown parameters, so that initial guesses on the true values of these parameters are needed for implementation of these procedures. For instance, optimal sample size formulas for testing a normal mean depend on the variance that must be replaced by arbitrary guesses. Hence the resulting sample size criteria are only locally optimal and can be quite sensitive to the values chosen.

The Bayesian approach allows the statistician to use all prior information on the parameters of the model including their uncertainty, so that the above mentioned problem is automatically overcome by using a prior distribution for all the unknown parameters in the model. This results in greater flexibility than the classical approach.

Although the literature on Bayesian sample size determination is not as large as the frequentist one, the problem has been considered by several authors. Adcock (1997) reviews both frequentist and Bayesian methods for choosing the sample size. Decision theoretic approaches to the sample size problem are considered, for instance, in Raiffa and Schlaifer (1961), Berger (1985) Piccinato (1996) and Lindley (1997), where choice criteria are obtained by maximizing a suitable expected utility. The problem of determining the sample size is also considered in testing problems, with particular attention to clinical trials (Spiegelhalter and Freedman, 1986; Verdinelli, 1996, DasGupta and Vidakovic, 1997; Weiss, 1997, Lee and Zelen, 2000) and in estimation problems (see, among others Pham-Gia and Turkkan, 1992). For an exhaustive overview of Bayesian experimental design see Chaloner and Verdinelli (1995).

In this paper we focus on sample size determination for interval estimation, from a Bayesian point of view. In this context, several methods have already been proposed: for an extensive overview, see, for instance, the special issue of *The Statistician* (1997, vol. 47 n. 2), dedicated to this topic.

The available procedures can be classified into two main categories: interval-based versus decision-theoretic-based criteria. The former methods (see, for instance, Joseph and Belisle, 1997) are essentially based on specific features of set estimators, such as their expected length and their frequentist coverage. Conversely, decision theoretic criteria (Bernardo, 1997; Lindley, 1997) are developed by formalizing the sample size determination task as a decision problem and by maximizing suitable expected utilities.

Of course, there are advantages and disadvantages in adopting either one of the two approaches. In this paper, however, we do not want enter this important controversy. Rather, we focus on a interval-type method, based on the probability of having credible sets with length not greater than a fixed threshold. In the following we will name this the *Length Probability Criterion* (LPC). This method has first been used by Joseph, Wolfson and du Berger (1995) in the binomial context and by Joseph and Belisle (1997) for sample size choice for interval estimation of normal means. In the following sections we also compare LPC to another criterion introduced by Joseph, Wolson and du Berger (1995), the *Average Length Criterion* (ALC).

The contributions of this paper are the following. First, in Section 2, we start the discussion on LPC and ALC, that are numerically compared in several examples throughout the paper.

Second, we revisit the special yet important settings, already considered by Joseph and Belisle (1997), of sample size choice for interval estimation of a normal mean (Section 3) and of the difference between two normal means (Section 4) using conjugate priors. This context is particularly relevant since explicit expressions of the probability distribution of the random length of the HPD sets can be found. These results are important not only because they give one the chance of straightforward implementation and comparison of alternative sample size determination methods, such as, for instance, LPC and ALC, but also because they allow one to check the accuracy of a numerical procedure for determining the sample size that we propose in Section 5, as a key contribution of the paper, for all those situations in which analytic results are not straightforward to determine. This numerical procedure is based on estimating the predictive distribution of the random length of the set estimators and prevents one from using standard computationally expensive search algorithms.

Finally, the numerical procedure is employed in Section 6 for sample size determination using LPC in survival analysis in the presence of censoring. This is a case in which analytic results on the length of HPD sets are not available. In this context, we also make use of LPC for evaluating the impact of censoring on the design of the experiment.

2. PROBLEM SETTING

We want to find the optimal size of a random sample $\mathbf{X}_n = (X_1, \cdots, X_n)$, whose joint density $f_n(\cdot|\theta)$ depends on the unknown parameter $\theta \in \Theta$.

For an observed sample $\mathbf{x}_n = (x_1, \cdots, x_n)$, the posterior density of θ is

$$\pi(\theta|\mathbf{x}_n) = \frac{f_n(\mathbf{x}_n|\theta)\pi(\theta)}{m_n(\mathbf{x}_n)} \tag{1}$$

where π is the prior density of θ and

$$m_n(\mathbf{x}_n) = \int_\Theta f_n(\mathbf{x}_n|\theta)\pi(\theta)d\theta$$

is the predictive density of $\mathbf{x}_n$. If the parameter θ is a multidimensional vector $\theta = (\theta_1, \theta_2)$, where $\theta_1 \in \Theta_1$ is the parameter of interest and $\theta_2 \in \Theta_2$ is a nuisance parameter, the posterior density of θ_1 is

$$\pi(\theta_1 \mid \mathbf{x}_n) = \int_{\Theta} \pi(\theta_1, \theta_2 \mid \mathbf{x}_n) d\theta_2$$

where $\pi(\theta_1, \theta_2 \mid \mathbf{x}_n)$ is the posterior density (1) of the whole parameter θ.

In the following we will suppose that the parameter of interest is one-dimensional and that, for each n and for each $\mathbf{x}_n$ its posterior density is unimodal, so that set estimates are intervals of the real line.

Given a sample $\mathbf{x}_n$, the most common Bayesian interval estimates for θ are equal-tails and HPD intervals: the $(1-\alpha)$-level equal-tails interval is the interval $[q_{\alpha/2}, q_{1-\alpha/2}]$ whose endpoints are the $\alpha/2$ and $1-\alpha/2$ quantiles of the posterior density. The $(1-\alpha)$-level HPD is defined as the subset of Θ with posterior density greater than some threshold

$$H_\alpha(\mathbf{x}_n) = \{\theta \in \Theta : \pi(\theta \mid \mathbf{x}_n) \geq k_\alpha\},$$

where k_α is the largest real number such that the posterior probability of $H_\alpha(\mathbf{x}_n)$ is greater than or equal to $1-\alpha$.

From the computational point of view, equal-tails intervals are much easier to work with than HPD's. This reason and the fact that HPD sets are not invariant under parameter transformations make the use of equal-tails intervals for interval estimation very common. Conversely, HPD intervals are of minimal size among all the sets with posterior probability equal to $1-\alpha$ and this renders HPD sets recommendable whenever a "preferred" parametrization can be identified. Of course HPD and equal-tails coincide when the posterior density is symmetric.

In sample size determination problems the idea is that, before performing the experiment yielding the data, we want to choose the minimal sample size that satisfies a selected criterion. We are then in a pre-experimental setting and thus both the interval estimator and its length are functions of the random sample $\mathbf{X}_n$ that has density m_n. Hence all pre-experimental computations should be done taking the randomness of $\mathbf{X}_n$ into account; moreover, the prior distribution π must be proper, otherwise the predictive density m_n would also be improper and thus useless for design purposes. In the following we will denote with P the underlying probability measure with respect to which the sample $\mathbf{X}_n$ has density m_n and with E the expectations computed through it.

The sample size choice criteria used in the following are based on features of interval estimates for the parameter of interest. We will focus our presentation on HPD sets, but it can as well be rephrased in terms of equal-tails intervals. For related frequentist methodologies see Beal (1989).

Among the several criteria proposed in the Bayesian literature we will focus on the so called *Average Length Criterion*, proposed by Joseph, Wofson and du Berger (1995). For ALC, the idea is to find, for a fixed α, the smallest sample size such that the expected length of the $(1-\alpha)$-level HPD is less than a chosen value, ℓ. Then, denoting by $L_\alpha(\mathbf{X}_n)$ the random variable corresponding to the length of the $(1-\alpha)$-level HPD set, we look for the smallest n such that

$$\mathsf{E}[L_\alpha(\mathbf{X}_n)] \le \ell,$$

where the expectation is with respect to the predictive distribution of the sample $\mathbf{X}_n$. Therefore, this criterion only requires an average control on the length of the HPD set, with no control on the variability of this length.

As an alternative to ALC we here consider the use of the *Length Probability Criterion*: we select n in order that the probability of having an HPD for θ with length greater than ℓ_0 is less than a chosen level γ. Then, we choose the smallest n such that

$$\mathsf{P}[L_\alpha(\mathbf{X}_n) \ge \ell_0] \le \gamma.$$

Joseph and Belisle (1997) have used what we call LPC as a special case the *Worst Outcome Criterion* (WOC), originally introduced by Joseph, Wolfson and du Berger (1995). The basic idea that leads to WOC is determining the minimal sample size so that both length and coverage of the posterior interval estimators are controlled. See also Joseph, du Berger and Belisle (1997) for further details on WOC.

Note that implementation of LPC requires one to fix (α, ℓ_0, γ). Therefore, the optimal sample sizes determined using this method depends on the values chosen for these three quantities. Note also that, under rather mild conditions, as $n \to \infty$ the posterior distribution of θ tends almost surely to a point mass, so that $L_\alpha(\mathbf{X}_n) \to 0$; this ensures the existence of some n satisfying the LPC. Moreover, asymptotic normality makes the use of HPD and equal-tails equivalent for large samples. In Example 4 it will be shown that for relatively small samples the use of LPC based on HPD results in saving a few experimental units with respect to the same criterion based on equal-tails intervals. This might be relevant whenever the cost of observations is high.

3. SAMPLE SIZE DETERMINATION FOR THE NORMAL MEAN

In this section we revisit the sample size determination problem for interval estimation of the normal mean, using conjugate priors. This context has been previously considered by Joseph and Belisle (1997), who provide closed-form expressions that can be used to implement both ALC and LPC. We here provide, in Appendix A1, a derivation of the probability distribution of the random variable $L_\alpha(\mathbf{X}_n)$ which is alternative and slightly more detailed than that given by Joseph and Belisle (1997).

Hence, let us suppose that the observations $X_1, \cdots, X_n$ are exchangeable, normally distributed with unknown mean μ and unknown precision λ. Here $\mu \in \Re$ is the parameter of interest and $\lambda \in \Re^+$ the nuisance parameter. We consider the usual conjugate prior for the parameter (μ, λ), *i.e.* a gamma distribution with fixed parameters (ν, β) for the precision λ and, conditionally on λ, a normal distribution for the mean μ with prior mean μ_0 and precision $n_0\lambda$. Using the notation in Bernardo and Smith (1994),

$$f_n(\mathbf{x}_n \mid \mu, \lambda) = \prod_{j=1}^{n} \mathrm{N}(\mathbf{x}_j \mid \mu, \lambda),$$

$$\pi(\mu, \lambda) = \mathrm{N}(\mu \mid \mu_0, n_0\lambda)\mathrm{Ga}(\lambda \mid \nu, \beta)$$

and, for a given sample $\mathbf{x}_n$ (with sample mean $\bar{x}$ and sample variance s^2), the posterior distribution of μ turns out to be

$$\pi(\mu \mid \mathbf{x}_n) = St\left(\mu \middle| \mu_n, \frac{(n_0+n)(2\nu+n)}{2\beta + 2g(\mathbf{x}_n)}, 2\nu + n\right)$$

where

$$\mu_n = \frac{n_0\mu_0 + n\bar{x}}{n_0 + n} \quad \text{and} \quad g(\mathbf{x}_n) = \frac{1}{2}\left(ns^2 + \frac{n_0 n(\bar{x} - \mu_0)^2}{n_0 + n}\right). \tag{2}$$

It follows that, *a posteriori*,

$$\frac{\mu-\mu_n}{\sqrt{\dfrac{2\beta+2g(\mathbf{x}_n)}{(n_0+n)(2v+n)}}}$$

has a standard Student distribution with $2v+n$ degrees of freedom (df). Since such a distribution is symmetric, the $(1-\alpha)$-HPD set coincides with the equal tails interval

$$H_\alpha(\mathbf{x}_n)=\left\{\mu\in\Re:|\mu-\mu_n|\le t_{2v+n;1-\alpha/2}\sqrt{\frac{2\beta+2g(\mathbf{x}_n)}{(n_0+n)(2v+n)}}\right\}$$

and its length is

$$L_\alpha(\mathbf{x}_n)=2t_{2v+n;1-\alpha/2}\sqrt{\frac{2\beta+2g(\mathbf{x}_n)}{(n_0+n)(2v+n)}},$$

where $t_{2v+n;1-\alpha/2}$ is the $(1-\alpha/2)$ quantile of the Student distribution with $2v+n$ df (note that the HPD length does not depend on the prior mean μ_0).

In Appendix A1 we provide a detailed derivation of the exact expression of the probability that $L_\alpha(\mathbf{X}_n)$ is greater than any fixed value; this formula can be used to choose the sample size according to LPC.

In particular, if we want to select the smallest n such that $\mathrm{P}[L_\alpha(\mathbf{X}_n)\ge\ell_0]\le\gamma$ from (A3) in Appendix A1, it follows that we need to find n such that

$$\mathrm{P}[L_\alpha(\mathbf{X}_n)\ge\ell_0]=\int_0^u \mathrm{Be}(t\,|\,v,\tfrac{n}{2})dt\le\gamma \quad \text{with} \quad u=\frac{8\beta}{\ell_0^2(n+2v)(n+n_0)}t^2_{2v+n;1-\alpha/2} \tag{3}$$

where $\mathrm{Be}(\cdot\,|\,v,\tfrac{n}{2})$ is the Beta density with parameters $(v,\tfrac{n}{2})$.

Example 1 Joseph and Belisle (1997, Table 1) and Ibrahim, Chen and Sinha (2001, Example 9.5) compute sample size according to ALC in the 6 cases corresponding to the parameters settings summarized in Table 1.

The top part of Table 2 contains the optimal sample sizes obtained through ALC, the corresponding expected length and the probability of obtaining of HPD sets larger than ℓ.

Table 1. Prior parameters, confidence levels and length thresholds in the 6 cases considered by Joseph and Belisle (1997) and Ibrahim, Chen and Sinha (2001).

	Case					
	1	2	3	4	5	6
n_0	10	10	10	10	100	10
ν	2	2	2	2	100	100
β	2	2	2	2	100	100
$1-\alpha$	0.99	0.95	0.80	0.50	0.95	0.95
ℓ	0.5	0.2	0.2	0.2	0.2	0.2

It is clear that using ALC does not prevent one from having credible intervals larger than the threshold ℓ. The second part of Table 2 contains the same quantities, but the optimal sample size is now obtained through LPC (with the same length threshold $\ell_0 = \ell$ and with $\gamma = 0.10$). This choice of the thresholds makes LPC a more strict requirement than ALC, resulting in larger sample sizes. From this example it is clear that the expected length is inadequate to summarize the distribution of $L_\alpha(\mathbf{X}_n)$: in cases 5 and 6 a moderate increase in the sample size (14.5% and 11.5% respectively) produces a dramatic decrease in the probability of large intervals (from 0.48 to 0.10) while the expected length is almost insensitive to the change.□

Table 2. ALC and LPC: optimal sample size and the corresponding expected length and probability of obtaining large set estimates.

	Case					
	1	2	3	4	5	6
n_{ALC}	160	595	248	61	288	378
$\mathbf{E}[L_\alpha(\mathbf{X}_{n_{ALC}})]$	0.50	0.20	0.20	0.20	0.20	0.20
$\mathbf{P}[L_\alpha(\mathbf{X}_{n_{ALC}} \geq \ell)]$	0.36	0.36	0.36	0.36	0.48	0.48
n_{LPC}	391	1435	607	160	330	421
$\mathbf{E}[L_\alpha(\mathbf{X}_{n_{LPC}})]$	0.32	0.13	0.13	0.13	0.19	0.19
$\mathbf{P}[L_\alpha(\mathbf{X}_{n_{LPC}} \geq \ell_0)]$	0.10	0.10	0.10	0.10	0.10	0.10

Finally note that, as an alternative to (3), one could control the probability of obtaining a large set estimate using Markov inequality. In fact

$$P[L_\alpha(\mathbf{X}_n)\geq \ell_0]\leq \frac{E[L_\alpha(\mathbf{X}_n)]}{\ell_0}$$

and, in order to select n such that $P[L_\alpha(\mathbf{X}_n)\geq \ell_0]\leq \gamma$, one can use ALC with $\ell=\gamma\ell_0$. In general this results in a unnecessary large sample size: for instance in case 1 of Example 1, the sample size required would be 16668 instead of $n_{LPC}=391$.

4. SAMPLE SIZE DETERMINATION FOR THE DIFFERENCE OF NORMAL MEANS

Suppose now that we are interested in determining the HPD set for the difference between the means of two normal distributions. This problem is especially relevant since it covers many practical situations, as, for instance, the comparison of the effects of two treatments in clinical trials.

We consider two random samples $\mathbf{X}_{n_1}^{(1)}$ and $\mathbf{X}_{n_2}^{(2)}$ for which we make the same distributional assumptions of Section 3: for r=1,2

$$f_{n_r}(\mathbf{x}_{n_r}^{(r)}\mid\mu_r,\lambda)=\prod_{j=1}^{n_r}\mathrm{N}(\mathbf{x}_j^{(r)}\mid\mu_r,\lambda)$$

$$\pi(\mu_r,\lambda)=\mathrm{N}(\mu_r\mid\mu_{0r},n_{0r}\lambda)\mathrm{Ga}(\lambda\mid\nu,\beta)$$

We assume $\mathbf{X}_{n_1}^{(1)}$ and $\mathbf{X}_{n_2}^{(2)}$ independent conditionally on all the parameters and the two prior means μ_1 and μ_2 independent conditionally on the common unknown prior precision λ. The parameter we are interested in is $\delta=\mu_1-\mu_2$. Note that the above prior assumptions are equivalent to assigning

$$\pi(\delta,\lambda)=\mathrm{N}(\delta\mid\mu_{01}-\mu_{02},(n_{01}+n_{02})\lambda)\mathrm{Ga}(\lambda\mid\nu,\beta)$$

The posterior distribution for δ is such that

$$\frac{\delta-(\mu_{n_1}^{(1)}-\mu_{n_2}^{(2)})}{\sqrt{\dfrac{2\beta(n_1+n_{01}+n_2+n_{02})}{(n_1+n_2+2\nu)(n_1+n_{01})(n_2+n_{02})}}\sqrt{1+\dfrac{g^{(1)}(\mathbf{x}_{n_1}^{(1)})+g^{(2)}(\mathbf{x}_{n_2}^{(2)})}{\beta}}}$$

has a standard Student distribution with $n_1+n_2+2\nu$ df, where $\mu_{n_r}^{(r)}$ and $g^{(r)}(\mathbf{x}_{n_r}^{(r)})$ are defined as in (2), $r=1,2$.

The length of the HPD interval is then

$$L_\alpha(\mathbf{x}_{n_1}^{(1)},\mathbf{x}_{n_2}^{(2)})=2t_{2\nu+n_1+n_2;1-\alpha/2}\cdot$$
$$\cdot\sqrt{\frac{2\beta(n_1+n_{01}+n_2+n_{02})}{(n_1+n_2+2\nu)(n_1+n_{01})(n_2+n_{02})}}\sqrt{1+\frac{g^{(1)}(\mathbf{x}_{n_1}^{(1)})+g^{(2)}(\mathbf{x}_{n_2}^{(2)})}{\beta}}$$

and, as for the single normal mean problem, it does not depend on the prior means μ_{0r}.

In Appendix A2 the exact formulas needed to determine sample size according to either LPC or ALC are given (see also Joseph and Belisle, 1997, for an alternative derivation on of these results). From (A6) it is easy to check that the distribution of the random component of $L_\alpha(\mathbf{X}_{n_1}^{(1)},\mathbf{X}_{n_2}^{(2)})$ depends on the sum n of n_1 and n_2 but not on their separate values. Once the total size n is fixed, the only component of $L_\alpha(\mathbf{X}_{n_1}^{(1)},\mathbf{X}_{n_2}^{(2)})$ affected by the allocation of n in n_1 and n_2 is

$$\sqrt{\frac{2\beta(n_1+n_{01}+n_2+n_{02})}{(n_1+n_2+2\nu)(n_1+n_{01})(n_2+n_{02})}}$$

that attains its minimum when $n_1+n_{01}=n_2+n_{02}$, so that it is always convenient to choose

$$n_1=\frac{n+n_{02}-n_{01}}{2}\quad\text{and}\quad n_1=\frac{n+n_{01}-n_{02}}{2}.$$

Taking into account the above constraints, $L_\alpha(\mathbf{X}_{n_1}^{(1)},\mathbf{X}_{n_2}^{(2)})$ depends on the total size n only, which can be determined according to either LPC or ALC.

Example 2 Spiegelhalter, Freedman and Parmar (1994) consider the following example based on Errington *et al.* (1991) regarding a clinical trial for comparing high energy neutron therapy (r=1) versus conventional radiotherapy for treatment of pelvic cancers (r=2).

Under proportional hazards assumption, if R_{n_r} is the log-rank test statistics relative to n_r events observed in group r, then $Y_{n_r}=R_{n_r}/n_r$ has approximately a normal density centered at the log-hazard ratio μ_r with variance σ^2/n_r. We can think of Y_{n_r} as the average of n_r exchangeable normal random variables. The interest is on $\mu_1 - \mu_2$ that is the difference between the log-hazard ratios in the two groups. Thus we are in the setting considered in this section.

Interviews with experts of neutron therapy lead to consider (0, 0.355) as the range of equivalence for the two therapies; thus for $\delta \in (0,0.355)$ we would be unable to make a definitive choice of treatment, while $\delta \leq 0$ or $\delta \geq 0.355$ provide decisive evidence in favor of treatment 2 or 1 respectively. Therefore, in order that the $(1-\alpha)$-level HPD does not contain simultaneously values for δ in the two decisive regions, it may be desirable that $L_\alpha(\mathbf{x}_{n_1}^{(1)}, \mathbf{x}_{n_2}^{(2)}) < 0.355$.

Spiegelhalter, Freedman and Parmar (1994) consider a fixed variance $\sigma^2 = 4$ (equivalently $\lambda = 1/4$) and, according to information collected interviewing specialists, a normal prior for δ with $\mu_{01} - \mu_{02} = 0.169$, $n_{01} = 22$ and $n_{02} = 26$. In order to avoid such a sharp assumption on the precision λ, we consider here it unknown with a gamma prior density with $\nu = 1602$ and $\beta = 6404$ (so that the variance σ^2 has mean 4 and standard deviation 0.1).

Using LPC with the requirement $\mathsf{P}[L_\alpha(\mathbf{X}_{n_1}^{(1)}, \mathbf{X}_{n_2}^{(2)}) \geq 0.355] \leq \gamma$, for $\alpha = \gamma = 0.05$ we obtain n=1952 as the total sample size, with $n_1 = 978$ and $n_2 = 974$.

The high number of observations required in this example might be reduced by increasing α and/or γ, but of course this would result in a growth of the probability of having decisive evidence towards both treatments at the same time.

5. NUMERICAL PROCEDURE

For dealing with the criteria introduced in Section 2, one needs to study the sampling distribution of the length of the HPD set. When the posterior density is symmetric, finding the HPD set is quite easy (the endpoints of $H_\alpha(\mathbf{x}_n)$ are the $\alpha/2$ and $(1-\alpha/2)$ quantiles of the posterior distribution) and determining the sampling distribution of $L_\alpha(\mathbf{X}_n)$ might be feasible.

When the posterior density is not symmetric, finding an analytic expression for the HPD set is not easy and studying the sampling distribution of $L_\alpha(\mathbf{X}_n)$ turns out to be awkward. In order to use our criterion for determining the sample size, we propose a simple numerical procedure to approximate HPD sets and to simulate the distribution of the length $L_\alpha(\mathbf{X}_n)$.

To approximate the HPD set for a given sample $\mathbf{x}_n$

a) generate a large sample $\Theta_N = (\theta_1, \cdots, \theta_N)$ of i.i.d. observation from the posterior distribution of the parameter of interest θ;
b) compute the corresponding values of the posterior density $\Pi_N = (\pi(\theta_1 \mid \mathbf{x}_n), \cdots, \pi(\theta_n \mid \mathbf{x}_n))$;
c) choose $k_\alpha(\Theta_N)$ as the $N\alpha$-th ordered element of Π_N so that the proportion of elements of Π_N greater than $k_\alpha(\Theta_N)$ is equal to $(1-\alpha)$;
d) define the approximated HPD set as the interval containing all the points in Θ_N with posterior density greater than $k_\alpha(\Theta_N)$,

$$\left[\min\{\theta \in \Theta_N : \pi(\theta \mid \mathbf{x}_n) > k_\alpha(\Theta_N)\}, \max\{\theta \in \Theta_N : \pi(\theta \mid \mathbf{x}_n) > k_\alpha(\Theta_N)\}\right]. \tag{4}$$

The idea leading to this procedure for approximating the HPD set is that, since $k_\alpha(\Theta_N)$ is the $N\alpha$-th ordered element of Π_N, as $n \to \infty$ the random variable $k_\alpha(\Theta_N)$ converges almost surely to the α quantile of the posterior distribution of the random variable $\pi(\theta \mid \mathbf{x}_n)$ (viewed as a transformation of the random parameter θ) and then the posterior probability of the set (4) tends to $1-\alpha$.

The procedure sketched above avoids both bisection and integration steps needed by standard numerical algorithms for determining HPD intervals; moreover it allows to approximate HPD sets even when the posterior density is cumbersome and equation $\pi(\theta \mid \mathbf{x}_n) = k_\alpha$ is difficult to solve. The procedure only requires sampling from the posterior distribution (step (a)), which can almost always be done directly or using Metropolis-Hastings or other techniques based on Monte Carlo Markov Chains.

To simulate the whole sampling distribution of $L_\alpha(\mathbf{X}_n)$

1. generate a sample $\mathbf{x}_n$ from the predictive distribution: sample θ from the prior π and $\mathbf{x}_n$ from $f_n(\cdot \mid \theta)$;
2. compute the approximated HPD set through steps (a)-(d) listed above;
3. repeat the operation for a sufficiently large number of samples.

This procedure is used to generate a large number of 'observations' of the random variable $L_\alpha(\mathbf{X}_n)$ so that expectations and probabilities can be easily computed using Monte Carlo techniques.

The procedure described above can be used to determine the sample size according to either LPC or ALC. For testing the numerical procedure, in the following example we find numerical results for the normal mean problem and compare them with the analytic ones. In Section 6 we use the numerical procedure in models for censored survival data where analytic results are not easily obtainable.

Example 3 To check the accuracy of the numerical procedure, we consider the case 1 setting (first column of Table 1) of Example 1. For each n in $\{10,\cdots,410\}$, we generated 1000 samples of size n from the predictive distribution and, for each sample, we computed the approximated HPD according to steps (a)-(d) with N=10000.

In Figure 1 both the exact value and the numerical approximation of $\mathsf{P}[L_\alpha(\mathbf{X}_n)\geq 0.5]$ are plotted as functions of n. Similarly in Figure 2 for $\mathsf{E}[L_\alpha(\mathbf{X}_n)]$. In both figures the two curves overlap almost perfectly.

6. SAMPLE SIZE DETERMINATION FOR SURVIVAL DATA

We are here interested in estimating the expected lifetime of a group of individuals. The problem is again to decide on the sample size necessary in order to obtain, with a given probability, HPD sets with length less than a fixed value.

Under type I censoring, the exact lifetime $\mathbf{X}_j$ of individual j is observed only if the subject presents the event during the observation time $(0,t_j^*]$, where t_j^* is the censoring time for the j-th subject.

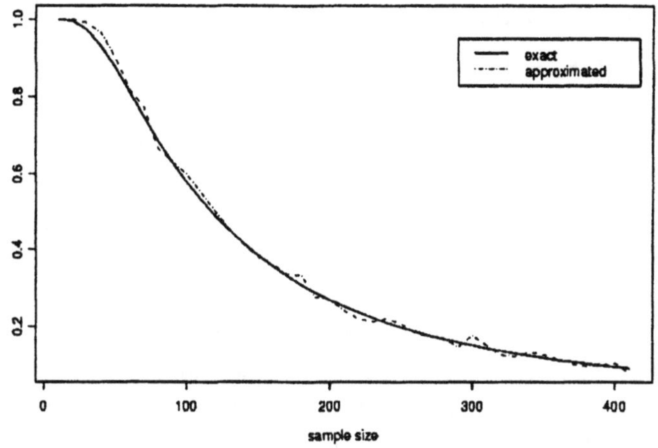

Figure 1. Exact value and numerical approximation of $\mathrm{P}[L_\alpha(\mathbf{X}_n) \geq 0.5]$.

Let us suppose that $X_1, \cdots, X_n$ are exchangeable and, conditionally on the unknown expected survival time θ, exponentially distributed. Using standard notation the likelihood function of θ relative to the observed vectors $(\mathbf{t}_n, \boldsymbol{\delta}_n)$ is

$$f_n(\mathbf{t}_n, \boldsymbol{\delta}_n) = \prod_{\{j:\delta_j=1\}} \frac{1}{\theta} \exp(-t_j/\theta) \prod_{\{j:\delta_j=0\}} \exp(-t_j^*/\theta)$$
$$= \theta^{-\sum_{j=1}^n \delta_j} \exp\left(-\frac{1}{\theta} \sum_{j=1}^n t_j\right)$$

where $t_j = \min\{x_j, t_j^*\}$ denotes the effective observation time of subject j and $\delta_j = 1$ if $x_j \leq t_j^*$ and $\delta_j = 0$ otherwise.

Assuming that θ has the conjugate inverse gamma prior, with fixed parameters ν and β; the posterior distribution of θ is thus inverse gamma

$$\pi(\theta \mid \mathbf{t}_n, \boldsymbol{\delta}_n) = \mathrm{Ig}(\theta \mid \nu + \sum_{j=1}^n \delta_j, \beta + \sum_{j=1}^n t_j).$$

Analytic expressions for HPD sets cannot easily be found and, in the following example, we resort to the numerical procedure of Section 5.

Example 4 Freireich *et al.* (1963) report the result of a study on the effect of the drug 6-Mercaptopurine on the ability to maintain remission in acute leukemia patients. The drug is administered to 21 patients and at the end of the experiment, after one year, the observed results are $\sum_{j=1}^{21} t_j = 359$ (in weeks) and $\sum_{j=1}^{21} \delta_j = 9$.

Suppose now we are interested in planning a new experiment to estimate the mean survival time θ for patients submitted to 6-Mercaptopurine therapy. We consider here a common censoring time $t^* = 52$ weeks (corresponding approximately to an expected censoring fraction of $1/4$).

We use data from the experiment reported by Freireich *et al.* (1963) to elicit the parameter of the prior distribution for θ. We first fix the prior mean of the unknown expected survival time equal to the MLE of θ determined in the previous experiment. Furthermore, assuming that our prior belief about θ is worth 9 observations (the number of uncensored survival times in the previous experiment), standard elicitation techniques for conjugate distributions (Bernardo and Smith, 1994, Section 5.2) yield $\nu = 10$ and $\beta = 359$. This prior elicitation implicitly assumes a sort of exchangeability between data of the old and the new experiment. This assumption might be questionable but it is a reasonable starting point.

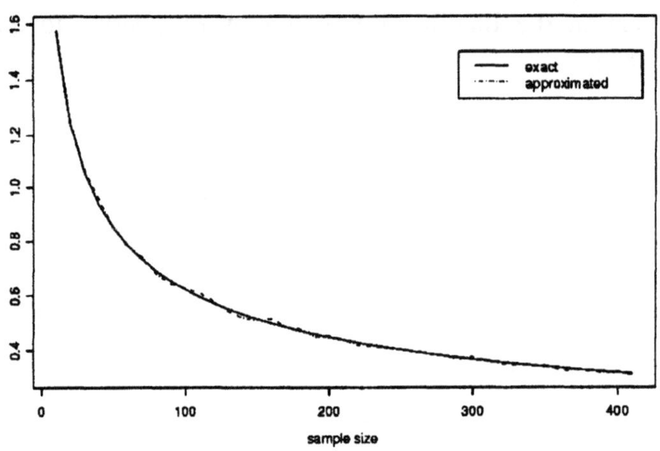

Figure 2. Exact value and numerical approximation of $\mathsf{E}[L_\alpha(\mathbf{X}_n)]$.

Figure 3 shows, for the 0.90-level HPD and equal-tails intervals of θ, the estimated values of $\mathsf{P}[L_\alpha(\mathbf{T}_n, \mathbf{\Delta}_n) \geq 30]$ as functions of *n*. In this case, according to LPC (with HPD sets), *n* = 26 observations are sufficient in order to have $\mathsf{P}[L_\alpha(\mathbf{T}_n, \mathbf{\Delta}_n) \geq 30] \leq 0.20$; using equal tails instead of HPD sets would require 3 additional observations with the same level of uncertainty.

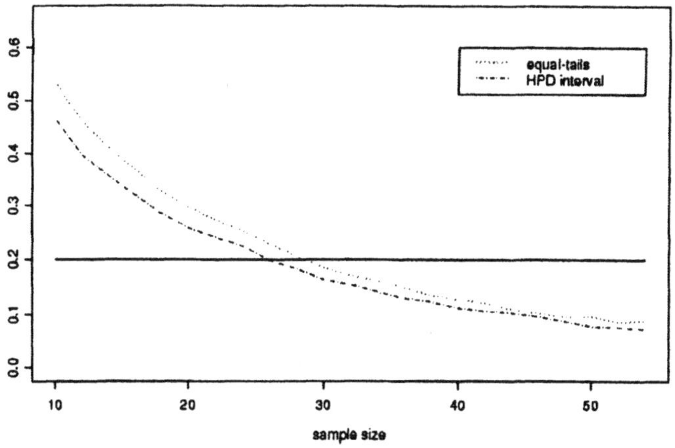

Figure 3. Numerical approximation of $\mathsf{P}[L_\alpha(\mathbf{X}_n) \geq 30]$ for equal-tails and HPD sets.

Suppose now that, a change in the budget forces us to consider a shorter observation time $t^* = 21$ weeks (corresponding to an expected censoring fraction of 3/7). Figure 4 shows the change in $\mathsf{P}[L_\alpha(\mathbf{T}_n, \boldsymbol{\Delta}_n) \geq 30]$ due to decreasing the observation time. In this case, LPC with the same values $\alpha = 0.10$, $\ell_0 = 30$ and $\gamma = 0.20$, gives $n = 52$.

7. FINAL REMARKS

Bayesian methods for sample size choice overcome the typical limitations of frequentist criteria of requiring initial guesses for nuisance parameters and of not taking into account the available prior information.

Unlike Bayesian criteria previously introduced as ALC, based only on the expectation of the length of credible sets, the LPC criterion considered here takes into account the whole distribution of $L_\alpha(\mathbf{X}_n)$.

We have revisited the problem of sample size determination for interval estimation of the normal mean and of the difference between two normal means using conjugate priors. In these cases exact expressions of optimal sample sizes can be derived. This task was first pursued by Joseph and Belisle (1997). In Appendixes A1 and A2 alternative proofs are given. These results are particularly relevant since, in the practice, even in complex setups, sample size is often calculated using the normal approximation to the actual model.

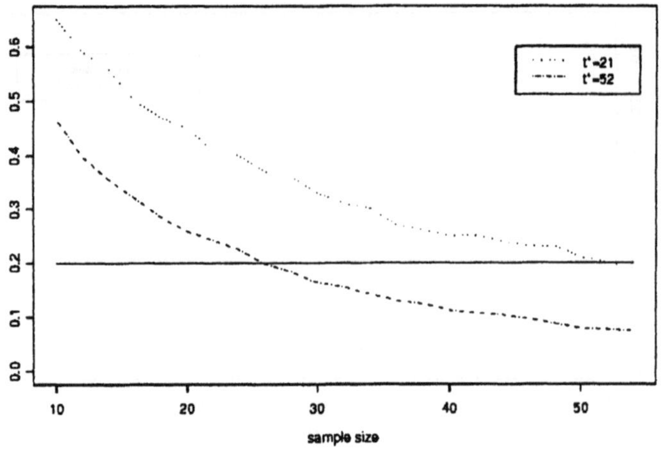

Figure 4. Numerical approximation of $\mathsf{P}[L_\alpha(\mathbf{X}_n) \geq 30]$ for two different censoring times.

We also propose a numerical procedure for LPC that can be exploited when exact formulas are not available; we check its accuracy in the normal model by comparing approximated to analytic results. The procedure makes it possible to use LPC in contexts more general than those described here since it only requires sampling from the predictive (which is always straightforward) and from the posterior (which is affordable, even in the non conjugate case, using MCMC techniques).

The use of LPC is illustrated in several examples, most of which are real design problems from the literature. For some of these examples, not only is the optimal sample size determined according to LPC, but the overall plot of $\mathsf{P}[L_\alpha(\mathbf{X}_n) \geq \ell_0]$ is given as a function of the sample size n. From a practical point of view these plots can be useful in order to visualize whether an increment in the sample size determines a significant decrease of $\mathsf{P}[L_\alpha(\mathbf{X}_n) \geq \ell_0]$.

LPC is also used in a survival analysis context. We claim that, in addition to its standard use for sample size choice, comparisons of the plots of $\mathsf{P}[L_\alpha(\mathbf{T}_n, \boldsymbol{\Delta}_n) \geq \ell_0]$ can give an idea, before the experiment is performed, of the impact of different censoring times (and hence of censoring fractions) on the analysis. In the paper we considered exponential survival data with type I censoring, however the use of LPC in more general survival contexts is straightforward.

APPENDIX

A1 Exact distribution of $L_\alpha(\mathbf{X}_n)$ for the mean in the normal case

We compute here the exact distribution of $L_\alpha(\mathbf{X}_n)$ under the hypotheses in Section 3. The length of the HPD set is

$$L_\alpha(\mathbf{X}_n) = 2t_{2v+n;1-\alpha/2}\sqrt{\frac{2\beta}{(n+2v)(n+n_0)}}\sqrt{1+\frac{G_n}{\beta}} \tag{A1}$$

where, according to (2), G_n can be written as

$$G_n = g(\mathbf{X}_n) = \frac{1}{2\lambda}\left(\lambda n S^2 + \lambda\frac{n_0 n(\overline{X}-\mu_0)^2}{n_0+n}\right) \tag{A2}$$

and $\overline{X}$ and S^2 are the sample mean and variance respectively. Conditionally on the precision λ, the two terms in parentheses are independent and have both χ^2 distribution, with n - 1 and 1 df respectively. It follows that $2\lambda G_n$ has χ^2 distribution with n df and G_n has gamma distribution with parameters $(\frac{n}{2},\lambda)$.

As in Bernardo and Smith (1994) we denote with $\mathrm{Be}(\cdot|\alpha,\beta)$ and $\mathrm{Ga}(\cdot|\alpha,\beta)$ the beta and gamma density respectively, and

$$\mathrm{Gg}(x|\alpha,\beta,n) = \int_0^\infty \mathrm{Ga}(x|n,\lambda)\mathrm{Ga}(\lambda|\alpha,\beta)d\lambda = \frac{\beta^\alpha\Gamma(\alpha+n)}{\Gamma(\alpha)\Gamma(n)}\frac{x^{n-1}}{(\beta+x)^{\alpha+n}}.$$

Since $\sqrt{1+G_n/\beta}\geq 1$ almost surely, then $\mathrm{P}[\sqrt{1+G_n/\beta}\geq x]=1$ for all $x<1$. Recalling that λ has gamma distribution with parameters (v,β), for $x\geq 1$ we have

$$\begin{aligned}
\mathrm{P}\left[\sqrt{1+\frac{G_n}{\beta}}\geq x\right] &= P[G_n\geq\beta(x^2-1)] \\
&= \int_0^\infty\left[\int_{\beta(x^2-1)}^\infty \mathrm{Ga}(g|\tfrac{n}{2},\lambda)dg\right]\mathrm{Ga}(\lambda|v,\beta)d\lambda \\
&= \int_{\beta(x^2-1)}^\infty\left[\int_0^\infty \mathrm{Ga}(g|\tfrac{n}{2},\lambda)\mathrm{Ga}(\lambda|v,\beta)d\lambda\right]dg
\end{aligned}$$

$$= \int_{\beta(x^2-1)}^{\infty} \mathrm{Gg}(g \mid \nu, \beta, \tfrac{n}{2})dg = \frac{\beta^{\nu}\Gamma(\nu+\frac{n}{2})}{\Gamma(\nu)\Gamma(\frac{n}{2})} \int_{\beta(x^2-1)}^{\infty} \frac{g^{\frac{n}{2}-1}}{(\beta+g)^{\nu+\frac{n}{2}}} dg$$

$$= \frac{\Gamma(\nu+\frac{n}{2})}{\Gamma(\nu)\Gamma(\frac{n}{2})} \int_{\beta(x^2-1)}^{\infty} \left(\frac{\beta}{\beta+g}\right)^{\nu-1} \left(\frac{g}{\beta+g}\right)^{\frac{n}{2}-1} \frac{\beta}{(\beta+g)^2} dg$$

$$= \frac{\Gamma(\nu+\frac{n}{2})}{\Gamma(\nu)\Gamma(\frac{n}{2})} \int_0^{x^{-2}} t^{\nu-1}(1-t)^{\frac{n}{2}-1} dt = \int_0^{x^{-2}} \mathrm{Be}(t \mid \nu, \tfrac{n}{2})dt \,. \qquad \text{(A3)}$$

The density of $\sqrt{1+G_n/\beta}$ is then, for $x \geq 1$,

$$f_{\sqrt{1+G_n/\beta}}(x) = -\frac{d}{dx}\mathrm{P}\left[\sqrt{1+\frac{G_n}{\beta}} \geq x\right] = \mathrm{Be}(x^{-2} \mid \nu, \tfrac{n}{2})2x^{-3}$$

and, for $k \leq 2\nu$, the k-th moment is

$$\mathrm{E}\left[\sqrt{1+\frac{G_n}{\beta}}^{\,k}\right] = \int_1^{\infty} x^k \mathrm{Be}(x^{-2} \mid \nu, \tfrac{n}{2})2x^{-3}dx = \int_0^1 t^{-\frac{k}{2}} \mathrm{Be}(t \mid \nu, \tfrac{n}{2})dt$$

$$= \frac{\Gamma(\nu+\frac{n}{2})}{\Gamma(\nu)\Gamma(\frac{n}{2})} \int_0^1 t^{\nu-\frac{k}{2}-1}(1-t)^{\frac{n}{2}-1} dt = \frac{\Gamma(\nu+\frac{n}{2})\Gamma(\nu-\frac{k}{2})\Gamma(\frac{n}{2})}{\Gamma(\nu)\Gamma(\frac{n}{2})\Gamma(\nu-\frac{k}{2}+\frac{n}{2})}$$

$$= \frac{\Gamma(\nu+\frac{n}{2})\Gamma(\nu-\frac{k}{2})}{\Gamma(\nu)\Gamma(\nu-\frac{k}{2}+\frac{n}{2})}$$

It follows that for $\nu > 1$ the mean and the variance of $\sqrt{1+G_n/\beta}$ are

$$\mathrm{E}\left[\sqrt{1+\frac{G_n}{\beta}}\right] = \frac{\Gamma(\nu+\frac{n}{2})\Gamma(\nu-\frac{1}{2})}{\Gamma(\nu)\Gamma(\nu-\frac{1}{2}+\frac{n}{2})} \qquad \text{(A4)}$$

$$\mathrm{V}\left[\sqrt{1+\frac{G_n}{\beta}}\right] = \frac{\nu+\frac{n}{2}-1}{\nu-1} - \left(\frac{\Gamma(\nu+\frac{n}{2})\Gamma(\nu-\frac{1}{2})}{\Gamma(\nu)\Gamma(\nu-\frac{1}{2}+\frac{n}{2})}\right)^2 . \qquad \text{(A5)}$$

Using representation (A1), equations (A3), (A4) and (A5) let us compute distribution, mean and variance of $L_\alpha(\mathbf{X}_n)$.Of course we get the same expression as Joseph and Belisle (1997) for the mean $\mathrm{E}[L_\alpha(\mathbf{X}_n)]$.

A2 Exact distribution of $L_\alpha(\mathbf{X}^{(1)}_{n_1}, \mathbf{X}^{(2)}_{n_2})$ for the difference between two means in the normal case

In the hypotheses of Section 4, the length of the HPD set can be written as

$$L_\alpha(\mathbf{X}^{(1)}_{n_1}, \mathbf{X}^{(2)}_{n_2}) = 2t_{2\nu+n_1+n_2;1-\alpha/2}\sqrt{\frac{2\beta(n_1+n_{01}+n_2+n_{02})}{(n_1+n_2+2\nu)(n_1+n_{01})(n_2+n_{02})}}\sqrt{1+\frac{G^{(1)}_{n_1}+G^{(2)}_{n_2}}{\beta}}$$

where $G^{(1)}_{n_1}$ and $G^{(2)}_{n_2}$ are defined as in (A2), but relatively to sample $\mathbf{X}^{(1)}_{n_1}$ and $\mathbf{X}^{(2)}_{n_2}$ respectively.

Considerations analogous to those in Appendix A1 lead to

$$\mathrm{P}\left[\sqrt{1+\frac{G^{(1)}_{n_1}+G^{(2)}_{n_2}}{\beta}} \geq x\right] = \int_0^{x^{-2}} \mathrm{Be}(t \mid \nu, \tfrac{n_1+n_2}{2})dt \qquad x \geq 1 \tag{A6}$$

$$\mathrm{E}\left[\sqrt{1+\frac{G^{(1)}_{n_1}+G^{(2)}_{n_2}}{\beta}}\right] = \frac{\Gamma(\nu+\frac{n_1+n_2}{2})\Gamma(\nu-\frac{1}{2})}{\Gamma(\nu)\Gamma(\nu-\frac{1}{2}+\frac{n_1+n_2}{2})}$$

$$\mathrm{V}\left[\sqrt{1+\frac{G^{(1)}_{n_1}+G^{(2)}_{n_2}}{\beta}}\right] = \frac{\nu+\frac{n_1+n_2}{2}-1}{\nu-1} - \left(\frac{\Gamma(\nu+\frac{n_1+n_2}{2})\Gamma(\nu-\frac{1}{2})}{\Gamma(\nu)\Gamma(\nu-\frac{1}{2}+\frac{n_1+n_2}{2})}\right)^2$$

which allow us to compute exactly distribution, mean and variance of $L_\alpha(\mathbf{X}^{(1)}_{n_1}, \mathbf{X}^{(2)}_{n_2})$.

REFERENCES

Adcock, J. (1997). Sample size determination: a review. *The Statistician, 46*, 261-283.

Beal, S. L.(1989). Sample size determination for confidence intervals on the population mean and on the difference between two population means. *Biometrics, 45*, 969-977.

Berger, J. O.(1985). Statistical decision theory and Bayesian analysis, 2nd edition. Springer-Verlag, New York.

Bernardo, J. M. and Smith, A. F. M. (1994). Bayesian theory. Wiley.

Chaloner, K. and Verdinelli, I. (1995). Bayesian experimental design: a review. *Statistical Science, 10*, 237-304.

DasGupta, A. and Vidakovic, B. (1997). Sample size problems in ANOVA: Bayesian point of view. *Journal of Statistical Planning and Inference, 65*, 335-347.

Errington, R. D. *et al.* (1991). High energy neutron treatment for pelvic cancers: study stopped because of increasing mortality. *The British Medical Journal, 302*, 1045-1051.

FREIREICH, E. J. *et al.* (1963). The effect of 6-Mercatopurine on the duration of steroidinduced remissions in acute leukemia: a model for evaluation of other potentially useful therapy. *Blood, 21*, 699-716.

IBRAHIM, J. G., CHEN, M. H., AND SINHA, D. (2001). Bayesian survival analysis. Springer-Verlag, Berlin.

JOSEPH, L. AND BELISLE, P. (1997). Bayesian sample size determination for normal means and difference between normal means. *The Statistician, 46*, 209-226.

JOSEPH, L., DU BERGER, R. AND BELISLE, P. (1997). Bayesian and mixed Bayesian/likelihood criteria for sample size determination. *Statistics in Medicine, 16,* 769-781.

JOSEPH, L., WOLFSON, D. AND DU BERGER, R. (1995). Sample size calculation for binomial proportions via highest posterior density intervals. *The Statistician, 44*, 143-154.

LEE, S. J. AND ZELEN, M. (2000). Clinical trials and sample size considerations: another perspective. *Statistical Science, 15*, 95-110.

LINDLEY, D. V. (1997). The choice of sample size. *The Statistician, 46*, 129-138.

PHAM-GIA, T. G. AND TURKKAN, N. (1992). Sample size determination in Bayesian analysis. *The Statistician, 41*, 389-397.

PICCINATO, L. (1996). Metodi per le decisioni statistiche. Springer-Verlag Italia.

RAIFFA, H. AND SCHLAIFER, R. (1961). Applied statistical decision theory. Boston: Harvard University Graduate School of Business Administration.

SPIEGELHALTER, D. J. AND FREEDMAN, L. S. (1986). A predictive approach to selecting the size of a clinical trial, based on subjective clinical opinion. *Statistics in Medicine, 5*, 1-13.

SPIEGELHALTER, D. J., FREEDMAN, L. S. AND PARMAR, M. K. B. (1994). Bayesian approaches to randomized trials. *Journal of the Royal Statistical Society, 157*, 357-416.

VERDINELLI, I., (1996). Bayesian design of experiments for the linear model. Ph.D. Thesis Department of Statistics, Carnegie Mellon University.

WEISS, R. (1997). Bayesian sample size calculations for hypothesis testing. *The Statistician, 46*, 209-226.

Chapter 8

ATTRIBUTING A PALEOANTHROPOLOGICAL SPECIMEN TO A PREHISTORIC POPULATION: A BAYESIAN APPROACH WITH MULTIVARIATE B-SPLINE FUNCTIONS

P. Frederic[1*], G. D'Amore[2] and E. Pacciani[3]
Dipartimento di Scienze Statistiche, Università di Bologna, Bologna, Italy[1]; Laboratori di Antropologia, Dipartimento di Biologia Animale e Genetica, Università di Firenze, Firenze, Italy[2]; Soprintendenza ai Beni Archeologici della Toscana, Firenze, Italy[3]

1. INTRODUCTION

Human bones were recovered in 1997 near Serra San Quirico in Ancona province (Marche, Central Italy) during archaeological excavations carried out by the Soprintendenza ai Beni Archeologici delle Marche. The site is located in a cave, 20 metres above the plane of the road, on the wall of a fluvial gorge called "Gola della Rossa". The remains consist of a cranial vault and a few non-articulated postcranial bones, possibly belonging to the same individual.

The cranial vault is represented by: an incomplete calotte (figures 1-2), better preserved on the left side, consisting of an almost complete frontal bone, the left parietal posteriorly incomplete, the right parietal limited to its anterosagittal part and a small posterolateral portion; the nasal bones lacking the inferior ends only; a small portion of the *processus frontalis* of the right maxilla; the *processus frontalis* of the left maxilla complete in its superior portion and articulating with the frontal bone and nasal bone; the left lacrimal bone; a portion of the *pars orbitalis* of the left maxilla; a portion of the orbital surface of the left greater wing of the sphenoid, including the superior margin of the orbit.

* For correspondence: frederic@stat.unibo.it

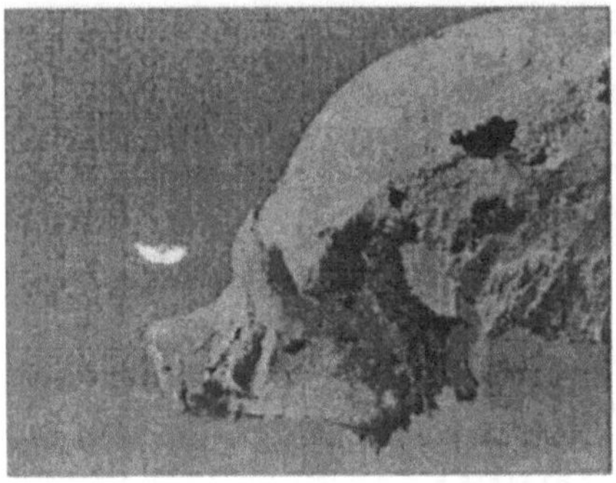

Figure 1. The cranial vault in left lateral view

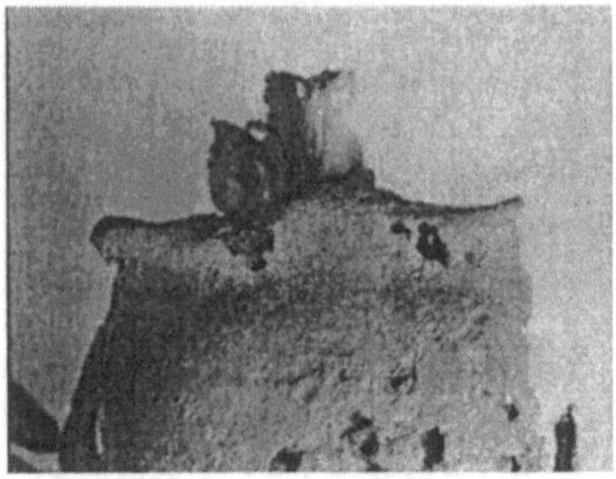

Figure 2. The cranial vault in superior view

The cranial vault shows a series of morphological features rather unusual in modern populations:

i) a marked prominence of the supraorbital region. The relief is not very thick, but is sagittally (anteroposteriorly) prominent for its entire extension; the projection is particularly evident in superior view (figure 1.2);

ii) a rather thick vault; maximum thickness at the parietal level is 10 mm;

iii) very prominent nasal bones. The prominence is further emphasized by a rather low and receding frontal profile in lateral view, although it appears rounded because of the presence of frontal eminences.

Since no archaeological finds were associated with the human bones, it is not possible to attribute them with certainty to a particular cultural group. Therefore, the aim of the present work is a comparative analysis to place the specimen in the context of different prehistoric human groups from Italy and, more generally, from Europe.

Two of the skeletal remains (the cranial vault and a clavicle) have been dated by Accelerator-Mass Spectrometry (AMS) ^{14}C, which produced the following calibrated dates: 4.717-4.360 b. C. and 5.225-4.893 b. C., respectively. Moreover, the cranial vault has been dated by ^{235}U-^{231}Pa Non-Destructive Gamma-Ray Spectrometry (NDGRS), with the following result: 8.000 $\pm$ 3.000 b. C. According to these dates and to geographical and topological considerations, three different cultural attributions are possible: Upper Paleolithic (Pa), Mesolithic (Me) and Neolithic (Ne).

The sex diagnosis was made on the basis of morphological features of the preserved anatomical parts. According to some of these qualitative features (e.g. supraorbital region development, receding frontal profile, rounded upper orbital margin, vault thickness), the cranial vault seems to belong to a male individual; other features (e.g. frontal eminences), instead, are more typical of a female.

Thus, some uncertainties remain, relating to both the chronological position and the sex diagnosis. These two aspects are also somewhat related, since sexual dimorphism can vary among populations. Therefore, it seems reasonable to restrict the hypotheses on the origin of the Gola della Rossa specimen (*GdR*) to six alternatives: Upper Paleolithic Male (PaM), Upper Paleolithic Female (PaF), Mesolithic Male (MeM), Mesolithic Female (MeF), Neolithic Male (NeM), Neolithic Female (NeF).

In order to assign a probability to the six alternative hypotheses, we shall carry out a Bayesian Data Analysis. Two kinds of information will be dealt with:

a) assessment of the probability of the origin of *GdR* by two of us (experts E.P. and G.D.), using our knowledge of the reliability of $AMS\text{-}^{14}C$ and *U-Pa* dating and our personal feelings based on inspection of the specimen. These probability assessments will have the role of "initial probabilities" (priors). Read section 3;

b1) the values of 13 metric characters surveyed on *GdR*;

b2) the values of the same metric characters surveyed on six groups of individuals; each group can be (and has been) considered to belong to one, and only one, of the six alternative populations.

Details concerning the b_1) and b_2) data are given in section 2.

With these data, the likelihoods were elicited by means of the Bayesian B-spline model described in section 5. Section 4 will deal with an explorative analysis of the data.

2. MATERIAL

2.1 Data collection methods

For comparative purposes, the anthropometric analysis was performed on the cranial vault. Six of the 13 possible measurements were chosen, i.e. the ones most frequently available in the comparative samples (see section 4): Minimum frontal width (WFB), Maximum frontal width (XFB), Frontal arc (M26), Frontal chord (FRC), Orbital width (OBB), Orbital height (OBH).

Definitions of these measurements are reported in the classical treatises of Martin and Saller (1957), Howells (1973) and Bräuer (1988). However, a short account is given here:

i) Minimum frontal width: the lesser transverse width of the frontal bone, i.e. the distance between the two points *frontotemporalia* (right and left) of the frontal bone. These "landmarks" are defined as the most medial points along the curve of the two temporal lines. This measurement is coded as WFB, following the treatise of Howells (1973);

ii) Maximum frontal width: the greatest transverse width of the frontal bone, i.e. the distance between the most lateral points along the coronal suture. These points are named *coronalia.* The coronal suture is formed by contact of the posterior margin of the frontal bone and the anterior margins of the right and left parietal bones. This measurement is coded as XFB, following the treatise of Howells (1973);

iii) Frontal arc: the curvilinear distance between the points *nasion* and *bregma* along the profile of the frontal bone in a longitudinal plane. The landmarks *nasion* and *bregma* are defined as the intersection of the frontonasal suture with the sagittal plane, and the intersection of the coronal suture with the same plane, respectively. This measurement is coded as #26 in the treatise of Martin and Saller (1957), and is indicated as M26 in the present study;

iv) Frontal chord: the straight distance between *nasion* and *bregma.* This measurement is coded as FRC, following the treatise of Howells (1973);

v) Orbital width: the transverse width of the left orbital opening (the eyeball cavity), i.e. the distance between the two points *maxillofrontale* and *ektoconkion.* These landmarks are defined as the intersection between the frontonasal suture and the medial orbital margin, and the most distant point from the previous one along the lateral orbital margin, respectively. This measurement is coded as OBB, following the treatise of Howells (1973);

vi) Orbital height: the vertical distance between the upper and lower margins of the left orbital opening, taken perpendicularly to measurement M51. This measurement is coded as OBH, following the treatise of Howells (1973).

The values of the 6 measurements (in millimeters) on GdR are presented in Table 1.

Table 1.

Minimum frontal width (WFB)	99.0
Maximum frontal width (XFB)	126.0
Frontal arc (M26)	123.0
Frontal chord (FRC)	109.5
Orbital width (OBB)	41.0
Orbital height (OBH)	34.0

Individual data for the comparative samples were obtained from various literature sources dealing with the geographical areas, chronological periods and cultures more or less close to the contexts to which our specimen could belong. These sources are: Aimar, Giacobini (1989); Blanchard *et al.* (1972); Borgognini Tarli (1969); Borgognini Tarli (1976); Borgognini Tarli *et al.* (1993); Canci *et al.* (1993); Cavagna *et al.* (1995); Constandse-Westermann (1974); Ferembach (1974a;b;c); Formicola (1988); Gambier (1989); Graziosi (1942); Graziosi (1947); Kidder *et al.* (1992); Mallegni, Parenti (1972-73); Mallegni, Fabbri (1995); Milanesi, Lombardi (1978); Paoli *et al.* (1980); Pardini, Lombardi Pardini (1981); Parenti (1960); Parenti, Messeri (1962); Sergi *et al.* (1980); Vallois, de Felice (1977); Vandermersch (1981).

The dating, cultural attribution and sex diagnosis of the individuals are drawn from the sources themselves.

The data-base is available on request.

3. THE PRIORS

As mentioned in section 1, two experts, E.P. and G.D., assigned the priors to the six alternative hypotheses (*PaM*), (*PaF*), (*MeM*), (*MeF*), (*NeM*), (*NeF*). They followed a Delphi Method procedure, which in the present situation was deemed more suitable than more technical methods (Least Expected Penalisation, Pooling Opinion Criteria, etc.) used on other occasions (see for example Cencetti *et al.*, 1995; Lad, Di Bacco, 2002). Here we give the assigned values together with a short account of the motivations that produced them.

Concerning the sex diagnosis, the probability of "Male" ("*M*") or "Female" ("*F*") was first assigned conditioned to the cultural period ("*Pa*", "*Me*", "*Ne*"). A higher probability was always attributed to "*M*" than to "*F*" within each possible cultural attribution on the basis of the morphological discriminant characters, which consisted mostly of robusticity features:

$$\begin{aligned} &\Pr\{M|Pa\}=0,70\\ &\Pr\{M|Me\}=0,80\\ &\Pr\{M|Ne\}=0,99\\ &\Pr\{F|Pa\}=0,30\\ &\Pr\{F|Me\}=0,20\\ &\Pr\{F|Ne\}=0,01 \end{aligned} \tag{3.1}$$

The probability of "*M*" increases from the Paleolithic to the Neolithic, since there is a well known trend towards lesser robusticity ("gracilization") from Paleolithic to Mesolithic and, even more, from Mesolithic to Neolithic.

As robusticity is generally a typical masculine feature, the robust appearance of the *GdR* specimen makes it more and more "masculine" over time.

Concerning the absolute dating, probabilities were assigned to the three possible cultural periods according to each of the two methods. *AMS-*^{14}C dating assigned the highest probability to the chronological limit between the Mesolithic and Neolithic; moreover, the "probability curve" did not include the Paleolithic. Hence equal probabilities were assigned to "*Me*" and "*Ne*" and null probability was assigned to the Paleolithic:

$$\begin{aligned} &\Pr\{Pa|AMS-C14\}=0{,}00\\ &\Pr\{Me|AMS-C14\}=0{,}50\\ &\Pr\{Ne|AMS-C14\}=0{,}50 \end{aligned} \tag{3.2}$$

However, *NDGRS* assigned the highest probability to the chronological limit between the Upper Paleolithic and Mesolithic, and the "probability curve" did not include the Neolithic. Hence equal probabilities were assigned to "*Pa*" and "*Me*", whereas null probability was assigned to the Neolithic:

$$\begin{aligned} &\Pr\{Pa|NDGRS\}=0{,}50\\ &\Pr\{Me|NDGRS\}=0{,}50\\ &\Pr\{Ne|NDGRS\}=0{,}00 \end{aligned} \tag{3.3}$$

Finally, we believe the *AMS-*^{14}C dating to be more reliable than the *NDGRS* dating: its reliability is widely accepted, and we obtained similar results when it was applied to two different bone samples. We quantify this difference, choosing the *AMS-*^{14}C response or – alternatively – the *NDGRS* response with the probabilities:

$$\begin{aligned} \Pr\{AMS-C14\}&=0{,}70\\ \Pr\{NDGRS\}&=0{,}30 \end{aligned} \tag{3.4}$$

Combining (3.1), (3.2), (3.2), and (3.4), we obtain

$$\begin{aligned} &\Pr\{M \cap Pa\} = 0{,}1050 \\ &\Pr\{M \cap Me\} = 0{,}4000 \\ &\Pr\{M \cap Ne\} = 0{,}3400 \\ &\Pr\{F \cap Pa\} = 0{,}0450 \\ &\Pr\{F \cap Me\} = 0{,}1000 \\ &\Pr\{F \cap Ne\} = 0{,}0035 \end{aligned} \tag{3.5}$$

which will be the assumed prior probability distribution for the Bayesian Analysis.

4. EXPLORATIVE DATA ANALYSIS

In this section, we will use some statistical data analysis tools to describe the missing data problem and to highlight some features of the data-set.

There are many missing values in the data-set, with several variables having few observations. This problem is graphically described in figure 3. Each plot represents the matrix of a given group (Neolithic, Mesolithic, etc.) whose rows and columns are first sorted by the number of missing values, then reordered to put columns and rows with similar missingness patterns together. The fill colours represent the presence-absence of observations: light grey means the observation is available, dark grey the observation is missing (details of this kind of graphic representation can be found in Shafer, 1997, and Schimert *et al.*, 2000). It is evident that some variables cannot be used. This imposes a drastic reduction of the dimensions, accomplished by ignoring a group of variables.

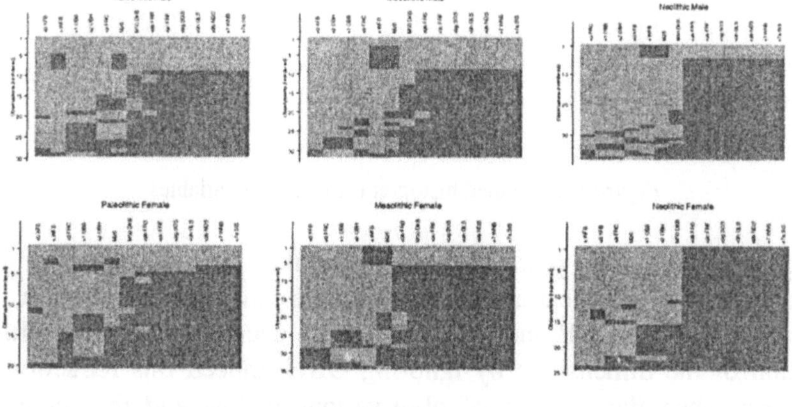

Figure 3. Position of missing data in the six groups

A preliminary explorative data analysis of marginal densities was conducted to choose an appropriate likelihood model. Many distributions seem to be poorly represented by a simple model like normal distribution. Figure 4 shows some smoothed empirical distributions over the respective normal quantile (quantile-quantile plot). The deviance in the tail of the distributions should be noted.

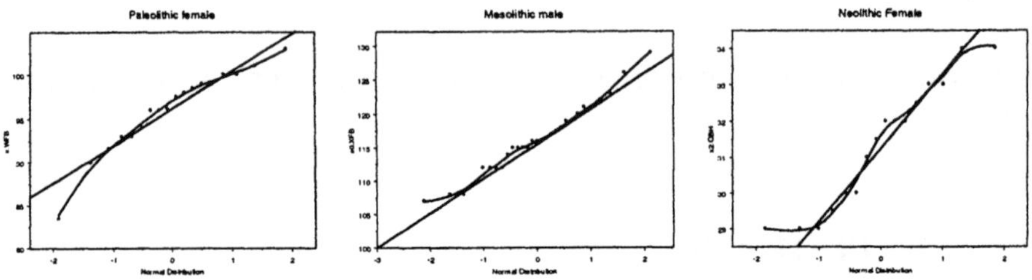

Figure 4. QQ-plot of some variables of several groups

Furthermore, figure 5 shows some smoothed (normal kernel smoothing) histograms for other variables. Note that they are not symmetrical but likely unimodal. Since it is hard to elicit a full probability model for the data, we opted for a *flexible* likelihood model using multivariate B-spline. Details of this model will be given in section 6.

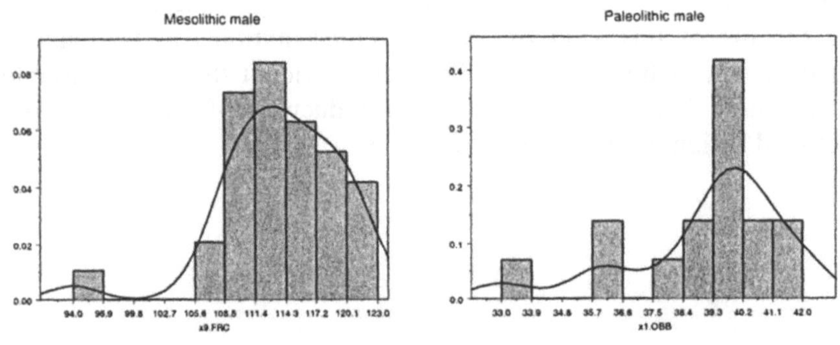

Figure 5. Smoothed histograms for several variables

Figure 6 shows the pairs plot for Mesolithic females (plots for other groups have similar features). An accurate analysis revealed a high correlation between OBB and OBH. Hence we decided to perform a further reduction of the dimensions by ignoring OBH. Indeed this reduction was necessary: when the number of observations is low and the number of dimensions is too high (as in the present situation), flexible models are not able to keep small features of data and tend to describe them with a flat distribution. Details of this problem, named the *curse of dimensionality*, can be found in Huber (1985).

Finally, a *grand tour* in the four-dimensional data space has been improved; since there are some reasons to exclude the presence of clusters, the data description using a unimodal distribution appears to be appropriate. The next section will deal with the likelihood model.

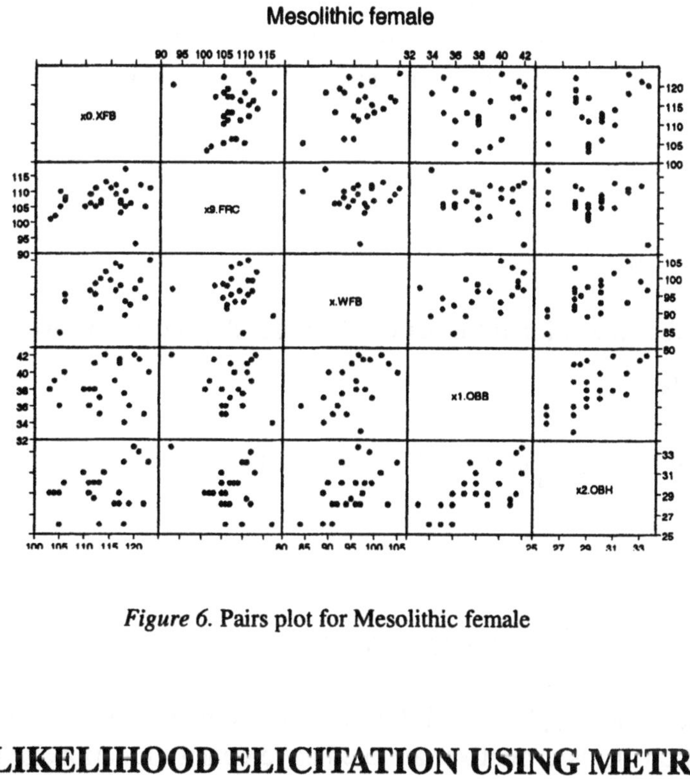

Figure 6. Pairs plot for Mesolithic female

5. LIKELIHOOD ELICITATION USING METRIC DATA

The goal is to assign the new observation to one of the populations $\mathcal{P}_1,\dots,\mathcal{P}_h,\dots,\mathcal{P}_H$ once its measures $y_{new} = \left(y_1^{(new)},\dots,y_k^{(new)}\right)$ and the available information $\mathbf{y}^{(1)},\dots,\mathbf{y}^{(h)},\dots,\mathbf{y}^{(H)}$ for any population h, are known:

$$\mathbf{y}^{(h)} = \begin{pmatrix} y_{11}^{(h)} & y_{12}^{(h)} & \cdots & y_{1k}^{(h)} \\ y_{21}^{(h)} & y_{22}^{(h)} & \cdots & y_{2k}^{(h)} \\ \vdots & \vdots & \ddots & \vdots \\ y_{n_h 1}^{(h)} & y_{n_h 2}^{(h)} & \cdots & y_{n_h k}^{(h)} \end{pmatrix}$$

As pointed out in section 4, the first serious problem is the presence of missing data. Thus, for every h, there are some couples i, j for which $y_{ij}^{(h)}$ is not available. This problem will be discussed later. At the moment, suppose $\mathbf{y}^{(h)}$ is completely known.

Let $\Pr\{\mathcal{P}_h\} = \pi_h$ be the prior information (discussed in section 3); we now want to model $\Pr\{\mathcal{P}_h \mid y_{new}, \mathbf{y}^{(h)}\}$. Let $\Pr\{\mathcal{P}_h\} = \pi_h$ be the prior information (discussed in section 3) we will use theme to model $\Pr\{\mathcal{P}_h \mid y_{new}, \mathbf{y}^{(h)}\}$. The discriminatory criterion used is: y_{new} is assigned to $\mathcal{P}_h$, if

$$\frac{\Pr\{\mathcal{P}_h \mid y_{new}, \mathbf{y}^{(h)}\}}{\Pr\{\mathcal{P}_l \mid y_{new}, \mathbf{y}^{(l)}\}} > 1, \qquad \forall l \neq h$$

Note that the prior information does not depend on measures y_{new} and $\mathbf{y}^{(h)}$. Then

$$\Pr\left\{\mathcal{P}_h \mid y_{new}, \mathbf{y}^{(h)}\right\} \propto \Pr\left\{\mathcal{P}_h \mid \mathbf{y}^{(h)}\right\} f\left(y_{new} \mid \mathbf{y}^{(h)}, \mathcal{P}_h\right)$$

consequently

$$\Pr\{\mathcal{P}_h \mid y_{new}, \mathbf{y}^{(h)}\} \propto \pi_h f_h(y_{new} \mid \mathbf{y}^{(h)})$$

where the symbol $f_h(\cdot) = f(\cdot \mid \mathcal{P}_h)$ is used to simplify the notation.

Function f_h is a multivariate predictive density function for population h, i.e.:

$$f_h(y_{new} \mid \mathbf{y}^{(h)}) = \int f_h(y_{new} \mid \theta_h) f_h(\theta_h \mid \mathbf{y}^{(h)}) d\theta_h \tag{5.1}$$

with θ_h a representation parameter according to standard exchangeability hypotheses (see De Groot, 1970; Berger, 1980). The goal is now to model the likelihood function $f_h(\mathbf{y}^{(h)} \mid \theta_h)$ and the prior probability density $f_h(\theta_h)$.

As pointed out in section 4, for every population h, $\mathbf{y}^{(h)}$ seems to be poorly represented by simple models like a multivariate normal distribution. For this reason, we used a "*flexible*" model, i.e. a mixed model of multivariate normalised B-spline densities and a uniform prior:

$$f_h(\mathbf{y}_i^{(h)} \mid \theta_h) = \sum_{m=1}^{M} \theta_{hm} \mathbf{B}_m(\mathbf{y}_i^{(h)}), \qquad \theta_{hm} \geq 0, \sum_{m=1}^{M} \theta_{hm} = 1, \qquad f_h(\theta_h) \propto 1$$

$$f_h(\mathbf{y}^{(h)} \mid \theta_h) = \prod_{i=1}^{n_h} \sum_{m=1}^{M} \theta_{hm} \mathbf{B}_m(\mathbf{y}_i^{(h)}), \ \mathbf{y}_i^{(h)} = (y_{i1}^{(h)}, \dots, y_{ik}^{(h)}) \in \mathbb{R}^k$$

where $\mathbb{R}$ represents the real field, and $\mathbf{B}_m : \mathbb{R}^k \to \mathbb{R}$ is the tensor product of some fixed normalized univariate B-spline base. This model is *flexible* in the sense that it provides a large variety of shapes for f_h. Further details about these tools will be given in the following subsections.

5.1 Spline functions and B-spline

A one-dimensional B-spline base is a finite set of continuous functions (spline functions) defined on a finite set of points called knots. The name spline was given by Schoenberg (1973) to identify piece-wise polynomial functions, also named univariate polynomial splines (*UPS*). A B-spline base is a set of splines used to generate a smooth-functions space. A detailed treatment of B-spline can be found in De Boor (1977) and De Boor (1978). To provide a multi-dimensional B-spline, we will use the tensor product of univariate spline functions.

Let $[a,b]$, $a > -\infty$ and $b < +\infty$, be a real interval, let $p \geq 0$ be an integer and let us consider a finite sequence of $p \leq m$ points $a < t_1 < \dots < t_m < b$, called knots. A real function g is a *UPS* of degree p, if $g : [a,b] \to \mathbb{R}$, so that:

$$\begin{cases} g(t) \in \pi^p, & t \in [t_i, t_{i+1}], \qquad i = 1, \dots, (m-1) \\ g(t) \in \mathscr{C}^{(p-1)}, & t \in [a,b] \end{cases}$$

where π^q is the class of polynomials of degree q, and $\mathscr{C}^q$ is the class of continuous differentiable functions with $q-1$ continuous derivatives. A *UPS* is unequivocally identified by specifying the parameter $2mq$ (see Schumaker, 1987, for details).

A B-spline is a specific spline. Let $p \geq 1$ be an integer, and let us consider a set of knots $a < t_1 < \dots < t_{p+2} < b$. If a function $B^{(p)} : [a,b] \to \mathbb{R}$ is a B-spline of degree p, then it has the following proprieties:

i) $B^{(p)}$ is a *UPS* of degree p

ii) $B^{(p)}$ is non-negative and a convex function

iii) $B^{(p)}(t) = 0, \quad \text{if } t < t_1 \text{ and } t > t_{p+2}$

Note that we have indicated some proprieties of B-spline functions that are useful for our task. More details can be found in De Boor (1978).

We can use these functions to generate a vector space. Figure 7 shows two B-spline functions for p=1 and p=2.

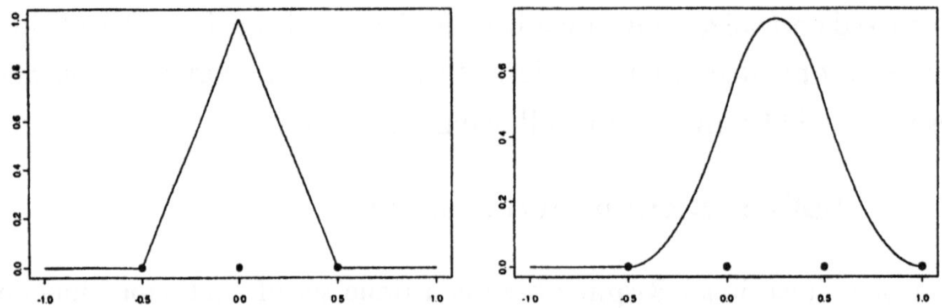

Figure 7. B-spline functions and their knots for p = 1 and p = 2

Once a set of m knots $a < t_1 < ... < t_m < b$ is fixed, a B-spline base $\mathcal{B}_{p;m}$ is a set of $M = m + p - 1$ B-spline functions, $\{B_1^{(p)}, ..., B_M^{(p)}\}$, such that the generic s-th B-spline $B_s^{(p)}$ is defined over the knots $\{t_s, ..., t_{s+p+2}\}$. A B-spline base is plotted in figure 8.

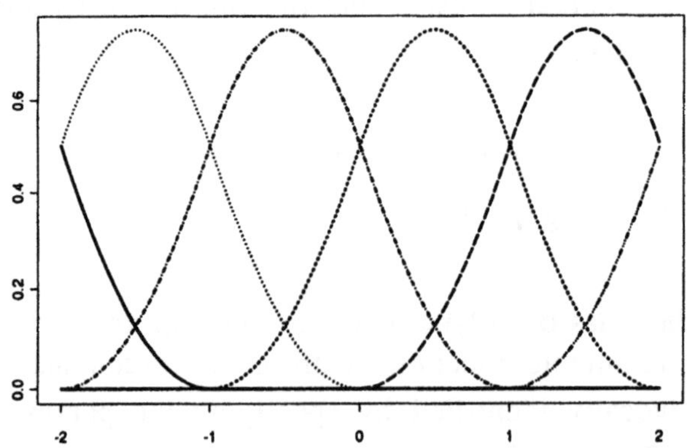

Figure 8. A B-spline base over the knots {-2, -1, 0, 1, 2} of degree p = 2

B-spline functions are easily computable. The following algorithm (De Boor, 1977) allows us to evaluate a B-spline for every t and p:

$$\frac{B_s^{(p)}(t)}{t_{s+p}-t_s}=\frac{t-t_s}{t_{s+p-1}-t_s}\frac{B_s^{(p-1)}(t)}{t_{s+p-1}-t_s}+\frac{t_s-t}{t_{s+p}-t_s}\frac{B_{s+1}^{p-1}(t)}{t_{s+p}-t_{s+1}}.$$

Since $B_s^{(0)}$ is the indicator function over $[t_s,t_{s+1}]$, this algorithm is easily implemented.

The set $\mathcal{B}_{p;m}$ is a base since its elements are linear independents, and they generate a vector space. A generic element of the space generated by $\mathcal{B}_{p;m}$ is: $f(t)=\sum_{s=1}^{M}\alpha_s B_s^{(p)}(t)$, where α_s, $s=1,\ldots,M$ are real values. Note that if we require that every element $B_s^{(p)}$ of $\mathcal{B}_{p;m}$ have integral units, then $f(t)=\sum_{s=1}^{M}\alpha_s B_s^{(p)}(t)$ can be reinterpreted as a probability density function if $\alpha_s>0,\forall s,\sum_{s=1}^{M}\alpha_s=1$. Some densities are plotted in figure 9 for different values of *p* and *M*.

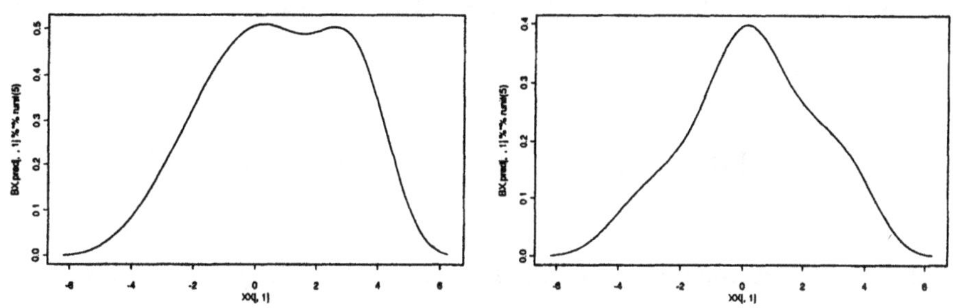

Figure 9. Two linear combinations of B-splines with positive coefficients

For our purpose, the degree of the B-splines used will be fixed (usually *p*=3); then, to simplify the notation, we will denote $B_s^{(p)}$ simply by the symbol B_s. Furthermore, we will be interested only in unimodal densities smoothly decreasing to zero at the extremity of the range. For this reason, we will only use the *m-p*-1 central B-spline. On the other hand, we will work with a restricted base rather than the complete one; see figure 10 to have an idea.

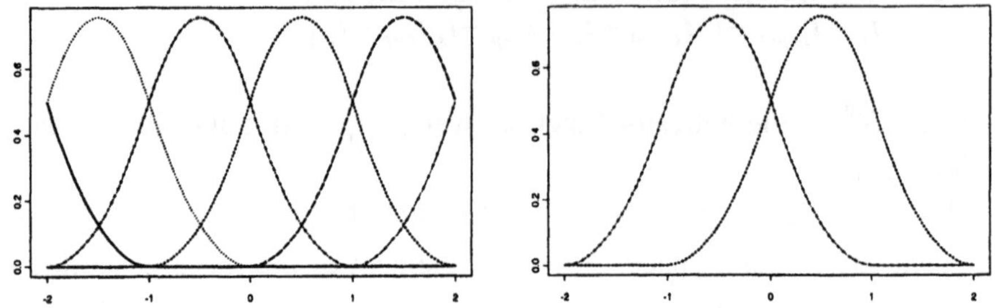

Figure 10. A complete B-spline base and the restricted one

5.2 Tensor Product of B-spline

Starting with k univariate B-spline bases, defined over the sets of knots $a_j < t_{j1} < \ldots < t_{jm} < b_j$, $j = 1,\ldots,k$, it is possible to build a k-dimensional one using the tensor product. Let $\mathcal{B}^k_{p;m}$ be a k-dimensional B-spline base, its generic element maps $\mathbb{R}^k$ in $\mathbb{R}$:

$$\mathbf{B}_{s_1,\ldots,s_k}(\mathbf{x}) = \prod_{j=1}^{k} B_{s_j;j}(x_j), \qquad \mathbf{x} = (x_1,\ldots,x_k) \in [a_1,b_1] \times \ldots \times [a_k,b_k]$$

where $B_{s_j;j}$ represents the s_j-th B-spline function of the j-th base. Clearly if every base has dimension M, the dimension of $\mathcal{B}^k_{p;m}$ will be M^k. To simplify the notation, we will enumerate each function $\mathbf{B}_{s_1,\ldots,s_k}$, $s_j = 1,\ldots,M$ using a single index s, i.e. $\mathbf{B}_s, s = 1,\ldots,M^k$; note the one-to-one correspondence between the two finite sets of indexes. In figure 11, the contours of the nine elements of a two-dimensional B-spline base of degree 3 are plotted.

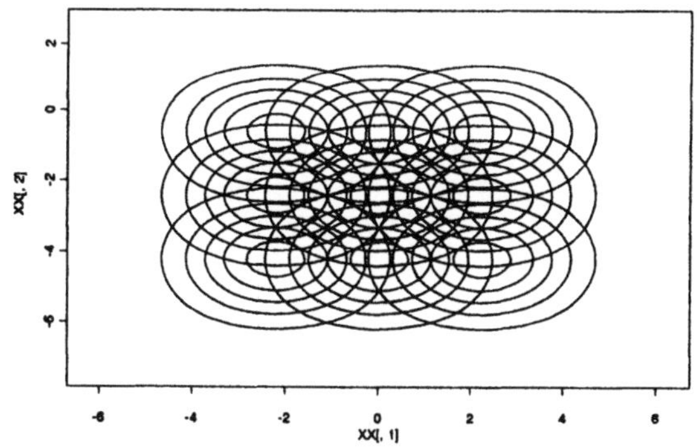

Figure 11. The contour plot of the 9 tensor products of a B-spline generating a two-dimensional functional space

Now given M^k real values $\theta_s, s=1,...,M^k$, the generic function generated by $\mathcal{B}^k_{p;m}$ is:

$$f(\mathbf{x}) = \sum_{s=1}^{M^k} \theta_s \mathbf{B}_s(\mathbf{x})$$

As pointed out in the previous subsection, if the initial B-splines are normalized and $\theta_s \geq 0, \Sigma_{s=1}^{M^k} \theta_s = 1$, then f can be viewed as a multivariate probability density function. Some examples, for k=2 and M=3,5, are shown in figure 12a and 12b. We will use this kind of function to perform the likelihood model for the data.

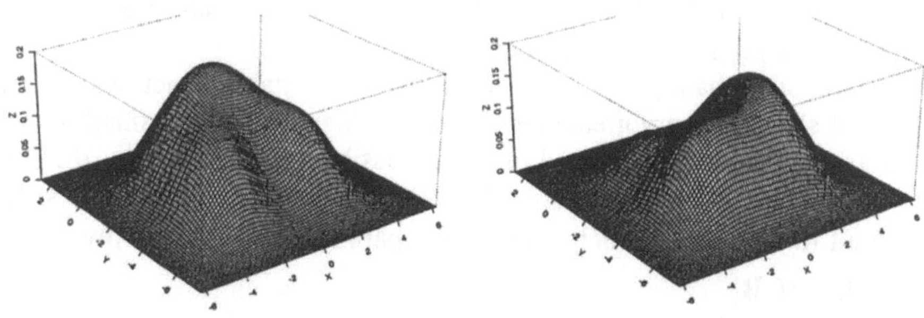

Figure12a Two densities obtained as linear combinations of B-splines of degree 3 for M=3

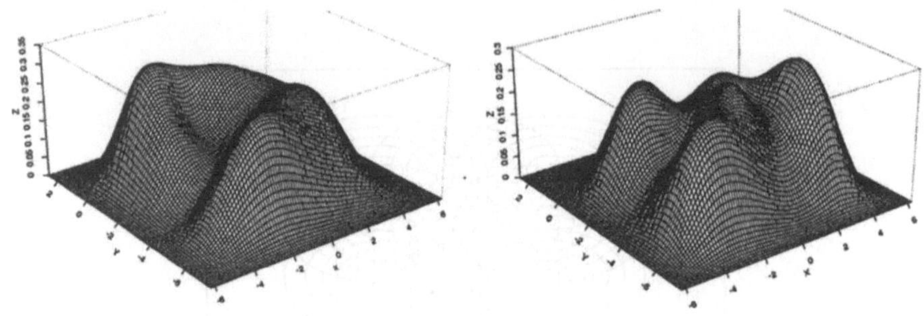

Figure 12b. Two densities obtained as linear combinations of B-splines of degree 3 for M=5

5.3 Why use B-splines to approximate densities?

Spline functions are intensively used in non-parametric statistical tools, and their use in non-Bayesian regression problems is now standard, see for example Eilers *et al.* (1996), Eubank (1982), Green and Silverman (1994) and Silverman (1984). However, less attention has been paid to their use in describing probability densities, see Boneva *et al.* (1971), Wahba (1971), de Montricher *et al.* (1975), Wahba (1975) and Gehringer and Redner (1992). All these works have a common goal: to *estimate the true* probability density or the *real* regression surface almost certainly when the sample size increases to infinity (see for example the earliest paper of Parzen ,1962, the point of view of Silverman, 1986, and recent developments in density estimation in Izeman, 1991). From the Bayesian point of view, it is obviously meaningless to talk about the *true density function*. Therefore, our interest is entirely devoted to choosing a B-spline model to elicit likelihoods using empirical data. In other words, our task is to reach a *smooth*, but *faithful*, description of the empirical distributions.

On the other hand, B-splines are easily computable functions and the variety of shapes is very great even for a low degree and for a small number of knots. As shown in figure 12a, it is possible to model many different density function shapes using only three B-splines on equidistant knots. It is important to note that in such a model the parameters θ_s do not involve the calculation of $\mathbf{B}_s$.

5.4 Missing data problem

As discussed above, a major problem is the presence of missing data in $\mathbf{y}^{(h)}$. Because of the nature of the observations, the missing data can be considered *missing at random* (in the sense of Gelman *et al.*, 1995). Let $\mathbf{I}^{(h)} = \{I_{ij}^{(h)}\}$, a matrix of the same dimension as $\mathbf{y}^{(h)}$ with the indicator for the observation of $\mathbf{y}^{(h)}$: $I_{ij}^{(h)} = 1$ if $y_{ij}^{(h)}$ is observed, $I_{ij}^{(h)} = 0$ if $y_{ij}^{(h)}$ is missing. Consider now $\mathbf{y}_{obs}^{(h)} = \{y_{ij}^{(h)}$ observed$\}$ and $\mathbf{y}_{mis}^{(h)} = \{y_{ij}^{(h)}$ not observed$\}$; clearly $\mathbf{y}^{(h)} = (\mathbf{y}_{obs}^{(h)}, \mathbf{y}_{miss}^{(h)})$. We assert that missing data can be missing at random if $\mathbf{I}^{(h)}$ does not depend on $\mathbf{y}_{mis}^{(h)}$. This is a sufficient condition to prove:

$$f_h\left(\theta_h \mid \mathbf{y}_{obs}^{(h)}\right) \propto f_h\left(\theta_h\right) f_h\left(\mathbf{y}_{obs} \mid \theta_h\right)$$
$$\propto \int f_h\left(\mathbf{y}^{(h)} \mid \theta_h\right) d\mathbf{y}_{miss}^{(h)} = \int f_h\left(\mathbf{y}_{obs}^{(h)}, \mathbf{y}_{miss}^{(h)} \mid \theta_h\right) d\mathbf{y}_{miss}^{(h)}$$

In other words, in such a situation the missing data are simply considered nuisance parameters. Consequently, instead of $f_h(\theta_h \mid \mathbf{y}^{(h)})$, we are now interested in $f_h(\theta_h \mid \mathbf{y}_{obs}^{(h)})$ and in using this quantity in model 5.1.

5.5 Computation

Since the functions B_{ij} are easy computable in any standard mathematical package, the first step consists in evaluating the $n \times M^k$ matrix **b** whose generic element is $b_{im} = \mathbf{B}_m\left(\mathbf{y}_i^{(h)}\right)$. Note that the evaluation of these functions does not involve parameter θ. For this reason, a Gibbs sampling algorithm (see Gilks *et al.*, 1996; Gelman *et al.*, 1995; Robert and Casella, 2000) was easily implemented, i.e. sampling from the univariate conditional distributions of θ_h. Note that, by using a standard one-dimensional sampling technique, this can be done up to the normalizing constant. Once N vectors $\left(\theta_h^{(0)}, \theta_h^{(1)}, \ldots, \theta_h^{(N)}\right)$ have been sampled using a Gibbs sampling algorithm, the predictive density function can be approximated by

$$f_h\left(y_{new} \mid \mathbf{y}_{obs}^{(h)}\right) \approx \frac{1}{N - N_0} \sum_{s=N_0}^{N} f_h\left(y_{new} \mid \theta_h^{(s)}\right) = \frac{1}{N - N_0} \sum_{s=N_0}^{N} \sum_{m=1}^{M} \theta_{mh}^{(s)} \mathbf{B}_m(y_{new}) \tag{5.2}$$

where N_0 is a threshold parameter.

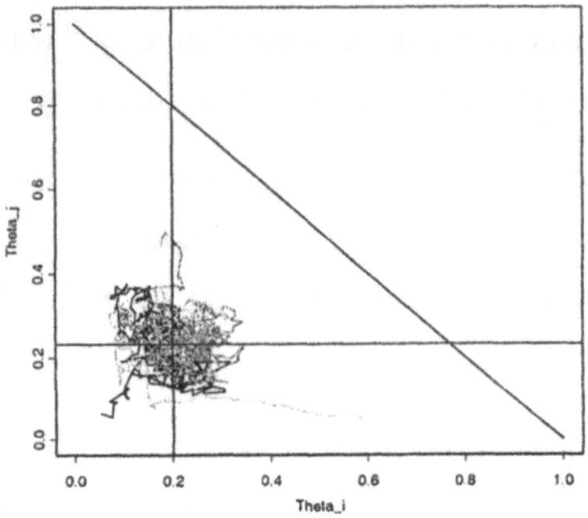

Figure 13. In a few iterations, three different chains converge to the posterior distribution, whose maximum coordinates are indicated

To check the convergence, we used graphical inspections, proceeding in the following way. It is easy to prove that $\log f_h\left(\theta_h \mid \mathbf{y}^{(h)}\right)$ is a convex function, i.e. it has only one absolute maximum and no relative one. Consequently we implemented an EM algorithm to evaluate $\arg\max_{\theta_h} f\left(\theta_h \mid \mathbf{y}_{obs}^{(h)}\right)$. Three different chains were then used to evaluate equation 5.2. Figure 13 shows trajectories for the three chains for a given pair of θ_{mh}. We can see that the convergence of the trajectories is very fast (around $N_0 = 20$ iterations): they suddenly run around the maximum (indicated by its coordinates).

6. CONCLUSIONS

Table 2 summarizes the prior values (shown in the first column), the Bayes factor values which represent likelihood in a normalized form (second column), and the posterior values (third column). The table suggests the following observations:

i) concerning the likelihood values, both Paleolithic groups have to be excluded because the four measurements indicate small cranial dimensions, outside the range of Paleolithic ones;
ii) the measurements indicate the greatest probability for the Neolithic period, because of the reduction in cranial dimensions characterizing this period; this finding contradicts our priors;

iii) the measurements also appear to capture a non-dimensional factor for the Mesolithic, as the probabilities between sexes are similar;

iv) finally, concerning the posterior values, the most important observation is that our initial opinion had such a decisive weight on the final sex attribution that it inverted the results of the comparative metric analysis. This evident disagreement is produced because we assign much greater significance to morphological characters than metric ones in the sex diagnosis.

In summary, we initially attributed the Gola della Rossa specimen to the Mesolithic male group on the basis of a set of morphological observations. While the metric analysis has changed our opinion about the chronological period, it has not altered our initial opinion about the sex of the individual.

Table 2

Population	Prior	Bayes factor	Posterior
Paleolithic male	0,1050	0,0000	0,0000
Paleolithic female	0,0450	0,0000	0,0000
Mesolithic male	0,4000	0,4390	0,1756
Mesolithic female	0,1000	0,5390	0,0539
Neolithic male	0,3400	2,1865	0,7434
Neolithic female	0,0035	7,7429	0,0271

ACKNOWLEDGEMENTS

The authors wish to thank Mario Di Bacco (Università di Bologna) for his valuable suggestions; Vera Caramella Crespi (Centro CNR per la Radiochimica e l'Analisi per Attivazione, Università di Pavia) for the U-Pa Gamma-Ray Spectrometry dating; Mara Silvestrini (Soprintendenza ai Beni Archeologici delle Marche) for allowing us to study the specimen.

REFERENCES

BERGER, J. O. (1980), Statistical Decision Theory. Springer-Verlag, New York.

BONEVA, L. I., KENDAL, D., STEFANOV, I. (1971), Spline Transformations: Three new diagnostic aids for the statistical data-analyst. *J. of the Roy. Stat. Soc.*, B 33-1, pp. 1-70.

BRÄUER, G. (1988), Osteometrie. a. Kraniometrie. In: Knussmann R. (Ed.) Anthropologie. Handbuck der vergleichenden Biologie des Menschen. Bd. I: Wesen und methoden der Anthropologie, G. Fischer-Verlag, Stuttgart-New York.

CENCETTI, S., D'AMORE, G., DI BACCO, M., PACCIANI, E. (1995), Visual diagnosis of the sex of a human skull and the wagers of de Finetti. In: Atti XI Congresso degli Antropologi Italiani, Isernia 13-16 Sept. 1995, A.B.B. C.O., Forlì, pp. 601-608.

DE BOOR, C. (1977), Package for calculating with B-splines. *SIAM J. numer. anal.* 14, pp. 441-472

DE BOOR, C. (1978), A Practical Guide to Splines. Springer, Berlin.

DE GROOT, M. E. (1970), Optimal Statistical Decisions. McGraw-Hill, New York.

DE MONTRICHER, G. F., TAPIA, R. A., THOMPSON, J. R., (1975), Non-parametric maximum likelihood estimation of probability densities by penalty function methods. *Ann. of Statist. 3-6*, pp. 1329-1348.

EILERS, P. H. C., MARX, B. D. (1996), Flexible smoothing with B-splines and penalties. *Statist. Sc. 11-2*, pp. 89-121.

EUBANK, R. L. (1982), Spline Smoothing and Non parametric Regression. Marcel Dekker, New York.

GEHRINGER, K. R., REDNER, R. A. (1992), Nonparametric probability density estimation using normalized B-splines. *Commun. Statist Simul. 21, 3*, pp. 849-878.

GELMAN, A., CARLIN, J. B., STERN, H. S., RUBIN, D. B. (1995), Bayesian Data Analysis. Chapman and Hall, London.

GILKS, W. R., RICHARDSON, S., SPIEGELHALTER, D. J. (1996), Markov Chain Monte Carlo in Practice. Chapman and Hall, London.

GREEN, P. J., SILVERMAN, B. W. (1994), Nonparametric Regression and Generalised Linear Models. A Roughness Penalty Approach. Chapman and Hall, London.

HOWELLS, W. W. (1973), Cranial Variation in Man. A Study by Multivariate Analysis of Patterns of Differences among Recent Human Populations. Papers of the Peabody Museum of Archeology and Ethnology, Harvard University, vol. 67. Cambridge, Massachusetts.

HUBER, P. (1985), On projection pursuit, *Ann. Statist. 13*, pp. 435-475

IZEMAN, A. (1991), Recent developments in nonparametric density estimation. *JASA* 86 (413), pp. 205-224.

LAD, F., DI BACCO, M. (2002), Assessing the value of a second opinion: the role and structure of exchangeability. *Annals of Mathematics and Artificial Intelligence 35(1-4)*, pp. 227-252.

MARTIN, R., SALLER, G. (1957), Lehrbuck der Anthropologie. 3 ed., G. Fischer-Verlag, Stuttgart.

PARZEN, E. (1962), On estimation of probability density function and mode. *Ann. of Math. Statist.* 33, pp. 1065-1076.

ROBERT, C. P., CASELLA, G. (2000), Monte Carlo Statistical Methods (Springer Texts in Statistics). Springer, Berlin.

SCHAFER, J. L. (1997), Analysis of Incomplete Multivariate Data. Chapman and Hall.

SCHIMERT, J., SCHAFER, J. L., HESTERBERG, T., FRALEY, C., CLARKSON, D. B. (2000), Analysing Data with Missing Values in S-plus. Insightful Corporation, Seattle, WA.

SCHOENBERG, I. J. (1973), Cardinal Spline Interpolation. SIAM, Philadelphia.

SCHUMAKER, L. L. (1987), Spline Functions: Basic Theory. John Wiley & Sons, New York.

SILVERMAN, B. W. (1984), Spline smoothing: the equivalent variable kernel method. *Ann. of Statist. 12*, pp. 898-916.

SILVERMAN, B. W. (1986), Density Estimation. Chapman & Hall, London.

WAHBA, G. (1971), A polynomial algorithm for density estimation. *Ann. of Statist. 46-6*, pp. 1870-1886.

WAHBA, G. (1975), Interpolating spline methods for density estimation. I: Equi-spaced knots. *Ann. of Statist. 3-1*, pp. 30-48.

Sources for the comparative data

AIMAR, A., GIACOBINI, G. (1989), A new Upper Paleolithic human skull from the Cave of San Teodoro (Messina, Sicily). In: Hominidae (G. Giacobini, Ed.). Jaca Book, Milan, pp. 495-499.

BLANCHARD, R., PEYRONY, D., VALLOIS, H. V. (1972), Le gisement et le squelette de Saint-Germain-la-Riviere. *Archives de l'Institut de Paleontologie Humaine*, Mem. 34.

BORGOGNINI TARLI, S. (1969), Studio antropologico di uno scheletro di epoca mesolitica rinvenuto nella grotta Maritza presso Avezzano (Abruzzo). *Rivista di Antropologia 56*, pp. 135-156.

BORGOGNINI TARLI, S. M. (1976), Studio antropologico di un cranio mesolitico rinvenuto nella grotta della Molara (Palermo-Sicilia). *Archivio per l'Antropologia e l'Etnologia 106*, pp. 193-228.

BORGOGNINI TARLI, S., CANCI, A., PIPERNO, M., REPETTO, E. (1993), Dati archeologici e antropologici sulle sepolture mesolitiche della Grotta dell'Uzzo (Trapani). *Bullettino di Paletnologia Italiana 84*, pp. 85-179.

CANCI, A., REPETTO, E., MINOZZI, S., BORGOGNONI TARLI, S. M. (1993), Due scheletri di età neolitica dalla grotta delle Arene Candide (Liguria). Scavi 1973. *Rivista di Antropologia 71*, pp. 285-303.

CAVAGNA, P., BERZERO, A., D'AMORE, G., CRESPI, V. C. (1995), Un frontale umano di età wurmiana recente da Portalbera (PV): datazione gamma diretta, analisi morfologica e confronti. *Antropologia Contemporanea 18*, pp. 63-77.

CONSTANDSE-WESTERMANN, T. S. (1974), L'homme mesolithique du nord-ouest de l'Europe, distances biologiques, considerations genetiques. *Bull et Mem de la Soc d'Anthrop de Paris, T.1 serie XIII*, pp. 173-199.

FEREMBACH, D. (1974a), Le squelette epicastelnovien de la Baume de Montclus. *Bull et Mem de la Soc d'Anthrop de Paris, T.1 serie XIII*, pp. 109-127.

FEREMBACH, D. (1974b), Les hommes de l'Epipaleolithique et du Mesolithique de la France et du nord-ouest du bassin mediterranéen. *Bull et Mem de la Soc d'Anthrop de Paris, T.1 serie XIII*, pp. 201-236.

FEREMBACH, D. (1974c), Le gisement mesolithique de Moita do Sebastiao. Muge, Portugal. II. Antropologie. Direccao-General dos Assuntos Culturais, Lisboa.

FORMICOLA, V. (1988), The triplex burial of Barma Grande (Grimaldi, Italy). *Homo* 39, pp. 130-143.

GAMBIER, D. (1989), Fossil hominids from the early Upper Palaeolithic (Aurignacian) of France. In: The Human Revolution (P. Mellars, C. Stringer, Eds). Edinburgh University Press.

GRAZIOSI, P. (1942), L'uomo fossile della Barma Grande ai Balzi Rossi del Museo di Mentone. *Archivio per l'Antropologia e l'Etnologia 72*, pp. 22-51.

GRAZIOSI, P. (1947), Gli uomini paleolitici della Grotta di S. Teodoro (Messina). *Rivista di Scienze Preistoriche 2*, pp. 123-223.

KIDDER, J. H., JANTZ, R. L., SMITH, F. H. (1992), Defining modern humans: A multivariate approach. In: Continuity or Replacement? (G. Brauer, F.H. Smith, Eds). A.A. Balkeema, Rotterdam.

MALLEGNI, F., PARENTI, R. (1972-73), Studio antropologico di uno scheletro giovanile d'epoca gravettiana raccolto nella grotta Pagliacci (Rignano Garganico). *Rivista di Antropologia 58*, pp. 317-348.

MALLEGNI, F., FABBRI, P. F. (1995), The human skeletal remains from the Upper Paleolithic burials found in Romito Cave (Papasidero, Cosenza, Italy). *Bull et Mem de la Soc d'Anthrop de Paris, n.s. T.7*, pp. 99-137.

MILANESI, Q. F., LOMBARDI, E. C. (1978), Antropologia e antropometria di uno scheletro neolitico antico della Liguria occidentale (Arma di Nasino). *Archivio per l'Antropologia e l'Etnologia 108*, pp. 89-129.

PAOLI, G., PARENTI, R., SERGI, S. (1980), Gli scheletri mesolitici della Caverna delle Arene Candide (Liguria). *Memorie dell'Istituto Italiano di Paleontologia Umana, n.s. 3*, pp. 33-154.

PARDINI, E., LOMBARDI PARDINI, E. C. (1981), I Paleolitici di Vado all'Arancio (Grosseto). *Archivio per l'Antropologia e l'Etnologia 111*, pp. 75-119.

PARENTI, R (1960), Calvario cromagnonoide trovato in un deposito mesolitico del bacino fucense (Abruzzo). *Archivio per l'Antropologia e l'Etnologia 90*, pp. 5-99.

PARENTI, R., MESSERI, P. (1962), I resti scheletrici umani del Neolitico Ligure. *Palaeontographia Italica* n.s., *vol. 20*.

SERGI, S., PARENTI, R., PAOLI, G. (1980), Il giovane paleolitico della caverna delle Arene Candide. *Memorie dell'Istituto Italiano di Paleontologia Umana, n.s. 2*, pp. 13-38.

VALLOIS, H. V., DE FELICE, S. (1977), Les mesolithiques de France. Etude anthropologique. *Archives de l'Institut de Paleontologie Humaine* Mem. *37*.

VANDERMERSCH, B. (1981), Les hommes fossiles de Qafzeh (Israel). Paris: Centre National de la Recherche Scientifique.

Chapter 9

AN EXAMPLE OF THE SUBJECTIVIST STATISTICAL METHOD FOR LEARNING FROM DATA: WHY DO WHALES STRAND WHEN THEY DO?*

Frank Lad†‡
Department of Mathematics and Statistics, University of Canterbury, Christchurch, New Zealand/Aotearoa.

1. PRELUDE

Attending the Asti summer school where the papers in this book were presented were some thirty graduate students writing empirical theses using applied statistics. Their topics ranged from the monitoring of commercial fishing stock around Sardinia, to learning about the situation of current Nigerian immigrants to Italy, and to comparing the nutrition and weight gain of children of Chinese immigrants in Italy with children of their non-emigrating cohort in a Chinese village. The thesis students were attending the course to improve their practical statistical skills. Having been involved in the modern development of subjective Bayesian methods for some thirty years myself, I was somewhat surprised by how little was known of these major developments which have transformed statistical thinking throughout

* Some of the research printed in this article has previously been published. Permission to reprint Figures 4,5 and 6 has been granted by Springer-Verlag Publishers.

† For correspondence: F.Lad@math.canterbury.ac.nz

‡ This article was prepared while he was a visiting professor at the University of Bologna Institute for Advanced Studies. Thanks to Dimitri Giunchi for helpful discussions.

the world over this period. They had received major impetus from the research of the noted Italian probabilist, Bruno de Finetti, and his followers.

Nonetheless, the students were avidly interested to learn of the foundational motivation for these developments as well as their practical implications for data analysis. In the early 1980's many statisticians involved in the Bayesian movement expressed dissatisfaction with foundational discussion because it seemed to go on and on, impeding the application of the newly touted methods to practical problems. As a result of the great array of practical work that has flourished during the subsequent twenty years, to many people Bayesian statistical procedures provide methods for improved estimates of the same kind of "models" that have been long addressed by objectivist methods. This is a grave misstatement of the affair.

The present paper is designed to provide a practical example of a sophisticated statistical analysis of a real zoological question that is understandable to a mathematically unsophisticated audience, and to present the results in a context of discussion that highlights the foundational differences from objectivist methods rather than ignoring them.

We shall first discuss a startling zoological phenomenon of natural history, the mass stranding of whales on land, and develop it to a point that statistical evidence should be useful to improve our understanding of the situation. The fundamental difference between the attitudes toward statistical analysis of the data motivated by the objectivist methods of the twentieth century and by the remerging subjectivist methods will be presented in a separate Section. This will be followed by a description of Bayes' Theorem as it is used in subjective analysis, presented in a general way that highlights how the theorem models the change in scientific uncertainty about a problem when we have the chance to learn from newly acquired data. Using the general framework that is developed there we shall first examine a very simple but real application to see how the subjectivist method differs specifically from maximum likelihood methods, familiar to most routine users of statistical software. We shall then be ready to display the statistical analysis of data on whale strandings.

Although the details of the whale data analysis are more complicated, they should be understandable to any educated reader with the background achieved earlier in the article. Particular attention will be given to a databased function, which is commonly called a "likelihood function" for historical reasons. Substantive argument will be made to motivate a change in the name of the function to an "information transfer function." Although the function is abused in a misleading way in common statistical practice, it is a powerful mathematical form for summarising the data, as it is relevant to a scientific understanding of historical events. Moreover, it is central to the important computation of a predictive distribution for future observations based on this data. We shall conclude with some suggestions for contemporary statistical practice by applied researchers.

2. A PRACTICAL PROBLEM IN UNDERSTANDING NATURAL HISTORY

One of the most impressive phenomena of natural history to a fortunate observer is the live stranding of whales on a beach. Even the observation of a single live stranded whale is intriguing, affording one the chance to observe at close quarters a leviathan of the deep. But among certain species of whale, herd strandings of animals occur in the hundreds with some regularity in specific places, and they can even number more than one thousand at a time. Such an observation inevitably raises myriad questions to a naturalist. Professional zoologists study this phenomenon with respect to its size, seasonality, regularity, oceanic geography, coastal topography and physiological function among the many distinct species of whales. A useful literature review of research on this subject has been provided by Brabyn (1990), much of which is more easily accessible in the report of Brabyn (1991) and in the article of Brabyn and McLean (1992).

It turns out that stranding phenomena differ in regular ways among different species of whale. In some species only single live animals have ever been observed stranding, while in others the animals are observed stranding only in groups. Moreover, some species will commonly be found to strand in locations that exhibit a long tidal flat of sandy beach, while others strand commonly along shorelines that exhibit a precipitous drop from a stony beach. In each type of species-specific case, strandings are common enough at some locations to be even more or less "expected" every few years.

The statistical research presented in this article concerns a concomitant issue of the *timing of strandings*, specifically among pilot whales, *Globicephala melaena*. Much of the detail was first presented in the article of Lad and Brabyn (1993) which is now out of print. Springer-Verlag publishers have granted permission for the reprinting particularly of Figures 4, 5 and 6 which will appear later in this article. A very useful series of papers presenting applied statistical work using Bayesian methods appear in the subsequent volumes of *Case Studies in Bayesian Statistics* edited by Gatsonis et. al. (1995, 1997, 1998, 2001 and 2002).

Pilot whales are an offshore species of whale, spending most of their time in the deep seas off the continental shelf. They are known to strand in herds of sizeable numbers, commonly in the hundreds, and typically located at a tidal-flat with sandy beach topography. Because such locations feature rather large differences between the lengths of their spring tides and neap tides, some zoologists have speculated that the strength of the tides (and thus lunar cycles) have something to do with the timing of the strandings. Spring tides are tides that display a large difference between the high tide and low tide extremes, while neap tides are tides where this difference is minimal. Spring tides follow a semi-monthly cycle: they tend to occur in most locations within one to four days after a full moon and again after a new moon, while neap tides occur similarly within one to four days after the quarter moons.

A related consideration is that a range of natural phenomena are known to occur more frequently during the full moon nights than during new moon nights, or vice versa. Relevant to the stranding of whales for example, movements of squid along the shore have been reported to accentuate during new moon periods as opposed to full moon phases. See Gilmore (1957). But a wide array of natural phenomena is understood to vary with lunar phases. See for examples, Hedd, Gales, and Brothers (1992), De Casamajor, Bru, and Prouzet (2001), or Elangovan and Marimuthu (2001). Similar research is fairly extensive.

However, the relevance of lunar and tidal periods to whale strandings is a controversial subject. Most zoologists have felt that the difference between the forces of spring tides and neap tides is minimal when compared with the strength and swimming agility of a massive whale. Moreover they typically doubt the relevance of lunar periods of night light to whales who commonly hunt the deeps of the ocean for prey.

It should be evident from this brief zoological introduction to the issue that a systematic study of whale stranding data should provide some evidence to clarify our understanding and expectations of this phenomenon.

2.1 The New Zealand Whale Stranding Data Base

Situated as it is among the most southerly landmasses of the western Pacific Ocean north of Antarctica, the shores of New Zealand/Aotearoa make a readily accessible location for the stranding of whales. Many species are known to migrate to the food-rich waters of Antarctica during the antipodean summer months (November-March) and return to more northerly Pacific waters during the Antarctic winter. Indeed many specific locations of deep ocean troughs around New Zealand such as Kaikoura are well-known feeding grounds during wintertime. Furthermore, perhaps fortuitously for the questions of zoological concern, differences between spring and neap tidal extremes in New Zealand are among the largest observed anywhere on the globe. Thus, it is not surprising that many whale strandings have been observed live by humans over the course of modern history when detailed records have been kept. From the time of early European settlers (who appropriately enough included many attracted by whaling expeditions around the two major islands) informal written records were kept by the New Zealand Museum of Natural History. By the twentieth century, systematised records were kept by the country's Ministry of Agriculture and Fisheries. In the late 1980's the responsibility for tracking the stranding phenomena was transferred to the Department of Conservation. The complete record history has by now been formatted into a publicly accessible D-Base file, allowing a recording of unusual observational details as well as standard information. It is known as the New Zealand Whale Stranding Data Base, or NZWSDB.

The database contains records of strandings by some 35 of the world's known 75 or 80 species of whale in 1140 distinct episodes. In all, 8287 whales have been observed, most of which arrived in herds of many at a time. Pilot whales and sperm whales are the most common of the herd stranding species. More extensive summary of the database content appears in Lad and Brabyn (1993). Recordings since 1970 are considered to be the most precisely documented as to timing.

2.2 Transforming the records to usable data

The data we shall discuss here numbers 49 distinct herd stranding events by pilot whales, which were observed live by a reporting observer since 1970. On account of the live observation, the exact date of each stranding is known. The heights of the high and low tides surrounding the strandings were not recorded. However, knowledge of the exact date of occurrence allows us to identify relatively precisely the phase of the moon at the time of each stranding, a characteristic of both the lunatic and tidal theories that have been proposed as relevant to its timing. We need to explain briefly how this has been done.

Firstly, the precision of identifying the phase of the moon on the stranding date is limited by the fact that the period of a complete lunation is not fixed. While the mean duration of a complete lunar cycle is known fairly precisely to be 29.5306 days, the length of any particular lunation may differ by up to 8 hours more or less. A difference of this magnitude relative to more than 700 hours in a lunar month would not be great enough to affect greatly the following lunar dating procedure. For each of the stranding events, the date of each observed stranding was compared to the date of the nearest full moon. If the stranding occurred on a full moon day, the lunar date was coded as 15. If it occurred one day before or after the full moon, the lunar date was recorded as 14 or 16, respectively. Two days before and after would be coded 13 and 17. Extending this coding procedure in both directions before and after a full moon would determine the dating of the first day of a cycle as 1 and the last day of a cycle as 29. The extreme "half-day case" in which the nearest full moon occurred both 15 days before and 15 days after the stranding was arbitrarily defined to specify a recording of 30.

By this lunar dating procedure, the detailed recordings of information regarding the observed strandings has summarised the features relevant to the contestable theories of timing by a sequence of 49 numbers, each an integer between 1 and 30. How can statistical methods allow us to learn from this data what there is to be learned? Before engaging the details of an answer, we need to digress a bit about foundational controversies that have motivated a re-emergence of subjective Bayesian statistical methods during the latter half of the twentieth century. In developing the details necessary to analyse this data, we shall focus on their difference from the objectivist methods that dominated the century, and still dominate both introductory textbook presentations and widely marketed computational software.

3. FUNDAMENTAL QUESTIONS ABOUT STATISTICAL METHODS

Inspired both by new possibilities of astronomical observation allowed by the telescope and by the extension of mechanical engineering technique, renaissance science bequeathed to subsequent scientific understanding the image of Nature as a machine. In the early days the machine was imagined to be so precise and regular as to generate the heavenly "music of the spheres" as well as even the natural history of the "Tiger, tiger burning bright." While irregularities of measurement were recognised as problematic to understanding the mechanism of the machine already in the eighteenth and nineteenth centuries, the intensive atomic experimentation of the early twentieth century led to the specification of a supposed "randomness" as an intrinsic feature of the generating machine. Estimating procedures of "statistical mechanics" came to be seen as central to scientific inference, invading the imagination of theoreticians in virtually every field of physical and social science.

The understanding of Nature as a random generating device with stochastic laws that can be tamed by attention to an impersonal, sceptic and objective statistical method became virtually universal by the mid-twentieth century. See Hacking (1990). Statistical procedures for performing this task progressed from the crude method of moments to so-called maximum likelihood methods. The accessibility and practicality of these methods for achieving useful results have ensured that they have not only survived but still flourish among statistical practitioners in our new millennium. They are typically the methods of statistical practice and imagination that are presented as computational prescriptions to students of applied sciences. Researchers focusing their studies on the sciences are typically not conversant with mathematics at the level required to learn that at their foundation these proposed methods are riddled with circularities and contradictions. However, it should be known that among the current generation of leading statistical theorists and practitioners they have been forsaken for methods of statistical forecasting based on a completely different view of Nature and the foundation for our scientific understanding of it.

This is not the place to survey the developments of the subjectivist understanding and practice of statistical science as it remerged during the past fifty years, led by the works of L.J. Savage (1954) and Bruno de Finetti (1937, 1970, 1994, 1995). Instead, for such a survey I refer you to the generally readable Preface and first Chapter of the text of Lad (1996). Here, instead, we shall merely consider some sensible questions regarding a standard" statistical treatment of the whale stranding data, and propose that a different method of analysis makes much more realistic sense.

Proponents of the objectivist statistical method would have us believe that the stranding of whales occurs as an outcome of a Monte-Carlo type gaming machine. The machine yields a random result of a "success" (a whale stranding) or a "failure" (no whale stranding) on a New Zealand beach on any given day of a lunar month with a specific probability. Objectivists see the goal of statistics as discovering the statistical mechanics of this machine. This is to be achieved by firstly identifying a complete array of all the possible stochastic generating structures, or mathematical models, that could appropriately drive the machine. Then, on the basis of observed data, the random generating structure of the machine is estimated to be that structure for which the observed data outcome is specified to be the most probable. This is called the maximum likelihood estimate of the generating structure. Recognising that this maximum likelihood structure may not be the "true generating structure," but that some other structure may have generated the outcome as an unlikely outcome, the objectivist method proposes a relevant variance of the estimated generating parameters. Nonetheless, when using the method to make a statistical forecast of the lunar date of the next whale stranding to be observed, the maximum likelihood estimated generating model is used.

Rather than quibbling about technical details of such an estimation procedure, the subjectivist statistical outlook challenges the entire understanding of cosmology and science that lies beneath it as bizarre. A progressive understanding of science is to recognise Nature as a living organism, not as a machine at all. As a living organism it has a beginning (the so-called big-bang), a lifetime in which it develops, grows, and decays (natural history) and an end (the burnout of a star). Scientists, who are participants in this Nature, are individually and collectively uncertain to a greater or lesser extent about virtually every aspect of its course. Probability, and the statistical method of inference that derives from its structure, is a representation of a scientist's uncertainty about the course of the history rather than a feature of the history itself. The goal of scientific method is to face calmly our uncertainty about natural history by expressing it logically in terms of probabilities. This formalised uncertainty allows us to make sensible judgments about how to design appropriate experiments and historical investigations to reduce the uncertainty, increasing our understanding and appreciation of Nature as we do.

We do not presume that whale strandings arise as randomly generated outcomes from a gaming machine. Rather, cetacean behaviour is respected as an aspect of natural history that has emerged by the evolution of these thinking animals who make risky choices just as humans do. Why they make the dangerous choices they do is not precisely known to us. Thus, our uncertain opinions about their behaviours are representable only by probabilities. This is not unusual, since uncertainty and thus probability modifies our knowledge of virtually every topic that concerns us. In the remainder of this article we shall return to the study of the whale stranding data to see how this can be done, but only after we introduce the procedure by an examination of a central component of the method, Bayes' Theorem, along with a simpler example.

The divergence of this new contemporary understanding of Nature and of science from the stochastic epicycles of the received imagination of Nature as a machine is a liberating achievement of the past fifty years of struggle in the foundations of statistics. It is time for the dissemination of the method and the imagination to become widespread and commonplace in the understanding of applied scientists who are not necessarily expert in the language of mathematics. It would be particularly appropriate for this realisation to gain acceptance in Italy, where scientists should learn about and be especially proud of the great methodological achievements of their compatriot, Bruno de Finetti, 1906-1986. Through countless regular publications over the past century, he cheerfully and laboriously worked against the tide of international opinion in developing the most important aspects of the subjectivist statistical outlook and method. We are ready to display one of its practical details.

4. BAYES' THEOREM AND ITS RELEVANCE

At an advanced level of statistical study, one can learn that Bayes' theorem is only one useful component of more general methods organised via principles of coherent (non-contradictory) inference under uncertainty. But at any level of understanding, and surely at an introductory level for the scientist who knows only of objectivist methods and software, the theorem of Bayes for learning from data is crucial to a sensible understanding of statistical prospects.

In our first pass at understanding Bayes' Theorem, I shall present it in a symbolic fashion, almost as a dance. Hopefully the flow of its logic should become evident to anyone who has learned the most rudimentary elements of probability and its notation, no matter how they have been presented. To facilitate the exposition, we shall not belabour any fine details of interpretation nor notation here. Please read, enjoy, and think.

In pondering an observable feature of Nature, the scientist eventually surmises a limited array of hypotheses regarding its proliferation. Suppose we list them and denote them by the symbols $H_1, H_2, \ldots, H_N$. Presumably, each of these hypotheses has some degree of credibility to its proponent, or else it would not merit listing. Since the list is meant to be exhaustive of the ideas that we entertain, a scientist's total belief in the reasons for the phenomena would be distributed among these N hypotheses. Norming the total belief to a unit of 1, relative beliefs in these hypotheses are expressed by the scientist's probabilities $P(H_1), P(H_2), \ldots, P(H_N)$, which sum to 1.

The idea behind our formalisation to this point is that each proponent's understanding of the natural phenomena is a mixture of an array of hypothesized understandings. The weight of importance of each hypothesis within the scientific imagination is denoted by the proponent's probability value. The probabilities attached to the hypotheses are numbers personally assessed and asserted by a particular scientist based on related observations and conjectures, rather than numbers somehow merited objectively by the hypothesis itself. It is surely a well-known feature of science that scientists can and do disagree with one another in their assessments of the course of natural phenomena. We have already presented an example of this in proposing the lunar cycle as relevant to the timing of strandings of herds of whales on land. In some cases, disagreement can be great, blatant and emotional; in others it is only on matters of fine detail. Sometimes two, sometimes many scientists may *agree in their uncertainties*. In such cases they would assert the same probabilities; in others, not. So be it.

When designing a new experiment or historical investigation that will hopefully be informative on matters of concern or even contention, we typically can enumerate the possible observable outcomes of the experiment, at least in the form that they are summarised by numbers. For example, having developed the spectre of the whale strandings to the extent we have, we could enumerate all the distinct possibilities of what we might observe when we examine the records in the NZWSDB. For examples, we might observe

a) Every stranding occurs on the same day as a full moon, so the string of 49 numbers is a string exclusively of 15's.
b) The strandings occur uniformly across all the possible days of a lunar month. That is, the string of 49 numbers includes one of each integer between 1 and 30, while 19 of these integers appear twice in the sequence in whatever order.
c) The strandings usually occur a few days after new moons and full moons, in about equal proliferation. That is, the 49 numbers include a relatively large numbers of 1's, 2's, 3's and 4's, and also 16's, 17's, 18's and 19's in about the same abundance, in whatever order.
d) Actually, any sequence of 49 numbers, each an integer between 1 and 30, is *possible* to be observed. In fact, there are 30^{49} such possible ordered sequences of numbers, an immense number.

Suppose we denote the numerical data that summarises the outcome of an experiment by a letter D. The letter D could represent, for example, any one of the strings of numbers for the whale strandings that we have listed as possibilities just above. One of the central goals of scientific activity as a process is for scientists to accumulate telling evidence to an extent that all would agree in their probabilities, that is, in their uncertain knowledge. This would not preclude their remaining uncertain about what precisely may occur in the next experiment of observation. Even when scientists disagree, they obviously feel driven to communicate with each other regarding their procedures of observation/experimentation and with their conclusions regarding what they hope to infer from them. Bayes' Theorem provides a logical framework for calibrating how this can occur, yielding numerical values for the conditional probabilities

$$P(H_1 \mid D), P(H_2 \mid D), \ldots, P(H_N \mid D)$$

that are based on their initial information sources *augmented by the new observed data,* D. The numerical differences between the probability distribution $P(H_1), P(H_2), \ldots, P(H_N)$ and the conditional distribution $P(H_1 \mid D), P(H_2 \mid D), \ldots, P(H_N \mid D)$ display what we can rightfully learn about our assessment of the hypotheses from this data. This assessment, in the long and the short of statistical theory, is the goal of scientific experimentation and data analysis. These two probability distributions differ for any specific person on account of the fact that the latter distribution is informed beyond the former by the experimental observation of the data, D. For this reason, the former is called a "prior" distribution, and the latter a "posterior" distribution. The adjectives prior and posterior are relative to the public data D that is the common basis for all scientists' inference. Even the prior distributions, it should be noted, are posterior to other information and considerations that are specific to each deliberating scientist.

The computational application of Bayes' theorem requires that we assess how likely each of the possible new experimental observations might be under the scenarios of the various specified hypotheses. For each possible value of D, the data to be observed, we need to assess how likely it would be that this result would emerge according to the prescriptions of the hypotheses $H_1, H_2, \ldots, H_N$ that we entertain. The assessment of each $P(D \mid H_i)$ amounts to an evaluation of how likely the observation of this data D might be if it were driven according to the tenets of hypothesis H_i rather than some other hypothesis in the list. (Using the subscript i on the hypothesis H_i in this statement merely conveys that this evaluation of probability for the observed data must have been made relative to the context of *each* of the hypotheses, not merely for one specific one.) In fact, once we observe the actual data that result from the experimental observation, only one of these "possible" data values is relevant to our inference. Suppose we have assessed the probability of this data result given each of the relevant hypotheses according to the numbers

$$P(D \mid H_1), P(D \mid H_2), \ldots, P(D \mid H_N) \,.$$

The relative sizes of these numbers for the various possible hypotheses based on the same data are commonly referred to as the likelihoods for the hypotheses. We shall discuss important aspects of this list when considered as a function of the hypotheses, and the appropriateness of this nomenclature, later in this article.

Having assessed these probabilities for the observed data on the basis of each of the tendered hypotheses, Bayes' theorem allows the computation of each of the posterior probabilities $P(H_1 \mid D), P(H_2 \mid D), \ldots, P(H_N \mid D)$ according to the computational formula

$$P(H_i \mid D) = \frac{P(D \mid H_i)P(H_i)}{P(D \mid H_1)P(H_1) + P(D \mid H_2)P(H_2) + \ldots + P(D \mid H_N)P(H_N)} \tag{1}$$

for each hypothesis H_i.

Rather than dwell further on this computational formula at the moment, let us turn immediately to a simple computational example, and then re-examine the formula in the applied context to discern its precise content.

5. BAYES' THEOREM: A SIMPLE APPLICATION

By the conclusion of this article we shall be able to understand the use of Bayes' Theorem for statistical inference in the rather complicated case of the whale strandings data, without displaying every detail of the computation. To understand the computational strategy, we need to present first a simpler application. I shall be brief, but hopefully informative.

Developments in the technology of artificial insemination have been oriented toward designing a procedure whereby ejaculated sperm of a bull carrying an X-chromosome, the female sperm, can be separated from the male sperm, carrying a Y-chromosome. The financial benefits of such a technique can be immense, since the assurance of a female calf via the artificial insemination of the appropriate sperm would benefit the development of a milking herd without the cost of producing male calves, which are typically culled for veal. The production costs of the undesirable males, useless for dairy milk producers, are "wasted." Steers raised for beef are generally sired from different breeds of cows than dairy cows.

In devising a technique of sperm separation, various methods based on chemical and centrifugal separation have been attempted. Of concern in the practicality of any method is the *fecundity* of the mother cow when inseminated with the sex-strained female sperm. Will a cow inseminated with sperm produced by a specific sex-separation method conceive a healthy calf upon the first attempt via insemination? Or would her fecundity be reduced on account of the stress induced upon the sperm by its processing through the straining procedure? Animal breeders who develop such separation methods cannot be certain, though they surely have some ideas regarding the efficacy of the methods they have devised to date. This is the context in which the following example of a computation using Bayes' theorem is appropriate.

Suppose we are to inseminate ten 2-year-old (plus 3 months) Holstein dairy cows with X-chromosome sperm that has been separated by a specifically designed method. (A dairy cow is designated a "2-year-old" upon her delivering her first calf, and three months are normally allowed before inseminating her for her next conception. Animals in this state are ideal receptors for insemination experimentation, since it is known that they are capable of successful gestation.) One month after insemination it will be determined via a blood test whether conception has occurred, and one more month later it will be determined via sonogram whether the foetal development is healthy. The data to be recorded, D, is the number of the cows who are determined to be carrying a healthy foetus after this two-month check.

In this experiment, and in many experiments in which several individuals receive the same "treatment," the subjects are almost universally regarded symmetrically with respect to the *order* in which they achieve success or failure. This is to say that if the inseminated cows were arbitrarily designated to be cows number 1 through 10, experimentalists would typically assign equal probabilities to any ordered sequence of successes and failures among the 10 cows for which the total number of successes is the same. For example, if there were to be only one failure, it would be judged equiprobable that each of the cows would be the one to fail. If there were to be two failures, any selection of two cows to fail would be deemed equilikely as any other selection, . . . and so on to any larger number of failures through 9. This is a situation of uncertainty that is said to characterise *exchangeable* opinions regarding the experiments, an opinion structure that was illuminated in the previously mentioned works of de Finetti. In such a case, the uncertainty about every detail of the sequence of experiments is reduced to uncertainty about the sum of the successes to be achieved. What is called "de Finetti's representation theorem" is a theoretical result in probability that motivates the following method of analysis using Bayes' theorem.

Of concern to the designers of the sperm separation technique may be a variety of possible distortions to the potency of the sperm. There is no way of knowing for certain the gravity of these concerns and the incidence of infecundity they would induce, without experimentation. The hypothesized gravities of distortion could be denominated according to the possible fractions of all cows who would be fecund according to our two-month measurement procedure if a very large number of cows were inseminated with such sperm. Suppose we would designate this unknown proportion by a Greek letter, θ. Using this nomenclature, a list of exhaustive hypotheses entertained by the separation-procedure designers might be constructed as $(\theta=.1),(\theta=.2),(\theta=.3),...,(\theta=.9)$, where the value of the proportion is tracked merely to the first positive decimal place. Two brief comments are in order.

Firstly, why not study the fecundity of a large number of cows straight away using the sperm separation procedure in the first place? The answer, of course, is a matter of cost. The costs of breeding in the experimental setup are great in themselves. Before becoming involved in the large-scale application of a new procedure, a dairy would like to be fairly sure that the proportion of healthy conceptions would be high, more than half the conception rate of unseparated sperm in the very least. The costs of a wasted insemination round on an entire herd could be disastrous. We shall hopefully learn about the proportion of healthy conceptions achieved in a large number of attempts from the results we achieve in a smaller number of attempts, here only 10. Secondly, a numerical question concerns the validity of limiting the possible values of θ merely to the nine one-placed decimals from .1 to .9. This feature of this example is designed merely to ensure the reader's clarity in understanding the structure of the computational method. I shall remark later upon the relevance of this limitation to the accuracy of results we shall display, and also to the meaning of mathematical "integration" notation you will surely meet up with as you extend your study of Bayesian statistical methods. They can be found even within other articles appearing in this book.

5.1 The numerical routine of Bayes' theorem

Table 1 presents all the numerical results needed to compute the details and to understand the relevance of Bayes' theorem to the fecundity question. We can study the application of the theorem by describing the construction and manipulation of the various rows and columns of the table. These computations can be performed easily using Excel.

Across the first row of the table is a list of the nine hypotheses regarding the proportion of conceptions in a very large number of inseminations, listed only to the nearest first decimal place. Then the main block of columns at the top of the Table are headed by expressions such as $P(D|H=.1)$ and $P(D|H=.2)$. It turns out that a theorem of de Finetti requires that if a sequence of experiments is regarded exchangeably, then the probability distribution for the sum of successes achieved must be Binomial if the proportion of successes in a very large number of experiments is known to be the value specified by the hypothesis. We shall state this more formally in Section 6 below, when we expand our analysis to the more complicated whale stranding data. Here we should note only that the probabilities for the number of successes printed in each of these columns have been computed from binomial probability mass functions. So if the large proportion were known to equal θ, and the sequence of experiments is regarded exchangeably with respect to the order of successes, then the conditional probability of 0,1,..., or 10 successes out of 10 should be computed from $B(10,\theta)$.

However, the proportion of successes in a large number of attempts is not known! This is why we are doing the experiments with the 10 cows. The row of the table headed by "$P(H)=$" is an expression of the experimenter's probability assessments for the 9 possible proportion values. These probabilities result from the experimenter's assessments on the basis of uncertain knowledge about the aspects of the separation process that might be damaging to the sperms' potency. The assessment of such probabilities has been controversial in the acceptability of subjectivist statistical analysis mainly because of the received doctrine of objectivist statistical methods. According to this viewpoint, scientific method is supposed to allow us to achieve indubitable knowledge without any basis in private judgments based upon uncertainties. To the subjectivist viewpoint, such a claimed method is a chimera. If different scientists would assert different uncertain viewpoints, their different prior opinions need to be expressed. It is only by recognising such differences that the strength of the data in bringing different viewpoints into convergence can be assessed.

Table 1. The components for the computation of Bayes' Theorem. All probabilities have been rounded.

H =	.10	.20	.30	.40	.50	.60	.70	.80	.90
	$P(D\|H=.1)$	$P(D\|H=.2)$	$P(D\|H=.3)$	$P(D\|H=.4)$	$P(D\|H=.5)$	$P(D\|H=.6)$	$P(D\|H=.7)$	$P(D\|H=.8)$	$P(D\|H=.9)$
Data									
0	.3487	.1074	.0282	.0060	.0010	.0001	.0000	.0000	.0000
1	.3874	.2684	.1211	.0403	.0098	.0016	.0001	.0000	.0000
2	.1937	.3020	.2335	.1209	.0439	.0106	.0014	.0001	.0000
3	.0574	.2013	.2668	.2150	.1172	.0425	.0090	.0008	.0000
4	.0112	.0881	.2001	.2508	.2051	.1115	.0368	.0055	.0001
5	.0015	.0264	.1029	.2007	.2461	.2007	.1029	.0264	.0015
6	.0001	.0055	.0368	.1115	.2051	.2508	.2001	.0881	.0112
7	.0000	.0008	.0090	.0425	.1172	.2150	.2668	.2013	.0574
8	.0000	.0001	.0014	.0106	.0439	.1209	.2335	.3020	.1937
9	.0000	.0000	.0001	.0016	.0098	.0403	.1211	.2684	.3874
10	.0000	.0000	.0000	.0001	.0010	.0060	.0282	.1074	.3487
$P(H)=$	.03	.06	.11	.14	.14	.18	.18	.11	.05
$P(D=3\|H)$	.0574	.2013	.2668	.2150	.1172	.0425	.0090	.0008	.0000
	.002	.012	.029	.030	.016	.008	.002	.000	.000
$P(H\|D=3)$	.017	.122	.296	.304	.166	.077	.016	.001	.000
$P(H)=$	.03	.06	.11	.14	.14	.18	.18	.11	.05
$P(D=8\|H)$	.0000	.0001	.0014	.0106	.0439	.1209	.2335	.3020	.1937
$P(H\|D=8)$	.000	.000	.001	.013	.054	.190	.367	.290	.085

Once the experiments have been conducted, the observed data is used to identify which of the rows from the main block of Data probabilities is relevant to computing the appropriate inference from Bayes' theorem. We display the consequences of two such possibilities here. Our first computation will be based on a supposed result of achieving 3 conceptions out of 10 inseminations in the experiment. The row in the middle of the Table following "$P(H)=$" is headed $P(D=3|H)$. It is merely reprinted from the fourth row of conditional probabilities in the Data block of the Table above it. Note that the probabilities in this row do not sum to 1 (like the "prior probabilities" in the row headed $P(H)$ do.) For they are probabilities computed from different conditional probability distributions shown in those columns. The computation of Bayes' theorem requires that we multiply the components of these two rows, $P(D=3|H)$ with $P(H)$ to achieve the products shown in the next untitled row. Finally, this untitled row is summed (yielding 0.099 in this case) and each component of that untitled row is divided by this sum to yield the following row, headed appropriately by $P(H\,|\,D=3)$. This is the computational format of applying Bayes' Theorem as prescribed in the general formula (1). The "posterior probabilities" in this row do sum to 1, since they represent another probability mass function across the various possible hypotheses under consideration.

A second computation of Bayes' theorem completes this Table. It proceeds with the same computational process based on a supposition of observing 8 successes out of 10 inseminations, rather than 3.

5.2 Predictive probabilities : the theorem on total probability

What would be the assessed probability of a healthy conception in a single insemination attempt? A second important and relevant theorem is called the "theorem on total probability." In the context of this example it says that for any event F, your $P(F)$ can be computed as a weighted average of conditional probabilities:

$$P(F) = P(F|H_1)P(H_1)+P(F\,|\,H_2)P(H_2)+\cdots+P(F\,|\,H_N)P(H_N)$$

where the weights on the conditional probabilities are the prior probabilities on the conditioning hypotheses. A related statement of this theorem would allow us to compute your probability for F conditional on the Data, D, using the posterior probabilities as weights:

$$P(F|D) = P(F|H_1)P(H_1|D)+P(F|H_2)P(H_2|D)+\cdots+P(F|H_N|D).$$

To answer the question about the predictive probability for another conception, suppose we would designate this event of a conception on an 11th attempt by F. Using the theorem on total probability, there are two computations of interest to report. Before observing the data, the prior distribution over the hypotheses yields the weighted average $P(F) = .541$; conditioning on the data $D = 3$ would yield $P(F \mid D = 3) = .378$, while conditioning on the data $D = 8$ yields $P(F \mid D = 8) = .712$. These computations help to fill out our recognition that the experimenters are "of several minds" regarding the value of their separation efforts to this point. The theorem on total probability allows them to average their assessments of a conception numerically over these different states of mind, a perfectly reasonable thing to do.

A second worthwhile note is that this theorem of total probability can be used to specify prior probabilities for the 11 possible outcomes of the sum of successes in ten insemination attempts. In Table 1 we have displayed the conditional probabilities for these results given each of the possible hypotheses, computed as binomial probabilities. The theorem on total probability allows us to compute the unconditional probabilities for these outcomes via a weighted average of these columns, again using prior probabilities for the hypotheses as weights. Such computations yield the probabilities

.0210,.0484,.0749,.0990,.1188,.1331,.1401,.1351,.1145,.0795 and .0356

for 0 through 10 successes, respectively. This is *not* a binomial probability mass function at all, but is called a *mixture* of such functions. We shall comment on this again shortly.

5.3 Likelihood or information transfer?

As mentioned, the main columns of Table 1 were computed via a binomial probability mass function using the individual conception probability θ appropriate to each column of the table. If you have been introduced to the Binomial distribution in an objectivist context, you will have learned that it is the distribution for the sum of successes in a sequence of independent experiments, each generated according to the same probability. Objectivists think that unobservable "probabilities" are generating the successes and failures in the insemination experiment, and that the individual experiments are independent of each other because the conceptions by two different cows are causally unrelated to each other. In fact, objectivists think of the row of the table headed $P(D \mid H)$ corresponding to the observed data outcome as a function of the hypotheses that tells us how likely it is that the probability value represented in each particular hypothesis "generated" the data. In viewing the corresponding row as a function of the hypotheses, they call this function the likelihood function, informing us how likely it is that each of these probability values generated the data.

When asked to estimate the generating probability on the basis of the data, they have proposed an array of reasons why to estimate the probability by that value for which the likelihood is the greatest, calling this the "maximum likelihood estimate of the probability." In the cases of $D=3$ and $D=8$ shown in the Table, you can see that their estimates would be $p=.3$ and $p=.8$, respectively, by examining those rows to see where this likelihood is the greatest.

To the subjectivist who does not think that the data are generated by probabilities at all, this nomenclature for this important function misconstrues its role in the process of scientific inference. The rows of the table associated with $D=3$ and with $D=8$ are very important in the computation of Bayes' theorem for inference. However, it is not in the role of informing us about a chimerical "probability". Rather, it is in the role of combining the information in the new observations with other information available to experimenting scientists to compute the inferred probability distribution $P(H_1 \mid D)$ through $P(H_9 \mid D)$. For this reason, we regard it more appropriate to label this function $P(D \mid H)$ as an "information transfer function." It tells us how to transform the information in the data in combination with the other information available to us to derive our inferred posterior probabilities. The subjectivist has no qualms at all with asserting personally assessed probabilities for the hypotheses, neither before nor after observing the data from the experiment. These are merely the appropriate representation of the state of the observer's uncertainty. If you were to ask the subjectivist we have caricatured via the prior distribution displayed as $P(H)$ "what is the most likely hypothesis?" you would be answered according to the prior probability assertions before the experiment, with "$H=.6$ or H =.7 " since these were each assessed with probability .18. After observing $D=3$, you would be answered with "$H=.4$, assessed with $P(H=.4 \mid D=3)=.304$;" alternatively, after observing $D=8$ you would be answered with "$H=.7$, assessed with $P(H=.7 \mid D=8)=.367$." In neither case would the highest posterior probability be ascribed to the so-called "maximum likelihood estimate."

Moreover, the subjectivist does not regard the successes or failures among the individual experiments as independent at all. The outcome of each experiment tells us something about how to assess the other experiments. Observing successes tells us to regard the next experiment with a greater probability of success. Observing failures tells us to lower our probabilities for success in the next. This is what learning from data means. Precisely how the information is used is a consequence of the judgment to regard the sequence of experiments exchangeably.

We will have a chance to see these issues in operation more strongly in the complicated and real data situation of the whale strandings in Section 6.

5.4 The influence of distinguishing values of θ only to the nearest tenth

There are many computational issues associated with Bayes' theorem that we have smoothed over here, so to give a clear exposition of how scientific inference is seen to work from the subjectivist statistical perspective. One issue that could well have been provocative has been our consideration of the proportion of successes in a large number of inseminations to be denominated only to the nearest tenth. It is possible to make the computation to a finer degree of accuracy, but the Table would be much more difficult to "see" on account of its size. At this juncture, I will only report that if the recognised possibilities for the proportion were expanded to allow distinctions to the nearest second decimal place, the results differ very mildly. The computations would be structurally similar. When the probability results are summed once again to the nearest tenth, they differ from the numbers printed in the Table only in their third significant digit. They are closer in the case of $D=8$ than when $D=3$, being virtually identical.

Computational accuracy and feasibility in the application of Bayes' theorem has been the subject of extensive research development in recent years. Applications are now practical in even the most complicated models of opinion about complex data sets. It is worthy of mention that when hypotheses are refined to the finest extent possible, the summation that appears in the denominator of Bayes' equation (1) becomes replaced by an integral sign. In the case of the fecundity example, the infinite summation is expressed mathematically by the integral $\int_0^1 f(D|\theta)f(\theta)d\theta$. Practically understood, this means merely that the summation proceeds over *all* possible values of θ to the finest accuracy possible. This may be important merely for your feeling comfortable in reading articles that make use of the integral notation. Often the computational results are minimally different from those achieved with an adequately refined sum.

6. LEARNING FROM THE STRANDING DATA IS MORE COMPLICATED

The simplicity of the fecundity experiments is such that the formulation of the information transfer is determined exclusively by the judgment of exchangeability of the observed successes. This determination is via a theorem that is widely known as "de Finetti's representation theorem." This states that if you regard a sequence of success/failure experiments exchangeably no matter what is the number of experiments in the sequence, then your probabilities for the number of successes out of n experiments, S_n, must be computable in the form

$$P(S_n = x) = \int_0^1 \binom{n}{x} \theta^x (1-\theta)^{n-x} f(\theta) d\theta \tag{2}$$

for each value $x = 0,1,\dots,n$. Because of this theorem, it is required in such a simple problem that the information transfer function has the form of the binomial probability mass function $\mathrm{B}(\mathrm{n},\theta)$ that you can recognise within this formula. The function $f(\theta)$ expresses the prior distribution for the hypotheses denominated by all possible θ values between 0 and 1.

There are only two possibilities for the result of a single fecundity experiment, 1 and 0. Thus, the mixing parameter θ, which equals the assessed probability of a success in a single experiment according to a specific hypothesis, also determines the probability of a failure as $1-\theta$. In observing a whale stranding, the number of possible outcomes of the lunar date of the stranding is not two, but 30; for the coded lunar date of the stranding can be any number of 1 through 30. There is a generalisation of the exchangeability theorem (2) to allow for various hypotheses of 29 different probabilities (the thirtieth being required to make them sum to 1). But its application requires that we make summations (integrations) over possibilities in each of these 29 dimensions. It would require that we sum the number of successes observed on each of the 30 days of the lunar month, yielding. $S_1 = x_1, S_2 = x_2, \dots, S_{30} = x_{30}$ The generalised theorem states that

$$P\left[(S_1 = x_1)(S_2 = x_2)\cdots(S_{30} = x_{30})\right]$$

$$= \int_{S^{30}} \binom{\mathrm{n}}{x_1 x_2 \cdots x_{29} x_{30}} \theta_1^{x_1} \theta_2^{x_2} \cdots \theta_{29}^{x_{29}} \theta_{30}^{x_{30}} f(\theta_1, \theta_2, \cdots, \theta_{29}, \theta_{30}) d\theta_1 d\theta_2 \cdots d\theta_{29} d\theta_{30}. \tag{3}$$

The binomial mass function in equation (2) becomes a multinomial mass function in equation (3). The symbol $\int_{S^{30}}$ denotes that summation (integration) of this function must be computed over all possible vectors of $\theta_1, \theta_2, \cdots, \theta_{29}, \theta_{30}$ values that have non-negative components summing to 1. (This occurred automatically in expression (2) since in that equation the single θ and $(1-\theta)$ must sum to 1.) Not only are such extensive summations awkward, but also moreover no one who studies whale strandings would entertain seriously hypotheses of erratic sequences of occurrence on successive days of the lunar month in the long run. It is a requirement of mathematical modelling to devise a functional schema of hypothesised occurrence sequences over the days of a lunar month. These should not include crazy possibilities, but should still exhaust the styles of sequences that are motivated by zoological considerations. The first stage of modelling zoologists' attitudes is to construct a parametric family of functions in a form that can represent the complete range of hypothesised possibilities, but only that range. Thus, we want to devise a way to order the sizes of $\theta_1, \theta_2, \cdots$ and θ_{30} so they can fit only into the possible patterns that have been proposed. Furthermore we hope to design these functions using only a few recognised parameters rather than 30. We now describe how this family of functions can be designed for the whale stranding phenomena.

6.1 The structure of our attitudes: formulating the information transfer function

We will remember that one theory of strandings suggests that the time of their occurrence should be pro or counter-cyclic with the full moon phases. Fortunately, a well-known smooth cyclic function of this type is the trigonometric *cosine function*. Algebraically, the first function we shall need to consider can be written as a continuous function of time:

$$f_1(t \mid a_1) = a_1 \cos(2\pi t / 29.5306) + 1/29.5306 \quad \text{for } t \in [0, 29.5306] \quad (4)$$

Every piece of this function involves a number or the time variable, t, except for the coefficient a_1 that appears as a variable in front of the cosine function statement. When the argument of the function, t, varies from 0 to 29.5306, the argument inside the cosine statement varies from 0 to 2π, which equals the full circumference of a unit-circle. Thus, the cosine function component goes through one complete cosine cycle from 1 through 0, to -1, back through 0 and to 1 again. The constant 1/29.5306 added to the function ensures that the cosine cycles about this base rather than the usual 0 mean of a simple cosine function. Finally, the coefficient a_1 stands for an *amplitude* factor of the function, allowing the height of the cycling cosine to be great or small, even zero. Any specific numerical value of a_1 would specify a distinct function with that amplitude, so the "function" defined by (4) actually specifies a whole family of functions. The variable a_1, which identifies each member of the family, is called the "parameter" of the family. Let us look at two examples of family members.

Figure 1 displays two such cosine functions $f_1(t \mid a_1)$, one of them labelled with $a_1 = 8/295.306$ and the other labelled $a_1 = -4/295.306$. You should be able to see that the larger is the value of "a_1", the more extreme are the peaks and troughs of the function. Moreover, positive values of a_1 produce cosine functions that are pro-cyclic with the new moon, peaking at 0 and 29.5306. Negative values generate functions pro-cyclic with the full moon, peaking at 15. The idea of the mathematical modelling via this function is that the various values of a_1 correspond to varying strengths with which a zoologist might regard daily whale strandings as occurring pro- or counter-cyclic with the full moon phase of a lunation. Of course $a_1 = 0$ would correspond to a function that supports uniform probabilities over all dates in a lunar month, an attitude highly favoured by many zoologists. Finally, it should be recognised that since this functional form is being used to represent probabilities, the largest values of the amplitude parameter to be entertained would be 10/295.306 or -10/295.306, since probabilities can never be negative.

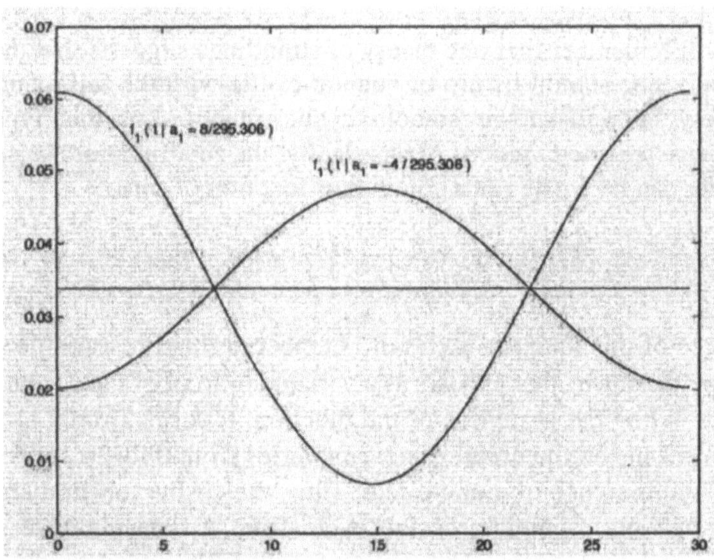

Figure 1. Two one-cycle sine functions of time, t, specified by different amplitudes.

Functions in the form of $f_1(t\,|\,a_1)$ can be used to represent opinions that stranding incidence varies largely in coincidence with the full moon (negative values of a_1) or the new moon (positive values of a_1), or not at all (value of $a_1 = 0$). However, they cannot represent the opinion that incidence varies with the strength of the tides, which cycle twice within a month. Fortunately, the cycle length of trigonometric functions such as cosine can be manipulated by a scale factor on its timing argument. Consider the function

$$f(t\,|\,a_2) \;=\; a_2 \cos(4\pi t/29.5306) + 1/29.5306 \quad \text{for} \quad t \in [0, 29.5306].$$

Notice the 4π in the cosine component as opposed to the 2π in the corresponding component of function f_1 in (4). This algebraic change has the effect that as the argument t of this function runs from 0 to 29.5306, the argument of the cosine component runs from 0 to 4π, twice around the circumference of a unit circle. By this means, for the various values of a_2 the cosine functions are forced to cycle twice within the prescribed lunar month rather than merely once.

There is one further complicating feature of the tidal hypotheses regarding the timing of the whale strandings. The spring tides do not occur on the full (or empty) moon day itself, but typically one to four days *after* the full/new moon. We are required to induce a *phase shift* on the two-cycle cosine functions, variable from 1 to 4 days. Algebraically, this is achieved by subtracting another parametric factor, denominated "p", from the argument t of the function f_2 as follows:

$$f_2(t\,|\,a_2, p) \;=\; a_2 \cos(4\pi(t - p)/29.5306) \;+\; 1/29.5306 \quad \text{for} \quad t \in [0, 29.5306]. \tag{5}$$

As with the single cycle function family, f_1, there are limits on the values of the parameters a_2 and p that we shall entertain in constructing the family of possible hypotheses. Again the value of a_2 is restricted to lie between 10/295.306 and -10/295.306. Positive values of the amplitude a_2 would represent attitudes that imagine stranding incidence as pro-cyclic with the spring tides. Negative amplitudes for a_2 would describe incidence as pro-cyclic with the neap tides. For someone who is willing to learn that tides *are* relevant, but does not really believe it, any prior weight on a positive a_2 amplitude would want to balance it by an equal weight on a corresponding negative amplitude value. We shall exemplify this in one of the prior distributions, shortly. The only phase shift values entertained will be the values of p at 1, 2, 3 and 4, since these are the feasible lag days for spring tides after a full or new moon.

Figure 2 displays four 2-cycle cosine functions, each specified by the amplitude $a_2 = 8/295.306$ but distinguished only by the four different values of the phase shift parameter, p.

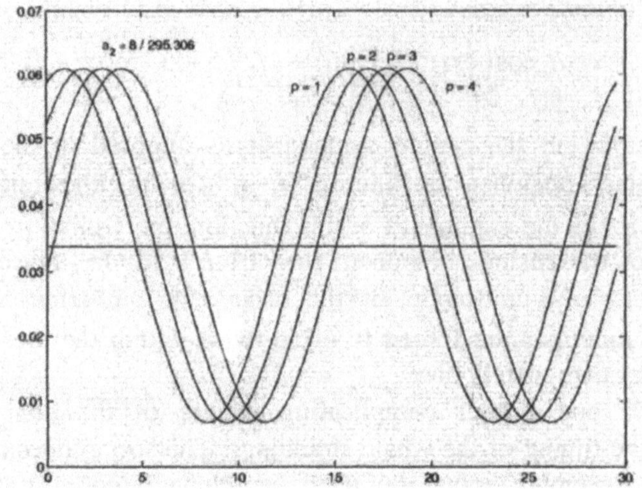

Figure 2. Two-cycle sine functions of time, t, with different phase shifts, p = 1, 2, 3 and 4.

Finally, we need to model the opinions of zoologists that *both* the single-cycle lunatic aspects of behaviour and the two-cycle per month tidal forces may be relevant to the stranding phenomena. This can be done algebraically by combining the two functions f_1 and f_2 into a single function using an array of possible weights on these two functional components, parameterised by the symbol γ. With this extensive background, we can now represent the relevant family of all realistic hypotheses of whale stranding timings under consideration by a family of functions in the form

$$f(t \mid a_1, a_2, p, \gamma) = \gamma f_1(t \mid a_1) + (1-\gamma) f_2(t \mid a_2, p) \text{ for } t \in [0, 29.5306]. \quad (6)$$

Each specific family member function is identified by four numerical values for the parameters a_1, a_2, p and γ. We shall exhaustively list the hypotheses specified by zoologists by enumerating an array of parameter possibilities: a_1 and a_2 can each range through the 21 possibilities $\{-10/295.306, -9/295.306, \cdots, 9/295.306, 10/295.306\}$; p ranges through

$\{1,2,3,4\}$ and γ ranges through $\{.1,.3,.5,.7,.9\}$. In all, there are 420 family members, each identified by a different specification of these four parameters.

We hope to learn about the amplitude of each cyclic factor and about the relative importance of these two hypothesised factors from the observed stranding data. The strength of the data in illuminating this situation can only be gauged relative to the strength with which various zoologists entertain the possibilities denominated by the parameter units. In the next Subsection we need to describe how this can be done.

A final technical comment is needed. The parametric function (6) of t is continuous in time. However, our measurements of the time of a whale stranding records only the day of the stranding. Thus, to identify the thirty θ values of equation (3) we need to integrate (sum) function (6) over the daily intervals of 24 hours. This has been done for the computations that follow, but the details are not important here. They are explained in Lad and Brabyn (1993) if needed. As a result, the information transfer function has the form of the product of the parameterised θ's according to a multinomial distribution:

$$f(x_1,x_2,\cdots,x_{30}\mid\gamma,a_1,a_2,p)=\theta_1(\gamma,a_1,a_2,p)^{x_1}\,\theta_2(\gamma,a_1,a_2,p)^{x_2}\cdots\theta_{30}(\gamma,a_1,a_2,p)^{x_{30}} \tag{7}$$

defined for each possible choice of γ,a_1,a_2 and p.

The functional modelling of the information transfer function we have constructed here amounts to a specification of the components of the stylised form of Bayes' theorem denoted in Section 4 by $P(D\mid H_i)$ for 420 different hypotheses H_i. In this case, each H_i is identified with an array of four parameter values, while the data D is to be identified with the specific data sequence of whale stranding dates found in the NZWSDB. They have been reduced to the statistics $x_1,x_2,\ldots,x_{30}$ that record the number of strandings that occur on the first, second, ... and thirtieth day of a lunar month. The last feature we need to discuss before inferential computations is the prior probability function to be applied to each parameter vector.

6.2 Assessing prior opinions about the possibilities

How large might the appropriate amplitudes and the phase shift be? Zoologists entertain and array of opinions. Of course, for someone who is belligerent in denying any possibility that lunar timing has any relevance to whale stranding phenomena, there is a simple prior and posterior probability mass function over the hypotheses we have identified. It is represented by a function which gives a total mass of 1 to the configuration $a_1 = 0$ and $a_2 = 0$. Expressing an attitude in this way means that for such a person, no amount of data of any content would change this opinion. It would imply that strandings are expected to occur uniformly over all possible days in a lunar month. In what follows we will develop a prior function over the hypothesis array specified by γ, a_1, a_2 and p that gives a large weight to the pattern of uniformity, but allows some possibility to amplitudes of various sizes, with probabilities diminishing as the size of the amplitude increases.

To begin the formulation, we shall specify that the prior mixing function is independent over the four parameter types. Formally this is to say that

$$m(\gamma, a_1, a_2, p) = m(\gamma)m(a_1)m(a_2)m(p).$$

Since the one-cycle and two-cycle hypotheses are quite distinct from each other, an independent mass function of this sort merely specifies that conditioning on a specific amplitude size for the one-cycle hypothesis would not influence one's opinions about the size of the amplitude for the two-cycle hypothesis, and vice-versa. For example, if one were to learn exclusively that the amplitude for the two-cycle tidal aspect of stranding phenomena were large, say $a_2 = -8/295.306$, one would still feel the same about the lunatic based amplitude, a_1, without separate evidence on that matter. Moreover, the attitude about the phase shift parameter of the two-cycle component is motivated merely by the fact that the spring tides occur between one and four days after the new and full moons, irrespective of the size of the amplitude of the tidal differences relevant to the stranding phenomena.

The numerical details of the specific prior distributions over these parameter configurations are most easily reported in the graphs of Figure 3. Let me explain their generation while you examine that figure. The top graph presents two identical mass functions, $m(a_1) = m(a_2)$, concentrated on the possible values of a_1 or a_2 running from -10/295.306 through 10/295.306. They express the attitude that the amplitudes probably equal 0, with $P(a_1 = 0) = .5$. However if the amplitudes are not 0, then they may be either positive or negative, with a weighting distribution that diminishes exponentially in both directions. The numerical sizes of these weights decline like .0990, .0601, .0364, .0221, .0134, .0081, .0049, .0030, .0018 and .0011 in both directions. The functions $m(a_1)$ and $m(a_2)$ thus represent the sceptical view that if there is a lunar component of stranding phenomena in either direction, it is counterbalanced by a reverse feature of the same magnitude. Nonetheless, this attitude is open to be influenced by observations if they are strong enough.

The second and third mass functions shown in the next two graphs express even a stronger probability mass on amplitudes of 0, with $P(a_1 = 0) = P(a_2 = 0) = .625$. However, if there is a lunar component to tidal phenomena for either lunatic or tidal reasons, the amplitudes are appropriate to be pro-cyclic with the full moon and with the spring tides in the two cases. Thus, the function $n(a_1)$ declines exponentially only to the negative side of 0, while $n(a_2)$ declines only to the positive side. These probabilities decline like .1486, .0901, .0546, .0331, .0201, .0122, .0074, .0045, .0027 and .0017. In each case, the alternately signed amplitudes are assessed with probability 0.

Finally, the mass function over the three values of p and the values of γ are uniform.

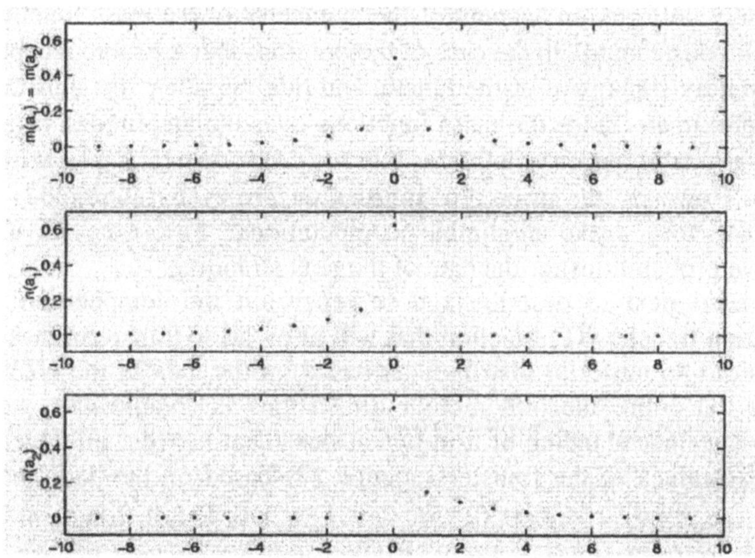

Figure 3. The top panel displays a prior probability mass function for the amplitudes of the one-cycle and two-cycle amplitudes corresponding to the views of a skeptic regarding lunar aspects of whale stranding phenomena. Nonetheless, this opinion is amenable to influence from data to some extent. The amplitude of 0 is assessed with probability .5, and remaining probability declines symmetrically to the left and to the right, massing mainly on small amplitudes. The next two panels describe opinions that are mildly supportive of pro-cyclic lunatic and tidal patterns. An even higher probability of .625 is accorded to the amplitude of 0, but the remaining probability declines only in favor of small pro-cyclic values.

6.3 Using the data to sharpen our understanding

We have described the details of zoologist's prior opinions to an extent that we have constructed two distinct prior mixing distributions over the parameters that identify the lunatic and tidal theories of the timing of whale strandings. Essentially, these prior mixing functions play the role of the $P(H_1),\dots,P(H_N)$ distribution in our generic discussion of Bayes' Theorem. We should note that both of these prior distributions (described by the functions $m(\gamma,a_1,a_2,p)$ and $n(\gamma,a_1,a_2,p)$ in Figure 3) would support a predictive distribution for the lunar date of the next whale stranding that is uniform over the days. Each parameter array (γ,a_2,a_2,p) specifies values for the thirty $\theta's$. Computing a weighted average of these values, with weights equal to the prior mixing function at the parameter array, would yield this predictive distribution.

In the case of the sceptical opinion represented by $m(\cdot)$ this distribution is precisely uniform, on account of the symmetry of the mass functions for the amplitudes about 0. In the case of the opinions that are more receptive to, if only mildly supportive of the lunatic and tidal theories, this uniformity is only approximate, since the mass functions over the amplitudes a_1 and a_2 put zero probabilities on amplitudes that would be counter cyclic with these theories. However, the prior probabilities on pro-cyclic amplitudes are so small that they make negligible computational difference to uniform predictive probabilities for the date of the next stranding.

We need next to describe and to report on the computation of the information transfer (IT) function that will allow us to transform these prior distributions to posterior distributions based on the data in the NZWSDB. Because the entire function in four dimensions is complicated, we shall develop our understanding of it in two stages. That is, we shall develop the numerical values of the transfer function (7) based on the data vector of $(x_1,x_2,\dots,x_{30})=$ (6, 1, 4, 0, 0, 0, 1, 1, 4, 1, 1, 3, 3, 0, 1, 1, 4, 1, 3, 6, 4, 2, 0, 0, 1, 0, 1, 0, 0, 0). The components of this vector merely sum the number of pilot whale herd strandings since 1970 that occurred on the thirty ordered days of a lunar month.

To begin, Figure 4 displays the computed values of the IT function (7) over a grid of values for a_1 and a_2 corresponding to the specific values of $p=3$ and $\gamma=.5$. It is easily seen that the largest values of this function occurs at $(a_1=-9/295.306, a_2=9/295.306)$. It is notable that these are values of the amplitudes that are strongly pro-cyclic with the full moon (since a_1 is negative) and pro-cyclic with the spring tides (since a_2 is positive.) While the function looms as a mountain, the scale of the function is such that its height at this peak is 81 times the value of the function at $(a_1 = 0, a_2 = 0)$. Counter-cyclic amplitudes receive negligible IT values.

Figure 4 is presented by itself here just for you to get your bearings in reading the following Figure 5, which displays the entire IT function over all four of its dimensions. The display of Figure 4 was achieved merely by arranging the function values in a matrix whose rows and columns correspond to the two-dimensional space of (a_1, a_2) pairs we are entertaining. To display Figure 5, I have stacked such matrices on top of one another in the order that at the top are the matrices for which $p = 1$, and then iteratively $\gamma = .1, .3, .5, .7$ and .9. Then follows the similar stack of matrices for which $p = 2, 3$ and 4, again iterating over values of γ in the same order. As a result, Figure 5 displays 20 ordered graphs similar to Figure 4, but corresponding to different values of the pair (p, γ). The graphs are compressed in the dimension of a_1 relative to Figure 4, but knowing how to read that Figure allows us to interpret this graph that displays the entire function of four variables.

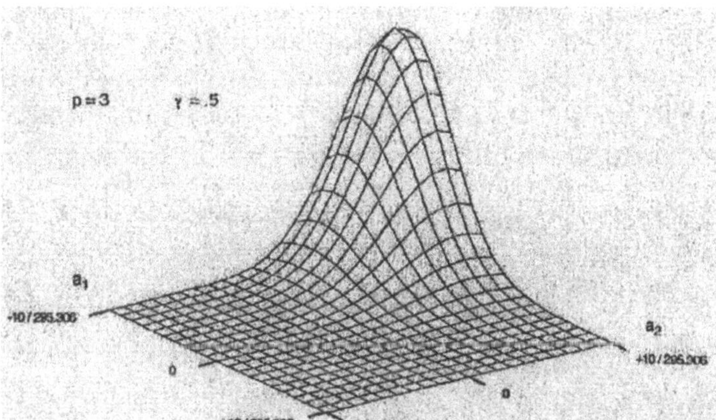

Figure 4. Information transfer (likelihood) function values for amplitude parameter pairs (a_1, a_2) concentrated at the weighting parameter on the one-cycle component, γ=5, and the phase shift for the two-cycle component, p=3. The maximum function value achieved relative to its value at (a_1=0, a_2=0) equals 81.

It is evident that the data transfers information almost exclusively supportive of amplitude values supported by tidal and lunatic theories. Negligible weights are easily seen for all negative values of a_2 by the low plain of the function there. In addition, each of the mountain ranges rising at the large a_2 values can be seen to peak at negative values of a_1, and decline quickly from there. The centring of the peaks in each range at $\gamma = .5$ shows that each of these theories receives about the same data support. The information function even seems to balance around the phase shifts of 2 and 3 days in preference to 1 and 4. Virtually all of the supported parameter configurations are among those specified by the contestable zoological theories!

Still, it must be said that the peaks of the information transfer function are not shocking relative to the height of the plains. As noted in the caption to Figure 4, the height of the function at its peak relative to the value for amplitudes $a_1 = a_2 = 0$ is only 81. The heights of the peaks, which look more like hills, are determined by the size of the data set. In this case there are only 49 observations. These are required to provide information about 4 parameters, which characterise 30 values of θ's. Precisely how to assess the weight of this evidence for practical purposes can only be determined by combining it with the prior expectation functions we have assessed. We can now look into this.

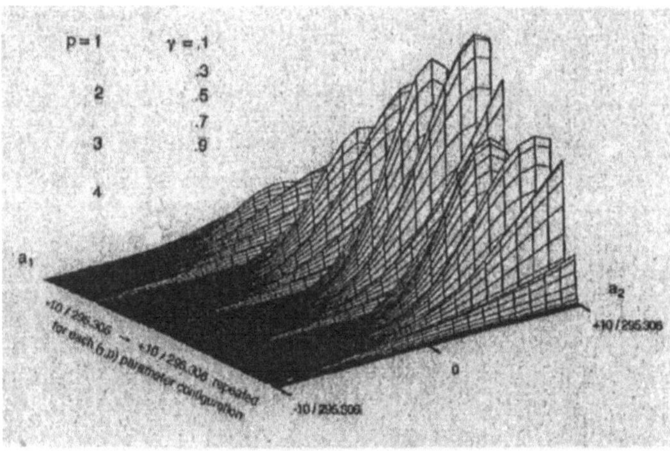

Figure 5. The information transfer function $f(x_1, x_2, \ldots, x_{30} | \gamma, a_1, a_2, p)$ based on 49 sharply dated whale strandings occurring since 1970, shown over the entire argument grid. In the a_2 direction, grid values run from -10/295.306 through +10/295.306 in twenty equal steps. In the a_1 direction, these same grid values are repeated in the grid for each combination of γ =.1, .3, .5, .7 and .9 with p=1, 2, 3, 4.

6.4 Predictive distributions, and the distortion provided by maximum likelihood methods

Having examined the information transfer function we have presented in Figure 5, it is easy to see how inappropriate are the maximum likelihood forecasts, and that they misrepresent what the data tell us. It is true that the information transfer (or so-called likelihood) function has its peak at the parameter configuration $(a_1, a_2, p, \gamma) = (-9/295.306, +9/295.306, 3, .5)$, but it is clearly evident from the graph of the function that other vectors are not greatly disfavoured by the data either.

The natural thing to do with the information provided by the data, and the formally correct thing to do as suggested by Bayes' theorem and the theorem on total probability, is to combine it with prior information to determine the strength of its content to effect scientific expectations regarding what will happen next. The results of these computations appear as predictive distributions for the lunar date of the next whale stranding in Figure 6. The prior mixing functions $m(a_1, a_2, \gamma, \mathrm{p})$ and $n(a_1, a_2, \gamma, \mathrm{p})$ were each multiplied by the IT function values displayed in Figure 5 to yield posterior mixing functions according to Bayes' rule. These mixing functions were then used to make a weighted average predictive probability for the lunar date of the next stranding, using the formalities of the theorem on total probability. These are the functions labelled $m(t \mid \mathbf{t}_{49})$ and $n(t \mid \mathbf{t}_{49})$ in Figure 6.

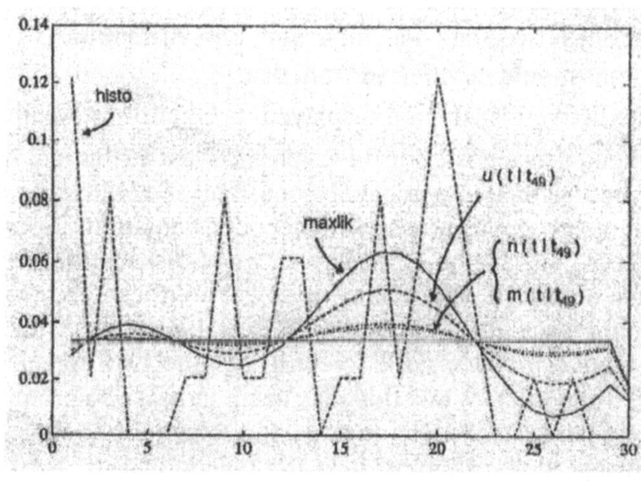

Figure 6. Posterior predictive distributions for the lunar date of the next pilot whale stranding, computed for three prior mixing functions, along with the connected histogram frequencies and the maximum likelihood forecast.

From the perspective of zoological theorists, it is notable that the forecasting distributions inferred by lunar theory supporters and sceptics are now so close together. True, neither distribution differs so markedly from the uniform assessment of probability 1/29.5306 for each day of the lunar month. Nonetheless, this little bit of data is strong enough to pull each of them into a mode of considering lunar periods as perhaps worthy of more serious consideration.

Proponents of objectivist methods do not like to make forecasting distributions that are weighted averages over an array of parameterised "models," because they think the weighting choices are arbitrary. Thus, in making forecasts based on data they are typically reduced to picking the forecasting distribution as the data distribution supported by the maximum likelihood estimates of their "model parameters." The function labelled "maxlik" in Figure 6 displays the forecasting function based on the pilot whale stranding data in this way. It is evident how distorted are the forecasting probabilities relative to those computed via Bayes' theorem and the posterior weighted average forecasts. This occurs because no weight is given to conditional forecasts based on opinion models that did not achieve the maximum likelihood based on the data. This is despite the fact that their likelihood function shows clearly that many other parameter configurations achieve high likelihood. The incongruous aspect of the distorted predictive probabilities their methods support is that their method can be interpreted as using a weighting function that gives all its mixing weight to only one parameter configuration. It is a regular feature of maximum likelihood forecasts that they overstate the high and low extremities of forecasting probabilities that should be inferred from data.

A third predictive distribution displayed in Figure 6 is labelled $\mathrm{u}(t \mid \mathbf{t}_{49})$. This was computed as a posterior Bayes predictive distribution, but based on a prior distribution that is completely constant at 1/420 over all the 420 possible parameter configurations under consideration. Some theorists favour the use of such "non-informative" prior distributions because they ostensibly give no prior favour to any theory at all. It can be seen that in this whale stranding case, the forecasting distribution this prior implies is intermediate between the maxlik forecast and the two agreeing posterior forecasts, $m(\cdot)$ and $n(\cdot)$. While this may seem to be a compromise position, it has two great demerits. Firstly, it gives no recognition to the great disdain with which many zoologists have held the lunatic and the tidal theories of stranding behaviour. That large amplitude theories of such behaviour should be given equal prior weight to zero amplitude theories would hardly be recognised by professionals as a compromise. Secondly, to impose uniformity for reasons of supposed objectivity at this late stage of the opinion modelling is to ignore the fact that already many many possible opinion distribution functions have been eliminated from the domain of such uniform opinions by our bold formulations of zoological theory. While virtually every thinking person would agree with the exchangeability properties of opinions about timing, we have already reduced the dimension of the required form of exchangeable distributions specified in equation (3) from the thirty θ's to the four parameters γ, a_1, a_2 and p. It appears that attempts to get rid of real prior opinions entertained by thinking professionals on the grounds that they are somehow arbitrary lead to far greater consequences of real arbitrariness.

7. THE CENTRALITY OF THE INFORMATION TRANSFER FUNCTION

A complete analysis of all the whale stranding data in the NZWSDB is beyond the scope of this article, and indeed is yet to be completed. The complexity of the analysis is increased by the fact that there are many species of whales involved. Some of these display rather different ocean-faring behaviours to those of the pilot whale, while other behaviours are shared. A complete analysis would involve assessments of groupings of species within what are called *hierarchical* structures of analysis. This topic would require much more extensive discussion. Nonetheless, it should be apparent from our presentation here that the information transfer function would be central to the understanding of the data content relevant to the issue of the timing of strandings in a lunar month.

It is only because this function, under the guise of a likelihood function, has been analysed by itself, and has been considered somehow to be "objective" that it can be used to support distortions to the inferences that can be made coherently from data. The subjectivist viewpoint in statistics offers a frank way to recognise the source of this important function itself in personal judgments, and to modify the function via mixture distributions to soften the harsh claims to forecasting power that rely on it exclusively.

8. CONCLUDING COMMENTS

There is a long tradition in statistical circles advising researchers to spend some time discussing their data design with a statistician prior to collecting the data. This has typically been an advice based on a notion that only data generated by properly randomised statistical designs is fit for rigorous statistical analysis. One of the recognised benefits of developments of subjectivist statistical theory is that it provides a logical structure in which inferences based on any data, however collected, can be coherently analysed. For probabilities are used not to model the intricacies of Natural processes themselves, but to characterise uncertain opinions about observable aspects of Nature. One must only be forthcoming and honest about the sources of the attitudes toward observations that are proposed.

The admirable dissemination of computational statistical software for data handling has been motivated by a feeling that statistical assessment should be taken out of the exclusive hands of professional specialists. Since everyone can learn from data, everyone should have the means at their disposal to make the computations required for this learning.

I think, nonetheless, that reasons for consulting a professional statistician on topics of importance, at least for a discussion, are more important than ever. It is easy to betray the value of one's data by relying on supposedly objective statistical methods that are available at the touch of a button. Somewhere in the analysis of statistical data it must be recognised that there are other sources of information regarding your problem than merely the data itself. Moreover, if the subject is controversial, the differing opinions need to be formalised to an extent that the strength of the data can be judged against an appropriate background. You will still need to touch a lot of buttons, but you will also need to think and make judgments for which only you are responsible. The presentation in this article has been designed to display the subjectivist foundation for the validity of making such judgments.

REFERENCES

BRABYN, M. (1990) Analysis of New Zealand Whale Strandings, University of Canterbury Department of Zoology Master's Thesis, Christchurch, New Zealand.

BRABYN, M. (1991) An analysis of the New Zealand Whale Stranding record, Wellington: New Zealand Department of Conservation, Science and Research Series No. 29.

BRABYN, M. and MCLEAN, I. (1992) The oceanography and coastal topography of herd stranding sites for whales in New Zealand, *Journal of Mammology*, vol. 73, 469-476.

DE CASAMAJOR, M.N., BRU, N., and PROUZET, R. (2001) Fluctuations of glass-eels (Anguilla anguilla L.) catches and variability of their catchability in the adour estuary. *Bulletin Francais de la Peche et de la Pisciculture*, 387-404.

ELANGOVAN, V. AND MARIMUTHU, G. (2001) Effect of moonlight on the foraging behaviour of a megachiropteran bat, Cynopterus sphinx, *Journal of Zoology*, vol. 253, 347-350.

DE FINETTI, B. (1937) La prevision, ses lois logiques, ses sources subjectives, *Annales de L'Institutes Henri Poincaré*, vol. 7, 1-68.

DE FINETTI, B. (1970) Teoria della Probabilità: sintesi introduttiva con appendice critica, Torino: G. Einaudi.

DE FINETTI, B. (1994, 1995) Theory of Probability: a critical introductory treatment, Volumes I and II, English translation by Antonio Machi and Adrian Smith of the 1970 Italian original, New York: John Wiley.

GATSONIS, C. *et. al* (1995, 1997, 1998, 2001, 2001) Case Studies in Bayesian Statistics, New York: Springer-Verlag, Lecture Notes in Statistics, Vols. 105, 121, 140, 162, 163.

HACKING, I. (1990) The Taming of Chance, Cambridge: Cambridge University Press.

HEDD, A., GALES, R. and BROTHERS, N. (1992) Foraging strategies of shy albatross (Thalassarche cauta) breeding at Albatross Island, Tasmania, Australia. *Marine Ecology Progress Series*, vol 4, 495-518.

LAD, F. (1996) Operational Subjective Statistical Methods: a mathematical, philosophical, and historical introduction, New York: John Wiley.

LAD, F. and BRABYN, M.W. (1993) Synchronicity of whale strandings with phases of the moon. *Case Studies in Bayesian Statistics*, edited by C. Gatsonis, J.S. Hodges, R.E. Kass, and N.D. Singpurwalla, New York: Springer-Verlag, 1993, 362-376.

SAVAGE, L.J. (1954) The Foundations of Statistics, New York: John Wiley.

Chapter 10

DEVELOPMENT AND COMMUNICATION OF BAYESAN METHODOLOGY FOR MEDICAL DEVICE CLINICAL TRIALS[*]

A. James O'Malley[†]
Department of Health Care Policy, Harvard Medical School, Boston, MA, USA.

1. INTRODUCTION

This paper presents Bayesian methods that have been proposed for the analysis (O'Malley, Normand, and Kuntz, 2003) and design (O'Malley, Normand, and Kuntz, 2002) of medical device clinical trials. Whereas the referenced papers are methodological, this paper is application oriented. This work is motivated by medical device trials, particularly those of coronary-artery stents (small metallic scaffolds used to enlarge coronary artery segments with plaque narrowing) .However, it has applications to all clinical trials.

Historically-controlled trials are studies in which investigators compare, retrospectively, current patients on a new treatment with previous or "historical" patients on the standard treatment. The FDA has recently approved the use of single armed historically-controlled trials for the clinical evaluation of some medical devices, such as prostethic heart valves and coronary-artery stents, in order to establish that the new device is safe and effective compared to approved stents (O'Malley, Normand, and Kuntz, 2003; Kereiakes *et al.*, 1999).

* This work was supported by the Advanced Medical Manufacturers Association (Washington, D.C.), a non- profit consortium of health care product manufacturers. The article uses material from joint work with Sharon-Lise T. Normand and Richard E. Kuntz presented elsewhere.

† For correspondence: omalley@hcp.med.harvard.edu

The motivation for historical-controls in the medical device industry stems from the ability to dramatically reduce the time reqluired to complete a trial. This is important in industries where technological advances are rapid. For exanlple, randornized trials of coronary-artery stents have a two-year timeline, much greater than the rate at which promising next generation stent designs continue to proliferate. In addition, because device modifications tipically result in only a small or local effect on patient outcome, conducting a randomized tria1 after each incremental improvement does not seem necessary.

The absence of randomization necessitates that hierarchical regression, propensity score methods, or other sophisticated models are used to account for heterogeneity among treatment groups which, if ignored, could bias the results. Therefore, a key issue in adopting historically-controlled trials is determination of a fair comparison between treatments, commonly referred to as an "objective performance criterion (OPC)". This term was introduced to the FDA approximately 10 years ago in the evaluation of prosthetic heart valves using single-arrm studies (Gersh *et al.*, 1986; Grumkemeier, Starr, and Rahimtoola, 1992; Grunkemeier, 1993). Aggregating data from all approved heart valve trials, the investigators calculated the complication rate per year and used this as a basis for an OPC. Like heart valves, there is an established pool of randomized trials of approved coronary stents that have been conducted in the US. Hovever, umlike heart valves, the reference population has changed appreciably in the past 10 years, several patient and tria1 characteristics impact the outcome, and two correlated endpoints are of interest. OPC for bivariate mixed outcomes were estimated using hierarchical regression methods inl O'Malley, Normand, and Kuntz (2003). This model based approach allows measures of OPC for a varied range of definitions to be developed. The broad classes of areas of application of the OPC will be discusses herein, and several examnples are provided.

In order for design calculations, such as sample size determination, to be meaningful, the intended analysis must be inbred within the calculation. If complexities of the intended analysis are not accounted for in the design of the trial, the study may be severely under-powered, increasing the likelihood that the recruitment of insufficient patients leads to a negative result, or over-powered; unnecessarily wasting financial resources, patient involvement, and time. Methodology for determining sample size for experiments involving hierarchical regression analysis was developed by O'Malley, Normand, and Kuntz (2002) in the context of a historically-controlled clinical trial. They adapted the algorithm for stochastic optimization in Müller and Parmigiani (1995) to compute power probabilities associated with Bayes decision rules. Unlike earlier work (for example, Self and Mauritsen, 1988 for generalized linear models; Vhittemore, 1981 and Hsieh, Bloch, and Larsen, 1998 for logistic regression;

Signorini, 1991 for Poison regression), analytic approximations are not utilized. Furthermore, in the spirit of Weiss (1997) and Spiegelhalter (1986) the uncertainty in unknown parameters propagates through the calculation of power and sample size. To retain familiarity with standard practices and henceforth assist in communications with the FDA, the *power* of the trial was the basis of all calculations; a tradition continued in this paper.

In this paper, we use the methodology in O'Malley, Normand, and Kuntz (2002) to estimate the relationship implied by coherence between an effect size or predicted value of an outcome of interest (e.g. the sample mean), power, the predictive probability of a hypothesis, and sample size. Such relationships may be displayed graphically, or specific values can be presented in tables. In this paper plots and tables for various permutations of these entities will be presented. To some extent this work is a response to the demands of trialists and regulators, who often rquest that information about the trial design be expressed in terms of an observable quantity (i.e. predicted outcome), or an effect (i.e. model parameter), of interest.

We introduce the motivating problem, and the historical stent data, in Section 2. We describe the methodology of O'Malley, Normand, and Kuntz (2003) for fitting a Bayesian hierarchical regression model to multivariate mixed outcome data in Section 3. The OPC is introduced and discussed in details in Section 3. The OPC for coronary-artery stents is estimated for various sub-populations in Section 4. Sample size determination is reviewed in Section 5, and used to derive the relationship between power, sample size, and predictive outcomes or model parameters in Section 6. Concluding remarks are presented in Section 7.

2. CLINICAL PROBLEM AND HISTORICAL DATA

Coronary disease results from lesions of fatty plaque that build up within the arterial wall. These plaque lesions may either rupture causing a heart attack, or gradually obstruct blood flow causing angina. Coronary stents are thin expandable metallic tubes that are delivered within the coronary artery by a catheter and are then expanded precisely at the site of an obstructive lesion. Typically up to two primary endpoints (measures of restenosis) are measured after coronary stenting. The first endpoint, which is obtained in all patients, is the incidence of clinically-driven repeat revascularization, denoted the target lesion revascularization (TLR) rate. TLR is designated by a clinical events committee, blinded to treatment assignment, who have access to clinical and angiographic laboratory data. The second end-point, obtained on a small randomly selected subset of patients, is defined as the degree of re-narrowing and is quantified by a computer based system that measures absolute and relative dimensions of the artery, including proportion diameter stenosis (PDS). Both measures are taken 9 months after stenting.

Table 1. Historical data for patients participating in 7 randomized coronary artery stent trials (1993-1999). Means (MN) and standard deviations (SD) are reported for the continuous variables; percentages are reported for binary variables. TLR = target lesion revascularization rate. PDS = Proportion diameter stenosis.-denotes not applicable.

Trial	Variable	Number Patients	Outcome Mn (SD)	Length (mm)	Diameter (mm)	Thickness (%)	Registry (%)	Diabetes (%)	Location (%)	Diseased Vessels (%) 2	Diseased Vessels (%) 3
1	TLR	1806	0.116	11.57 (6.27)	2.99 (0.49)	0.06 (0.13)	0	18	43	26	11
	PDS	0	- -	- -	- -	- -	-	-	-	-	-
2	TLR	1248	0.083	11.36 (6.05)	3.03 (0.48)	0.08 (0.11)	21	20	42	22	7
	PDS	357	0.342 (0.186)	10.93 (5.76)	3.03 (0.46)	0.08 (0.12)	0	18	44	18	6
3	TLR	201	0.100	14.72 (7.90)	3.02 (0.47)	0.09 (0.10)	100	21	40	24	11
	PDS	146	0.422 (0.181)	15.02 (7.90)	3.04 (0.46)	0.1 (0.10)	100	21	42	24	12
4	TLR	1087	0.107	13.97 (7.52)	3.03 (0.53)	0.08 (0.12)	26	24	40	28	13
	PDS	205	0.358 (0.217)	13.53 (7.11)	3.06 (0.51)	0.08 (0.11)	0	24	39	20	11
5	TLR	925	0.114	13.91 (8.47)	3.03 (0.49)	0.07 (0.13)	32	19	43	24	10
	PDS	206	0.368 (0.206)	11.44 (5.90)	3.05 (0.52)	0.07 (0.13)	0	21	44	22	6
6	TLR	313	0.099	12.74 (5.84)	3.11 (0.48)	0.1 (0.10)	0	19	38	23	11
	PDS	105	0.431 (0.173)	12.82 (5.20)	3.14 (0.51)	0.11 (0.11)	0	14	35	25	8
7	TLR	226	0.097	14.06 (7.08)	3.06 (0.59)	0.03 (0.13)	100	23	39	21	13
	PDS	99	0.384 (0.209)	13.28 (6.03)	3.16 (0.60)	0.06 (0.13)	100	21	37	26	7
All	TLR	5806	0.104	12.62 (7.04)	3.02 (0.50)	0.07 (0.12)	22	20	42	25	10
	PDS	1120	0.372 (0.198)	12.42 (6.49)	3.06 (0.60)	0.08 (0.12)	22	20	41	23	8

Outcomes for 5806 patient from seven historical trials of coronary stents conducted between 1993 and 1998 in the US are summarized in Table 1. These trials have been documented in refereed journals or are on record at the FDA (Serruys *et al.*,1994; Fischman *et al.*, 1994; Baim *et al.*, 2001a, 2001b; Leon *et al.*, 1998; Cutlip *et al.*, 1999 and FDA Pre-Market Approvals: P970020 and P970035). The stents comprising the trials have been approved for use, have very similar mechanical characteristics (all are balloon-expandable stainless steel 316 L stents), and are considered to be exchangeable.

The overall rate of TLR is 10.4% and the mean (standard deviation of) PDS is 0.37 (0.20). Seven patient covariates were considered important predictors of restenosis: the length of the lesion (Length); reference vessel diameter (Diameter); thickness of plaque as a fraction of diameter immediately after stent inflation (Thickness); enrolled as part of a single-arm Registry rather than as part of randomized two-arm trial (Registry); history of Diabetes-Mellitus (Diabetes); presence of diseaase in the left anterior descending coronary artery (location); and the number of diseased vessels (NumVes): 1, 2, or 3. Binary risk factors are coded 1 if true and 0 otherwise. Length, Thickness, and the binary risk factors are positively correlated with restenosis while Diameter is negatively correlated.

Note that Trials 1 and 6 do not contain registries, and in Trial 1 no patients were angiographically followed-up. Among patients with angiographic follow-up, the recruitment mode (Registry) was fixed within a, trials. In Trials 3 and 7, all patients followed-up were in a, registry, while in the other trials, no patient having angiographic follow-up was in a registry. Registry and the trial-level main effects are confounded with respect to PDS.

3. PROBLEM I: ESTIMATION OF THE OPC

Before design calculations can be considered, we firstly need to specify the model to be used for the analysis. The component of this model involving the data from the historical trials is the basis of the OPC.

3.1 Latent variable model for multivariate mixed outcomes

The preferred method of modeling multivariate mixed outcomes for medical device trials of coronary-artery stents is to specify independent models for the outcomes conditional on unobserved latent traits (O'Malley, Normand, and Kuntz, 2003). This avoids direct specification of a multivariate density, an onerous task when the multivariate normal distribution cannot be assumed. Each type of outcome may be related to its own latent trait, with the set of latent traits assumed to arise from a multivariate normal density (Dunson, 2000; Arminger and Küsters, 1988), or directly to a common latent trait (Samnel, Ryan, and Legler, 1997). Because latent traits can themselves depend on covariates a wide array of models are entertained. Latent variables can be incorporated at multiple levels of a model to account for correlation within clusters (Dunson, 2000). In this paper latent variables are only assumed at the patient level.

Let Y_{kij} and x_{kij} denote the kth $(k = 1,\dots,K)$ outcome variable and associated vector of covariates for the jth of m_i patients in the ith of n trials. The observations associated with the kth outcome concatenated across subjects and trials are denoted $\boldsymbol{Y}_k = (Y_{k11},\ldots,Y_{k1m},Y_{k21},\ldots,Y_{knm_n})$ and $x_k = (x_{k11},\ldots,x_{k1m_1},x_{k21},\ldots,x_{knm_n})$.

Hierarchical models are used to pool data from different trials and account for the clustering of the outcomes within trials. At the first level the outcome variable Y_{kij} is assumed to follow an exponential family

$$f(Y_{kij}|\eta_{kij},\phi_{ki}) = \exp\left\{\frac{Y_{kij}\eta_{kij} - d(\eta_{kij})}{\phi_{ki}} + c_k(Y_{kij},\phi_{ki})\right\},$$

where

$$E(Y_{kij}|\eta_{kij},\phi_{ki}) = d'(\eta_{kij}), \quad \text{and} \quad \operatorname{var}(Y_{kij}|\eta_{kij},\phi_{ki}) = \phi_{ki}d''(\eta_{kij});$$

ϕ_{ki} is a scaler dispersion parameter; $c_k(Y_{kij},\phi_{ki})$ is a function of Y_{kij} and ϕ_{ki}. The natural parameter η_{kij} can depend on covariates, other outcomes, latent variables, and unknown parameters. Let $h_k(.)$,a monotone function onto $(-\infty,+\infty)$, denote the link function in the model for the kth outcome.

Let b_{ij} denote an unobserved latent trait associated with the jth patient in the ith trial and $\boldsymbol{B} = (b_{11},\ldots,b_{1m_1},b_{21},\ldots,b_{nm_n})$. We assume that the outcomes are conditionally independent given (b_{ij},Θ); that is

$$f(Y_{1ij},\ldots,Y_{Kij}|x_{1ij},\ldots,x_{Kij},b_{ij},\Theta) = \prod_{k=1}^{K} f_k(Y_{kij}|x_{kij},b_{ij},\Theta).$$

Write $x_{kij} = (u_{kij},z_{ij})$ where z_{ij} is a vector of covariates common to all outcomes, and u_{kij} is a vector of additional covariates related to outcome k. The expectation of Y_{Kij} is related to u_{kij} via the link function

$$h_k(\eta_{kij}) = \theta_{ki} + \beta_k' u_{kij} + \gamma_k b_{ij} \tag{1}$$

and to z_{ij} by

$$b_{ij} = \lambda' z_{ij} + \varepsilon_{ij},$$

where ε_{ij} is an independent random variable with distribution $f(\varepsilon_{ij})$. The latent variable regression parameter λ measures the overall effect of z_{ij} on the outcomes, while the specific effect of u_{kij} on Y_{kij} is quantified by β_k. Under this model, the ratio of the effect of any two component of z_{ij} is the same for all outcomes.

3.1.1 Model identifiability

Model identifiability is a concern with latent variable models due to the abundance of parameters. In the model considered here, a unique parameter representing a latent variable is attached to every observation. Caution must be exercised to avoid non-identifiability by virtue of introducing too many unrestricted parameters. A model that is not identifiable by the data is one for which different choices of parameters lead to the same fit.

The model in (1) is clearly non-identifiable if u_{kij} and z_{ij} have covariates in common and the associated parameters are unconstrained. This problem can be avoided by requiring that u_{kij} and z_{ij} are disjoint. A weaker condition is to require that $\beta_{kj} = \beta_{1j}\,(k = 1,\ldots,k)$ for all covariates in u_{kij} that also appear in z_{ij}.

The rth moment of $h_k(\eta_{kij})$ is an affine function of $\gamma_k E\left[\varepsilon_{ij}^r\right]$. Therefore, the model is non-identifiable when $f(\varepsilon_{ij})$ depends on unknown parameters. We set $f(\varepsilon_{ij})$ equal to the parameter free standard normal density function. Because $\gamma = (\gamma_1,\ldots\gamma_k)$ and λ can be multiplied by -1 without affecting the model, the sign of one term must be fixed.

These conditions are usually sufficient to identify location-scale models such as the one considered here. However, if some outcomes have one-parameter distributions, such as the Bernoulli distribution, then at least one additional constraint will be required to identify γ (see Section 4).

3.2 Higher order components of model

The second level of the hierarchical model describes the relationship among the trial- main effects. We assume that the trial-main effects for outcome k, θ_k, are exchangeable conditional on the covariates. This means that $\Pr\left(\theta_{k1} < d_{(k1)},\ldots\theta_{kn} < d_{(kn)} \middle| x_{kij}\right)$ is the same for all permutations of $\{(k1),\ldots,(kn)\}$ (Berger, 1985; Lad, 1996), and is equivalent to assuming that θ_k contains a random sample of trial effects for trials of the same type. We assume that

$$\theta_{ki} \overset{ind}{\sim} f\left(\mu_k, \tau_k^2\right), i = 1,\ldots,n, \text{ for } k = 1,\ldots,K,$$

where μ_k and τ_k^2 are location and scale parameters respectively. Note that because the trial-main effects are surrogates for any unmeasured confounding variables, they are essentially trial-level latent variables (Dunson, 2000). Uncertainty in the model parameters is specified at the third stage of a three-level hierarchical model, and completes the specification of the prior distribution of the model parameters.

3.3 Model fitting

Let $\phi_k = (\phi_{k1},\ldots,\phi_{km}), \theta_k = (\theta,\beta,\phi,\gamma,\mu,\tau)_k$, and $\Theta = (\theta_1,\ldots,\theta_K,\lambda)$. By our earlier assumption the latent variables $\boldsymbol{B}$ are independent of Θ. Bayesian inference is, therefore, based on the posterior distribution of the unknowns given by:

$$f(\Theta,\boldsymbol{B}|Y,X) = \frac{f(Y|X,\Theta,\boldsymbol{B})f(\boldsymbol{B})}{f(Y|X)},$$

where $f(Y|X) = \int_{\Theta B} f(Y,X|\Theta,\boldsymbol{B})f(\Theta)f(\boldsymbol{B})d\Theta d\boldsymbol{B}$ is the marginal distribution of the data, $Y = (Y_1,\ldots,Y_k)$ and $X = (x_1,\ldots,x_K)$.

In general, analytic derivation of the posterior distribution is not possible because $f(Y|X)$ cannot be computed in closed form. This necessitates the use of numerical methods for model fitting. We use Markov Chain Monte Carlo (MCMC) implemented by the Gibbs Sampler (German and German, 1984; Gelfand and Smith, 1990) and the Metropolis-Hastings Algorithm (Metropolis *et al.*, 1953; Hastings, 1970).

3.4 Objective performance criterion (OPC)

The OPC is generically defined as a summary outcome measure for a population characterized by $X_{n+1} = \left(x_{1(n+1)},\ldots,x_{k(n+1)}\right)$, conditional on the parameters Θ from the historical trials. In this paper, the OPC is defined in terms of the marginal expected value of hypothetical outcomes at specific values of X_{n+1} or from associated populations of patients. Let $b_{n+1} = \left(b_{(n+1)1},\ldots,b_{(n+1)m_{n+1}}\right)$, and $Y_{n+1} = \left(Y_{1(n+1)},\ldots,Y_{K(n+1)}\right)$, where

$Y_{k(n+1)} = \left(Y_{k(n+1)1}, \ldots, Y_{k(n+1)m_{n+1}}\right)$, denote hypothetical latent variables, and hypothetical outcomes associated with these m_{n+1} patients.

There are two major scenarios under which OPC are computed. In the first instance $Y_{k(n+1)}$ is know, a situation that arises when X_{n+1} are covariates contained in the historical data (e.g. $X_{n+1} = X$), or at the completion of a trial. In this case the posterior distribution of b_{n+1} is used to compute the OPC, which summarizes the outcomes in the historical data in the former case, and predicts the outcome for patient enrolled in the new trial assuming that they had instead been enrolled in the historical trials, in the latter case. The other major scenario arises when nothing is known about b_{n+1}; it is then assumed that $b_{(n+1)j} \overset{ind}{\sim} f\left(b_{(n+1)j}\right)$. The resulting OPC tend to be used as industry standards as they are not specific to particularly patients but rather to the populations of all patients with a particular value of covariate.

Because the intercepts of the linear predictors, $\{\theta_{ki}\}_{1:n}$, vary across trials a model for weighting or sampling the trials is required in order to average over them. This renders a plethora of ways of defining the OPC. Ad-hoc methods such as assigning the trials equal weights could be used, yielding an external weighted average. Instead for the purpose of such averaging we may assume $\theta_{k(n+1)} = \sum_i^n \theta_{ki}/n, \theta_{k(n+1)} = \mu_k$, or $\theta_{k(n+1)} \overset{ind}{=\sim} f\left(\mu_k, \tau_k^2\right)$, depending on the intended application. In the latter case, $\theta_{k(n+1)}$ is assumed exchangeable with $\{\theta_{ki}\}_{1:n}$. However, this assumption may not be appropriate in the analysis of a new trial (see section 5).

3.4.1 OPC for a single patient

The OPC for patients with covariates equal to $x_{k(n+1)j}$ is defined as the marginal expected value of $Y_{k(n+1)}$. When nothing is known about $b_{(n+1)j}$, the OPC is

$$OPC_k\left(x_{k(n+1)j}, \Theta\right) = \int_{\theta_{k(n+1)}, b_{(n+1)j}} E\left[Y_{k(n+1)j} \middle| x_{k(n+1)j}, b_{(n+1)j}, \theta_{k(n+1)}, \Theta\right]$$
$$\cdot f\left(b_{(n+1)j}\right) f\left(\theta_{k(n+1)} \middle| \mu_k, \tau_k^2\right) d\theta_{k(n+1)} db_{(n+1)j}. \quad (2)$$

If the corresponding outcomes are observed and knowledge of $b_{(n+1)j}$ is to be used to compute the OPC, the posterior distribution of $b_{(n+1)j}$ given (Y_{n+1}, X_{n+1}) is used in (2).

The OPC for a specific covariate is useful when the covariate represents a standard patient. A regulatory agency such as the FDA might use such a patient to define a standard at which to monitor the performance of an industry over time.

3.4.2 OPC for multiple patients

The OPC for a specific group of patients in X_{n+1} is the average OPC over the associated covariates. Let S_g denote the set of patients in X_{n+1} corresponding to a subgroup g. The OPC for S_g is given by:

$$OPC_k\left(S_g,\Theta\right)=\frac{1}{N_g}\sum_{j=1}^{m_{n+1}} I\left(j\in S_g\right)OPC_k\left(x_{k(n+1)j},\Theta\right),$$

where $N_g=\sum_{j=1}^{m_{n+1}} I\left(j\in S_g\right)$ is the number of patients in S_g and $I(.)$ is the indicator function.

When $S_g = X_{n+1}$ the OPC measures the average expected outcome for a population of patients described by the empirical distribution of X_{n+1}. The OPC for a population in which the weight of S_g is $w_g\left(\sum w_g=1; w_g\geq 0\right)$ is defined as

$$\mathrm{OPC}_k\left(S_g,w_g,\Theta\right)=\sum_{g=1}^{m} w_g OPC_k\left(S_g,\Theta\right). \quad (3)$$

3.4.3 Transformed outcome OPC

The OPC may also be defined on the scale of the linear predictor. For example, take $\mathrm{OPC}=\mu=(\mu_1,\mu_2)$.For outcomes modeled using an identity link function, the OPC μ equals the expected outcome for a hypothetical patient with the average covariate. Because μ does not depend directly on the covariates, and henceforth applies simultaneously to all values of the covariates, it is a convenient measure to use in hypothesis testing. The value of this measure of OPC is largely for comparison, rather than setting industry standard for which measures of OPC that are on the scale of the outcome often make more sense.

3.4.4 Estimation of the OPC

The estimator of the OPC is its posterior mean, given by

$$\hat{\mathrm{OPC}}_k\left(x_{k(n+1)j},Y,X\right) = \int_{\Theta,\theta_{k(n+1)},b_{(n+1)j}} \mathrm{OPC}_k\left(x_{k(n+1)j},b_{(n+1)j},\theta_{k(n+1)},\Theta\right) \cdot f\left(b_{(n+1)j},\theta_{k(n+1)},\Theta \mid Y,X\right) d\Theta d\theta_{k(n+1)} db_{(n+1)j}.$$

The precision of the estimated OPC can be displayed using credibility ellipsoids (in two or three dimension), and is summarized by posterior standard deviation and correlations.

4. ESTIMATION OF THE OPC FOR CORONARY-ARTERY STENTS

We apply the latent variable model in (1) to the coronary stent data summarized in Table 1. Assign $k=1$ to target lesion restenosis (TLR), the binary outcome, and $k=2$ to proportion diameter stenosis (PDS), the continuous outcome distributions are Bernoulli and Gaussian respectively, and logistic identity link functions are assumed.

The vector x_{1ij} is comprised of the eight covariates summarized in Table 1 (Length, Diameter, Thickness, Registry Diabetes, Location, and Twoo and Three Diseased Vessels). Preliminary investigations (O'Malley, Normand and Kuntz, 2003) indicated that allowing β to vary among trials failed to improve the model fit. A random intercepts model (Atkinson,1997) appears adequate for these data.

The vector x_{2ij} is the same as x_{1ij} but with Registry omitted because it is confounded with the trial-main effects for PDS. Similarly, u_{1ij} and u_{2ij} differ only by the presence or absence of Registry. The covariates (including the latent variable) are centered, aligning the trial main-effects θ_{1i} and θ_{2i} with the expected outcomes for a hypothetical patient having the average covariate.

The first level of the hierarchical model is

$$f\left(Y_{1ij} \mid \pi_{ij}\right) = \pi_{ij}^{Y_{1ij}}\left(1-\pi_{ij}\right)^{1-Y_{1ij}},$$

$$f\left(Y_{2ij}\mu_{ij},\sigma_i^2\right) = \frac{1}{\left(2\pi\sigma_i^2\right)^{1/2}}\exp\left\{-\frac{\left(Y_{2ij}-\mu_{ij}\right)^2}{2\sigma_i^2}\right\}.$$

We estimate the model, denoted LVM, in which $\mu_{kij} = x_{kij}$ and $z_{ij}=0$. The resulting model is given by

$$\text{logit}\left(\pi_{1ij}\right)=\theta_{1i}+\beta_1'x_{1ij}+\gamma_1 b_{ij}$$
$$\mu_{ij}=\theta_{2i}+\beta_2'x_{2ij}+\gamma_2 b_{ij}$$
$$b_{ij}=\varepsilon_{ij}\sim N(0,1).$$

To make LVM identifiable by the data we set $\gamma_1=1$, thereby fixing the scale of the latent variable effects. Because PDS is not measured for any patients in trial 1, θ_{21} cannot be estimated from the data and is omitted from LVM. Finally, $b_{ij}=0$ and terms involving Y_{2ij} are omitted from the likelihood function if PDS was not measured for the jth patient in the ith trial.

4.1 Prior distributions

The components of θ_1 and θ_2 are assumed to be exchangeable between trials, implying no preference for any particular stent. For simplicity, prior independence is assumed between θ_1 and θ_2 even though it seems likely that these terms will be correlated (for example, a well conducted trial would be expected to led to better results on both outcomes than a poorly performed trial). Because prior independence does not imply posterior independence, this assumption had little effect on the analysis. The population from which θ_1 and θ_2 are drawn is represented by a normal probability distribution, given by

$$\theta_{ki}\overset{ind}{\sim}N\left(\mu_k,\tau_k^2\right),\text{ for } i=1,\ldots,n=7,k=1,2$$

The remaining parameters are assigned independent non-informative prior distributions: $p(\beta_k)\sim N(0,10^6)$, $p(\sigma_i^2)\sim IG(10^3, 10^3)$, $p(\gamma_2)\sim N(0,10^6)$, $p(\mu_k)\sim N(0,10^6)$, and $\tau_k^2\sim IG\left(10^{-3},10^{-3}\right),(i=1,\ldots,7;k=1,2)$. Gaussian and inverse-gamma priors are convenient because they are conjugate to Gaussian and gamma(chi-square) likelihood functions. The posterior distribution is well defined because the prior is a proper density, and dominated by the data because the prior variances are very large.

A non-informative prior was assumed because in practice it is easier to justify to regulatory agencies than a prior incorporating subjective prior information. The results were robust to the prior assumed for the patient level parameters $\left[\theta_k,\beta_k,\sigma_i^2,\gamma_k\left(i=1,\ldots 7;k=1,2\right)\right]$. This was understandable given by the large amount of data pooled within each trial. However , with only seven trials, the results were not surprisingly much more sensitive to the choice of prior for the trial-level parameters $\left[\mu_k \text{ and } \tau_k^2 \left(k=1,2\right)\right]$.

Techniques for model fitting are described in O'Malley, Normand, and Kuntz (2003), and the conditional posterior distributions are presented in Appendix A.

4.2 Results

4.2.1 Fitted models

The estimated posterior means and standard deviations of the model parameters revealed that where was relatively little variation in the trial main effects (O'Malley, Normand, and Kuntz,2003). This is understandable given that the stents tested in these trials previously satisfied equivalence tests. The posterior means were in the range -2.55 to -2.20 for TLR and 0.355 to 0.415 for PDS. The posterior means of τ_k^2 were 0.045 $(k=1)$ and 0.002$(k=2)$, providing further indication of the stability of the model between trials.

The strongest predictors of both outcomes were Thickness, Diameters, Length, and Diabetes. Relative effect sizes ranged from 3.1 to 10.5 for TLR and 2.23 to 7.2 for PDS (O'Malley, Normand, and Kuntz, 2003). Location was a moderately strong predictor with patients having disease in the left anterior descending coronary artery at greater risk than other patients. Patients with more diseased vessels were at more risk of TLR but did not have higher average . values of PDS. Only Registry did not have an impact on either outcome.

The correlation between the outcomes is reflected in γ_2; the posterior mean of $\gamma_2 = 0.173\,(0.005)$ indicating that a strong positive correlation persists between the outcomes. This makes if clear that multivariate modeling has the potential to yield results that are more precise than those from a univariate model.

4.2.2 Estimating the OPC

The OPC is computed for three scenarios that arise often in practice: 1) the OPC is required for a historical data set; 2) the OPC is required for a subgroup of patients in a historical data set; 3) the OPC is required for a population with a different distribution of patient characteristics than in a historical data set.

The OPC for the coronary stent data set is computed by setting $X_{n+1} = X$, the complete set of covariates from the historical trials. This is equivalent to computing the OPC based on the empirical distribution of the covariates for the historical trials. Because outcomes are available, the posterior distribution of the latent variables was used to compute the OPC.

The first scenario arises when a regulatory agency, such as the FDA, wants to establish industry standards that will be used for future stent trials. Such standards can be provided in the form of performance guidelines to potential trialists. The posterior mean of OPC (reported in Table 2) is (TLR,PDS) = (0.102,0.384), with posterior standard deviation (0.008,0.020), and posterior correlation 0.016.

Table 2 also contains the OPC for the six subgroups of patients in X formed from Diabetes and the Number of diseased vessels (NumVes). The posterior mean of the TLR component of the OPC is sensitive to both Diabetes and NumVes, while the PDS component is sensitive only to Diabetes. Diabetics with three diseased vessels have the greatest risk of TLR and experience the highest values of PDS, while non-diabetics with a single diseased vessel are al least risk. Figure 1 displays the 95% credibility ellipsoids of the OPC for each subgroup. The major axis indicates the direction of the correlation between the components (positive in each case), while the area of the ellipse measures the variability of the OPC (higher for Diabetics and increasing with Num-Ves).

Table 2. Estimated objective performance criteria (OPC) for coronary-artery stents. The OPC is the vector with first component and second components TLR and PDS respectively. The entries for each cell defined by the number of diseased vessels and diabetes status are: Row 1: Posterior mean of OPC [=(TLR,PDS)]; Row 2: Posterior standard deviation of OPC, and posterior correlation between the TLR and PDS components of the OPC; Row 3: the number of patients (total, followed-up) in the 7 historical trials. The bottom segment presents the OPC averaged over all patients directly using the historical data (unweighted), and for a population having different distribution of the number of diseased vessels and prevalence of diabetes (weighted).

Diseased Vessels		Non diabetics TLR	PDS	Correlation	Diabetics TLR	PDS	Correlation
One	Mean	0.086	0.375		0.122	0.424	
	SD	(0.008)	(0.020)	0.042	(0.013)	(0.023)	0.065
	N	3068	628		698	148	
Two	Mean	0.106	0.372		0.143	0.423	
	SD	(0.011)	(0.022)	0.058	(0.017)	(0.024)	0.116
	N	1133	197		312	60	
Three	Mean	0.110	0.368		0.163	0.427	
	SD	(0.014)	(0.027)	0.063	(0.0224)	(0.030)	0.080
	N	433	69		126	18	

Overall		Unweighted TLR	PDS	Correlation	Weighted TLR	PDS	Correlation
	Mean	0.102	0.384		0.117	0.398	
	SD	(0.008)	(0.020)	0.016	(0.010)	(0.020)	0.036
	N	5806	1120		5806	1120	

In practice, physicians can use tables and illustrations (like Table 2 and Figure 1 as a reference tool to help them to determine if coronary-artery stenting is in the best interest of the patient. Alternative therapies, for instance Brachytherapy, may be preferred if the patient has a high likelihood of experiencing a poor outcome. In addition to establishing risk strata for individual patients, clinical trialists may use this information to determine the expected outcomes under a variety of clinical conditions in order to design an adequately powered clinical trial.

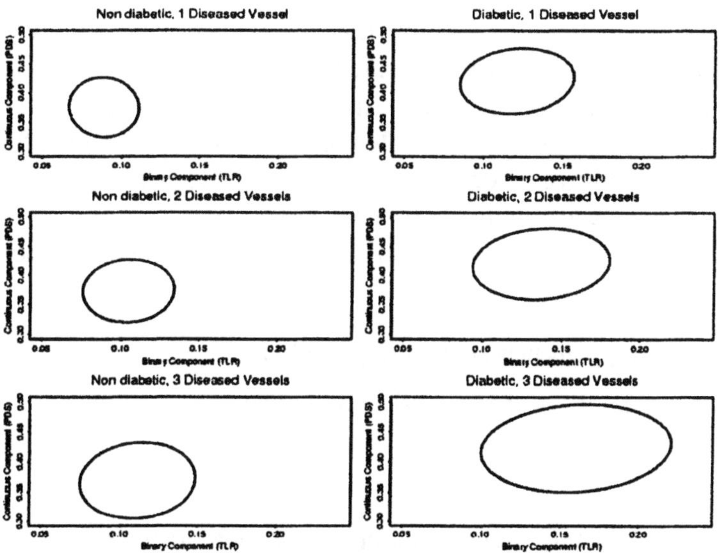

Figure 1.: 95% credibility ellipsoids of the OPC (with first and second components TLR and PDS respectively) stratified by diabetes and the number of diseased vessels for patients in the historical trials using LVM. The posterior mean, standard deviation, and correlation coefficient of OPC =(TLR,PDS) range from (0.086, 0.375), (0.008, 0.020), and 0.042 respectively for non-diabetics with 1 diseased vessel; to (0.163, 0.427), (0.022, 0.030), and 0.080 respectively for diabetics with 3 diseased vessels.

The methodology proposed provides a flexible solution to estimation of restenosis outcomes under conditions of varying reference populations and study samples. This will allow manufacturers and clinicians to evaluate important health care issues such as clinical utility and cost-effectiveness. For example, suppose that a stent manufacturer and clinical advisors wish to estimate the outcomes of a new coronary stent intended for a population characterized by heavy athersclerotic burden, in which 50% of the patients will have diabetes, and 20% and 10% will have 2 or 3 vessel coronary disease respectively. The posterior mean, standard deviation, and correlation of the binary and continuous components of the OPC for this new population are found (using Equation (3)) to be (0.117,0.398),(0.010, 0.20), and 0.036, respectively. Because the posterior means of the OPC are higher than when

$X_{n+1} = X$, a study involving such a population should allow for higher rates of TLR and values of PDS.

5. PROBLEM II: BAYESIAN SAMPLE SIZE AND POWER CALCULATIONS

To simplify matters, we assume that the analysis only involves a single binary outcome, namely TLR. Therefore, the indice for outcome is omitted, and because it cannot be identified , the latent variables b_{ij} is removed from the model. Furthermore, because Registry did not appear to influence the outcomes, it is removed from the model of the historical data. The model is otherwise the same as that in Section 3.1.

The outcomes for a new $(n+1)$th trial of m_{n+1} patients are described by

$$Y_{(n+1)j} \mid x_{(n+1)j}, \theta_{n+1}, \beta \overset{ind}{\sim} \text{Bernoulli}\left(Y_{ij} \mid \pi_{(n+l)j}\right) \text{ where}$$
$$\text{logit}\left(\pi_{(n+1)j}\right) = \theta_{n+1} + \beta' x(n+1j) \text{ for all } j \text{, and}$$
$$\theta_{n+1} \sim N\left(0, 10^6\right).$$

Because we ultimately want to compare the outcomes from the new trial with the outcomes from the historical trials and do not want to favor either hypothesis in the model specification, θ_{n+1} is a-priori independent of $\{\theta_i\}_{1:n}$.

In a generalized linear models framework, it is natural for hypotheses to be constructed on the scale of the linear predictor. The non-inferiority test

$$\mathcal{H}_0 : \theta_{n+1} \geq \bar{\theta}_h + \delta_0 \text{ versus } \mathcal{H}_A : \theta_{n+1} < \bar{\theta}_h + \delta_0 \text{,} \tag{4}$$

where $\bar{\theta}_h = \sum_{i=1}^{n} \theta_i / n$, and $\delta_0 > 0$ is the minimum clinically significant difference on the log-odds scale, is assumed. This designates $\bar{\theta}_h$ as the OPC. At a fixed value of the covariates, the log-odds ratio of the outcomes in the new and historical trials reduces to $\theta_{n+1} - \bar{\theta}_h$. Hence, the test in Equation (4) applies to all patients. Although (4) does not involve (β, μ, τ^2), these parameters affect the outcome and therefore impact the power of the test.

An alternative test is obtained by replacing $\bar{\theta}_h$ with μ in (4). This is appropriate when the historical trials represent a sample from a population of the same type of trials.

5.1 Decision rule

We use the test defined in Equation (4) with the decision rule: conclude $\mathcal{H}_A$ if the posterior probability of $\mathcal{H}_A$ exceeds $1-\alpha$. Let $\boldsymbol{D}_h$ denote all historical data, $\boldsymbol{D}_h = \{Y_{ij}, x_{ij}, i=1,...n, j=1,...m_i\}$. The trial main effects are concatenated in $\theta = (\theta_h, \theta_{n+1})$ where $\theta_h = (\theta_1, ...\theta_n)$ is the vector of random effects for the historical trials, and remaining parameters are denoted by $\xi = (\beta, \mu, \tau^2)$. Further, let $\Theta_A = \left\{\theta : \theta_{n+1} < \bar{\theta}_h + \delta_0\right\}$ be the set of values of θ for which $\mathcal{H}_A$ holds. Then $\mathcal{H}_A$ is concluded if

$$\Pr(\mathcal{H}_A \mid \boldsymbol{Y}_{n+1}, \boldsymbol{X}_{n+1}, \boldsymbol{D}_h) = \frac{\int_{\theta \epsilon \Theta_A, \xi} f(\boldsymbol{Y}_{n+1} \mid \boldsymbol{X}_{n+1}, \theta_{n+1}, \xi) f(\theta_{n+1}) f(\theta_h, \xi \mid \boldsymbol{D}_h) d(\xi, \theta)}{f(\boldsymbol{Y}_{n+1} \mid \boldsymbol{X}_{n+1}, \boldsymbol{D}_h)} \geq 1-\alpha,$$

where

$$f(\boldsymbol{Y}_{n+1} \mid \boldsymbol{X}_{n+1}, \boldsymbol{D}_h) = \int_{\theta, \xi} f(\boldsymbol{Y}_{n+1} \mid \boldsymbol{X}_{n+1}, \theta_{n+1}, \xi) f(\theta_{n+1}) f(\theta_h, \xi \mid \boldsymbol{D}_h) d(\xi, \theta)$$

is the marginal distribution of $(\boldsymbol{Y}_{n+1} \mid \boldsymbol{X}_{n+1}, \boldsymbol{D}_h)$. The set of values of $\boldsymbol{Y}_{n+1}$ for which $\mathcal{H}_A$ is concluded, given $(\boldsymbol{X}_{n+1}, \boldsymbol{D}_h)$, is denoted by

$$\mathcal{R}_A(\boldsymbol{X}_{n+1}, \boldsymbol{D}_h) = \{\boldsymbol{Y}_{n+1} : \Pr(\mathcal{H}_A \mid \boldsymbol{Y}_{n+1}, \boldsymbol{X}_{n+1}, \boldsymbol{D}_h) \geq 1-\alpha\}.$$

The space identified by $\mathcal{R}_A = \mathcal{R}_A(\boldsymbol{X}_{n+1}, \boldsymbol{D}_h)$ is often referred to as the rejection region.

5.2 Determining power

The power of the trial at $(\boldsymbol{X}_{n+1}, \theta, \xi)$ is the integral of $(\boldsymbol{Y}_{n+1} \mid \boldsymbol{X}_{n+1}, \theta, \xi)$, the likelihood function for the outcomes in the new trial, over $\mathcal{R}_A$. Is given by:

$$\text{pow}(\boldsymbol{X}_{n+1}, \theta, \xi \mid \boldsymbol{D}_h) = \int_{\boldsymbol{Y}_{n+1} \epsilon \mathcal{R}_A(\boldsymbol{X}_{n+1}, \boldsymbol{D}_h)} f(\boldsymbol{Y}_{n+1} \mid \boldsymbol{X}_{n+1}, \theta, \xi) d\boldsymbol{Y}_{n+1}. \tag{5}$$

The expression obtained in (5) is a function on unknown parameters (θ,ξ) and future covariates X_{n+1}. In a traditional power calculation, specific values would be substituted for (θ,ξ), and for terms involving X_{n+1}. Our approach is more general in that the uncertainty in these terms is incorporated.

Let $w(X_{n+1},\theta,\xi \mid D_h) = w(X_{n+1} \mid D_h)\, w(\theta,\xi \mid X_{n+1},D_h)$ be a probability distribution function, representing the importance of different values of (X_{n+1},θ,ξ). To avoid ambiguity with the probability distributions involved in the analysis of the trial, we refer to $w(.)$ as a parameter weighting distribution.

Uncertainty in (θ,ξ) is incorporated by integrating the product of $\text{pow}(X_{n+1},\theta,\xi \mid D_h)$ and $w(\theta,\xi \mid X_{n+1},D_h)$ over $\theta \in \Theta_A$ and ξ, yielding

$$\text{pow}(X_{n+1},D_h) = \int_{\theta\in\Theta_A,\xi} \text{pow}(X_{n+1},\theta,\xi \mid D_h)\, w(\theta,\xi \mid X_{n+1},D_h)\, d(\theta,\xi). \qquad (6)$$

Equation (6) computes power for fixed values of the covariate vectors in X_{n+1}, corresponding to hypothetical patients in the new trial. To incorporate uncertainty in X_{n+1}, $\text{pow}(X_{n+1} \mid D_h)$ is averaged over $w(X_{n+1} D_h)$ to give the power of the trial for sample size m_{n+1}:

$$\text{pow}(m_{n+1} \mid D_h) = \int_{X_{n+1}} \text{pow}(X_{n+1} \mid D_h)\, w(X_{n+1} \mid D_h)\, dX_{n+1} \qquad (7)$$

Figure 2 is a flow diagram describing the sequence of calculations used to compute power at a given sample size. This illustrates how the design problem is essentially transformed to an estimation problem. The historical data are first analyzed to determine prior distributions from which data for the new trial is generated. Both the historical and new arms of the trial are then analyzed simultaneously to yield a simulated outcome: conclude $\mathcal{H}_0$ or conclude $\mathcal{H}_A$. After multiple simulations power is estimated as Monte Carlo average of the simulated outcomes.

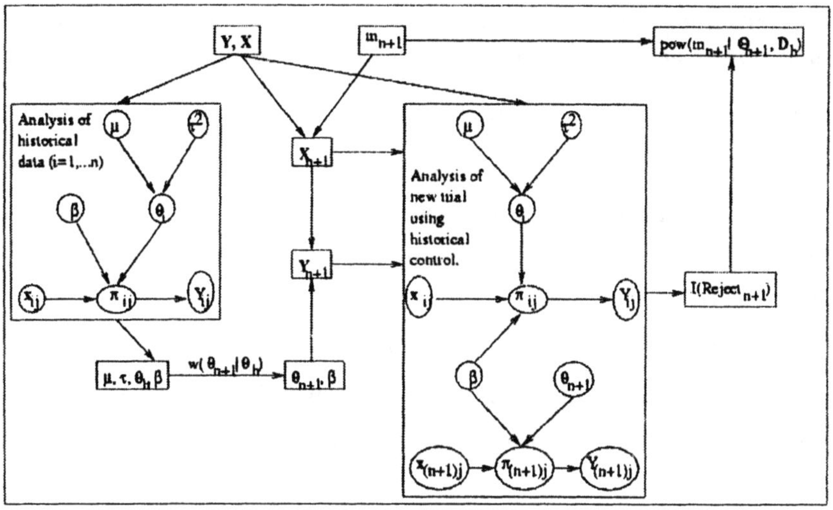

Figure 2. Power computation flow diagram. Ovals denote entities used to fit the model to either the historical data or to all of the data, while rectangles symbolize entities used to generate data for fitting the power function.

5.3 Parameter weighting distribution

In the trial of a new stent, θ_{n+1} (specifically the effect $\theta_{n+1} - \bar{\theta}_h$), is of primary interest while (X_{n+1}, θ_h, ξ) are nuisance terms. We weight (θ_h, ξ) by $f(\theta_h, \xi \mid D_h)$, the prior based on the historical data D_h, and take $w(X_{n+1} \mid D_h)$ to be the probability distribution of the covariates for the new trial, denoted by $f(X_{n+1} \mid D_h)$. This assumes that (θ_h, ξ) and X_{n+1} are independent given D_h, an assumption that seems reasonable. Thus, the parameter weighting distribution has the form

$$w(X_{n+1}, \theta, \xi \mid D_h) = f(X_{n+1} \mid D_h) f(\theta_h, \xi \mid D_h) w(\theta_{n+1} \mid X_{n+1}, \theta_h, \xi, D_h).$$

The covariate vectors in D_h may be used to determine $f(X_{n+1} \mid D_h)$. A simple, but often realistic choice, is defined by

$$\Pr(x_{(n+1)k} = x_{ij} \mid D_h) = \frac{1}{N}(i = 1, \ldots, n; j = 1, \ldots, m_i; k = 1, \ldots, m_{n+1}),$$

where $N = \sum_{i=1}^{n} m_i$.

In determining the sample size for a new trial, a common practice is to evaluate power at specific values of an effect size of interest, in this case $\theta_{n+1} - \bar{\theta}_h$. Let $\Theta_{n+1} \subseteq \Theta_A$ denote the set of values of θ for which $\theta_{n+1} - \bar{\theta}_h \in \delta_A(\theta)$. The set $\delta_A(\theta)$ can range from a single point δ_A (such that $\delta_A < \delta_0$), as for a traditional power calculation, to $(-\infty, \delta_o)$. The latter case yields the predictive power of Spiegelhalter and Freedman (1986) averaged over the uncertainty in ξ and X_{n+1}.

The parameter weighting distribution for θ_{n+1} is denoted $w(\theta_{n+1} | \theta_h)$ as it depends only on θ_h. This assigns positive weights to $\theta \in \Theta_{n+1}$ and zero weight to $\theta \notin \Theta_{n+1}$. In section 6 we assume that

$$w(\theta_{n+1} | \theta_h) = I(\theta \in \Theta_{n+1}), \tag{8}$$

where $I(.)$ is the indicator function, and consider point and interval specifications of $\delta_A(\theta)$.

5.4 Treatment effects and summary statistics decompositions

The relationship between power, sample size, and effect $c(\theta)$ or summary statistic $t(Y_{n+1}, X_{n+1}, D_h)$ of interest, may be computed using the same methodology as for general power and sample size calculation. This can be used to construct plots of power versus $c(\theta)$ or $t(Y_{n+1}, X_{n+1}, D_h)$ at fixed sample sizes, and plots of m_{n+1} versus $c(\theta)$ or $t(Y_{n+1}, X_{n+1}, D_h)$ at fixed power. The natural choice of $c(\theta)$ is $c(\theta) = \theta_{n+1} - \theta_h$. Plots involving summary statistics are generally most effective if $t(Y_{n+1}, X_{n+1}, D_h)$ is easy to understand and conceptualize; for example the mean outcome $\bar{Y}_{n+1}$.

To fit these plots, $c^S = c(\theta^S)$ and $t^S = \bar{Y}^S_{n+1}$ must be recorded at Step 1(c) of the algorithm presented in the section headed "Implementation" of O'Malley, Normand, Kuntz (2002); the revised algorithm is presented in Appendix B of these paper. To compute power as a function of $c(\theta)$, a smooth curve is fit to the data set $\{c^S, u^S\}_{1:S}$,while a power function depending on $t(Y_{n+1}, X_{n+1}, D_h)$ is obtained by fitting a smooth curve to

$\{t^S, u^S\}_{1:S}$. Plots whit $\Pr(\mathcal{H}_A \mid \Theta_{n+1}, D_h)$ as the dependent variable are obtained by substituting p^S (see Step 1(c) of the algorithm in Appendix B) for u^S.

5.5 Construction of plots

The outcome of the sth simulated analysis, u^S, is a Bernoulli random variable with expectation depending on the probability $\Pr(u^s = 1 \mid m_j^s) = \text{pow}(m_{n+1}^s, D_h \mid \Theta_{n+1})$. An analytic expression for the power function can be derived by fitting a regression model to $\{u^s, m_{n+1}^s\}_{1:s}$. The logistic regression model with

$$\Pr(u^S = 1 \mid m_j^s) = \frac{\exp\{\nu_0 + \nu_1 m_{n+1}^S + \nu_2 \log(m_{n+1}^S)\}}{1 + \exp\{\nu_0 + \nu_1 m_{n+1}^S + \nu_2 \log(m_{n+1}^S)\}} s = 1, 2, \ldots, S, \tag{9}$$

provides an accurate monotone-increasing estimate of the true power function for coronary stent trials. The parameter estimates of ν are substituted into (9) to evaluate power at different sample sizes. The smallest integer, $\hat{m}_{n+1}$, for which power is al least $1-\gamma$ is found by solving $\Pr(u = 1 \mid m_f) = 1 - \gamma$ for m_{n+1} and rounding upwards to the nearest integer. The solution typically needs to be obtained numerically.

Smooth curves describing the relationship between $\Pr(\mathcal{H}_A \mid Y_{n+1}, X_{n+1}, D_h)$ or the power of the trial and $t(Y_{n+1}, X_{n+1}, D_h)$ or $t(Y_{n+1}, X_{n+1}, D_h)$ are obtained by fitting the logistic regression models with

$$\text{pr}(p^S = 1 \mid t^s) = \frac{\exp(\nu_0 + \nu_1 m_{n+1}^S)}{1 + \exp(\nu_0 + \nu_1 m_{n+1}^S)}, \tag{10}$$

$$\text{pr}(u^S = 1 \mid t^s) \frac{\exp(\nu_0 + \nu_1 m_{n+1}^S)}{1 + \exp(\nu_0 + \nu_1 m_{n+1}^S)}, \tag{11}$$

respectively. Similarly, fitting the non linear regression models with

$$E(m_{n+1}^S \mid c^S) = \nu_0 c^S / (c^S + \nu_1)^{\mu_2}, \tag{12}$$

and

$$E\left(m_{n+1}^{S} \mid t^{S}\right) = \nu_0 t^{S} / \left(t^{S} + \nu_1\right)^{\mu_2}, \qquad (13)$$

yields smooth curves with $c(\theta)$ or $t(Y_{n+1}, X_{n+1}, D_h)$ as dependent variables. These equations are suggested from the fact that m_{n+1} increases asymptotically with $\theta_{n+1} - \bar{\theta}_h$ and $\bar{Y}_{n+1}$. The accuracy of the fit is remarkable (see Figure 4 and Figure 5).

Because $u(X_{n+1}, Y_{n+1}, \theta)$ typically cannot be evaluated analytically, numerical integration is required to determine if $Y_{n+1}^{S} \in \mathcal{R}_A\left(X_{n+1}^{S}, D_h\right)$. Appendix A in O'Malley, Normand, and Kuntz (2002) describes how samples are drawn from the posterior distribution of $\left(\theta_h, \theta_{n+1}, \beta, \mu, \tau^2\right)$. Monte Carlo methods can then be employed to compute $\Pr\left(\mathcal{H}_A \mid Y_{n+1}^{S}, X_{n+1}^{S}, D_h\right)$ and hence if $Y_{n+1}^{s} \in \mathcal{R}_A\left(X_{n+1}^{s}, D_h\right)$.

6. EXAMPLE: CORONARY- ARTERY STENTS

We assume a posterior probability of $1-\alpha = 00.95$ is required to conclude non-inferiority, take as $f\left(X_{n+1} \mid D_h\right)$ the empirical distribution of D_h given in (8), use $f\left(\theta_h, \xi \mid D_h\right)$ as the parameter weighting distribution for $\left(\theta_h, \xi\right)$, and as in (8) assume that $w\left(\theta_{n+1} \mid \theta_h\right)$ is the uniform distribution defined on the set Θ_{n+1}. Four specifications of $\delta_A(\theta)$ are used to illustrate the attainment of power as an unconditional function of m_{n+1}:

$w_1 : \delta_A(\theta) = \left\{\theta_{n+1} : \theta_{n+1} - \bar{\theta}_h\right\}$: the new stent is equivalent to the control stents.

$w_2 : \delta_A(\theta) = \left\{\theta_{n+1} : \theta_{n+1} - \bar{\theta}_h = 0.315\right\}$: the new stent is inferior to the control stents but not by an amount that is clinically significant.

$w_3 : \delta_A(\theta) = \left\{\theta_{n+1} : -1.50 \le \theta_{n+1} - \bar{\theta}_h < 0\right\}$: the new stent is better than the control stents.

$w_4 : \delta_A(\theta) = \left\{\theta_{n+1} : -0.87 \le \theta_{n+1} - \bar{\theta}_h < 0.63\right\}$: the new stent could be better or worse than the control stents.

Stochastic optimization was performed using data from two independent simulations. The simulation was conducted with 12 distinct values of m_{n+1} ranging from 5 to 800 (see Table 2) . the design points for the simulation experiment were skewed to the right because the power functions is more sensitive over small values of m_{n+1}. Precise estimates of the power were obtained by performing 1,000 simulations at each value of m_{n+1}, a total of $S = 12,000$ simulations. The standard error of estimates of power and sample size were evaluated using a non-parametric bootstrap (Efron, 1979) involving 250 bootstrap samples in which outcomes were sampled with replacement within the groups of 1,000 simulated outcomes associated with each distinct value of m_{n+1}.

6.1 Results

6.1.1 Estimates of optimal sample size

Point estimates of the optimal sample sizes based on Equation (9) are obtained by tracing the nominal level of power onto the m_{n+1} axis as depicted in Figure 3. The closeness of the fitted curve to the empirical estimates of power over the region $m_{n+1} > 50$, suggests that Equation (9) is a good model of the true power function. The power function under w_4 appears to have an asymptote around 0.9. because Equation (9) tends to 1 as $m_{n+1} \to \infty$, over-prediction of power is likely to occur at large m_{n+1}.

From Figure 3, the optimal sample size based on the Bayesian hierarchical covariate-adjusted model when $1-\gamma = 0.80$ is 136 subjects under w_1, and 234 subjects under w_4. The standard errors associated with these evaluations, 3.054 and 16.89 respectively, are due to lack-of-fit of the model given in Equation (9), and the use of a finite number of simulations.

6.1.2 Decomposition of power calculation

As previously noted $c(\theta) = \theta_{n+1} - \bar{\theta}_h$ and $t(Y_{n+1}, X_{n+1}, D_h) = \bar{Y}_h$ are the effect size and summary statistic under consideration. Figure 4 displays power and the predictive value of $\Pr(\mathcal{H}_A \mid D_h)$ in terms of $\bar{Y}_{n+1}$ when $m_{n+1} = 200$ and $m_{n+1} = 550$ respectively. The smooth curves presented in Figure 4 are obtained by applying logistic regression to the models in (10) and (11) respectively. The larger the value of $\bar{Y}_{n+1}$ the lower the power of predictive value of $\Pr(\mathcal{H}_A \mid D_h)$.

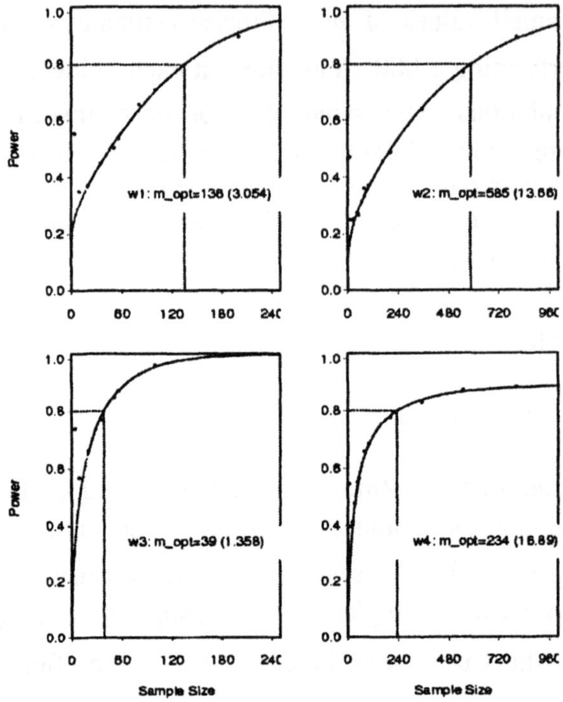

Figure 3. Bayesian power curve for the four uniform weight functions with positive weights over the regions; $\theta_{n+1} = \{\theta : \theta_{n+1} - \bar{\theta}_h = 0\}$ (w_1), $\theta_{n+1} = \{\theta : \theta_{n+1} - \bar{\theta}_h = 0.63/2\}$ (w_2), $\theta_{n+1} = \{\theta : -1.5 \le \theta_{n+1} - \bar{\theta}_h \le 0\}$ (w_3), $\theta_{n+1} = \{\theta : -0.87 \le \theta_{n+1} - \bar{\theta}_h \le 0.63\}$ (w_4). The historical control comprised of 5806 patients with $p_h = 0.104$. The optimal sample size at power 0.8 is displayed in each case. The power function has a broken line foe those values of m_{n+1} where the true power functions is highly disjointed.

The sensitivity of $\Pr(\mathcal{H}_A \mid D_h)$ to $\theta_{n+1} - \bar{\theta}_h$ or $\bar{Y}_{n+1}$ is much less than for the power probability because information is not dichotomized. If $\theta_{n+1} - \bar{\theta}_h = 0.4$, Figure 4 indicates that $\Pr(\mathcal{H}_A \mid D_h)$ is likely to be around 0.8, but that power will be less than 0.4. If $\bar{Y}_{n+1} = 0.120$ then power exceeds 0.8 and $\Pr(\mathcal{H}_A \mid D_h)$ is close to 1.

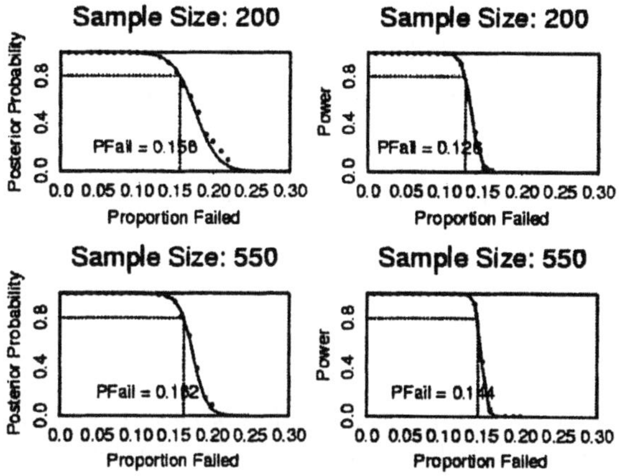

Figure 4. Plots of predictive probability of $\mathcal{H}_A$ and power versus $\bar{Y}_{n+1}$ when $m_{n+1} = 200$ and $m_{n+1} = 550$. The bullets denote the simulated probabilities used to fit the smooth curves. The values of $\theta_{n+1} - \bar{\theta}_h$ and $\bar{Y}_{n+1}$ corresponding to power 0.8 are displayed.

Table 3 presents the values of $c(\theta) = \theta_{n+1} - \bar{\theta}_h$ coherent with a given level of power at various m_{n+1}. If an organization was contemplating a trial of 200 patients, then to have power 0.8, they must assert that the effect is less than 0.119. If this is not the case, a larger sample size, such as 550 for which an effect as high as 0.341 is still coherent with power of at least 0.8, needs to be considered. A similar table can be constructed with m_{n+1} as subject. Our calculations revel that at $m_{n+1} = 200$ the predicted proportion of failures must be less than 0.127 in order for the trial at have power 0.8.

If power is fixed the relationship between $\theta_{n+1} - \bar{\theta}_h$ or $\bar{Y}_{n+1}$ and the value oh m_{n+1} required at given levels of power is more useful. The plots in Figure 5 display the relationship between m_{n+1} and $\theta_{n+1} - \bar{\theta}_h$ (top), and m_{n+1} and $\bar{Y}_{n+1}$ (bottom), for power 0.8 and 0.9; the smooth curves are obtained by applying linear regression to the models in (12) and (13) respectively. Plots of these form have been used to help determine appropriate values of m_{n+1} for coronary-artery stent trials. If $\bar{Y}_{n+1} = 0.13$, then $m_{n+1} = 236$ and $m_{n+1} = 289$ are necessary in order for the trial at have power at least 0.8 and 0.9 respectively. The value of m_{n+1} escalates as $\bar{Y}_{n+1}$ increases, until at near 0.16 it becomes impossible to conduct a trial with the required level of power. This happens because the outcomes associated with a predictive distribution for $\overline{Y}_{n+1}$ with mean 0.16 does not have a high likelihood of providing evidence sufficient to conclude $\mathcal{H}_A$.

Table 4 presents required values of m_{n+1} for more values of power. This depicts the fact that the required sample size for a specific level of power is very sensitive to prior expectation of $\overline{Y}_{n+1}$. If an organization predicted that $\overline{Y}_{n+1} = 0.11$, then a sample size of only 102 is required to achieve 0.8 power. However, if the new stent is such that $\overline{Y}_{n+1} = 0.15$ was expected, then a trial of 3603 patients is required.

Table 3 Values of $\theta_{n+1} - \theta_h$ (inner cells), the effect of interest, required to be coherent with the given sample size and power probability for the analysis of TLR.

Sample size	Power				
	0.5	0.6	0.7	0.8	0.9
5	-0.247	-0.543	-0.878	-1.294	-1.932
10	-0.212	-0.481	-0.778	-1.145	-1.7
20	-0.151	-0.374	-0.616	-0.909	-1.346
35	-0.075	-0.25	-0.435	-0.657	-0.985
50	-0.013	-0.154	-0.303	-0.48	-0.742
55	0.005	-0.127	-0.267	-0.433	-0.678
80	0.082	-0.018	-0.123	-0.249	-0.436
100	0.13	0.047	-0.04	-0.146	-0.304
200	0.276	0.232	0.181	0.119	0.022
350	0.375	0.345	0.309	0.263	0.192
550	0.436	0.41	0.379	0.341	0.28
800	0.474	0.448	0.419	0.384	0.328

Table 4. Sample sizes (inner cells) required for coherence with the given values of power and the predicted value of $\overline{Y}_{n+1}$, the sample proportion of TLR in a new trial.-indicates that based on the simulated data and conditional on the predicted sample mean being attained; it is not possible to obtain the required level of power at any sample size.

Y_{n+1}	Power				
	0.5	0.6	0.7	0.8	0.9
0.08	25	28	33	39	49
0.09	34	38	44	52	66
0.1	46	53	61	72	91
0.11	66	76	87	102	127
0.12	98	112	128	150	186
0.13	155	177	203	236	289
0.14	277	315	358	413	501
0.15	619	699	788	899	1075
0.16	2678	2935	3224	3603	4276
0.17	-	-	-	-	-
0.18	-	-	-	-	-

7. DISCUSSION

The current rapid pace of new technology turnover in the field of catheter-based coronary treatments is promising for both health care providers and patients who suffer from coronary disease. However, the randomized trial structure with its necessary lenghty duration cannot keep pace with the introduction and turnover of new stent generations.

The OPC is the expected outcome associated with approved devices, and may be used as the "control group" in the assessment of a new medical device. Grunkemeier, Starr, and Rahimtoola (1992); and Grunkemeier (1993) proposed exactly this in the area of heart valves. O'Malley, Normand, and Kuntz (2003) extended this idea in two directions: incorporating uncertainty in the OPC, and adjusting for confounding variables. We used a multivariate hierarchical regression model to estimate a bivariate OPC. Multivariate modeling permitted information to be shared between the outcomes. This was used to develop the OPC under a variety of scenarios. We have demonstrated that the OPC can be displayed graphically in the form of a confidence ellipsoid. It can be computed separately for soubgroups of a sample or population, or can be averaged over patients. Alternatively, the OPC for different types of patients can be presented on grids in which cells display the estimated OPC for the given type of patient.

The general methodology for sample size calculation can be adapted in several important directions. Most notably, criteria other than power may be used. Foe example, the probability of making a correct decision (between $\mathcal{H}_0$ and $\mathcal{H}_A$), or a utility function that offsets the cost of making an incorrect decision with the cost of sampling (see, for example, Müller and Parmigiani, 1995; Lindley, 1997), could serve as the basis of the calculations.

The strongest reasons for adopting our approach are practical rather than theoretical. Current methods for determining sample sizes often assume analyses that bear little resemblance to analyses that are appropriate for historically-controlled trials. This make the resulting calculations unreliable and can lead to trials that are either seriously under-or over-powered. Although analytic results are difficult to derive when intended analyses are complex, convenient solutions can be obtained through the use of large scale numerical integration.

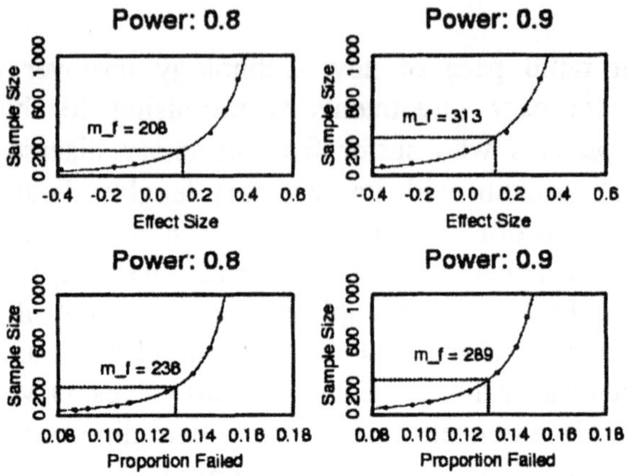

Figure 5. Plots of m_{n+1} versus $\theta_{n+1} - \overline{\theta}_h$ and versus $\overline{Y}_{n+1}$ for power 0.8 and 0.9. the bullets denote the empirical sample size values used to fit the smooth curves. The values of m_{n+1} corresponding to $\theta_{n+1} - \overline{\theta}_h = 0.13$ and $\overline{Y}_{n+1} = 0.13$ are displayed.

Finally we emphasize the importance of communicating the properties of a proposed trial to person with possibly little background in probability or statistics. Plots of power, or the predictive probability of $\mathcal{H}_A$, against an effect size or summary statistic of interest, have been suggested. Our experience with trials of coronary-artery stents has indicated that displaying the requirements or properties of a trial in terms of a summary statistic that is easy to conceptualize, such as the sample means, is most effective in obtaining internal and external approval for a trial. Like the general methodology, the uncertainty in nuisance parameters and unobserved covariates propagates through the computations, providing a platform for informed decision making.

Our work is ideally suited to trials of medical devices in which the time to realization of the primary endpoint is long relative to patient recruitment time, and where technological changes in the device proliferate at such a rate that the device life-cycle approaches that required for the conduct of a conventional randomized trial. However the approach has relevance to any field in which historical controls are used.

APPENDIX A: CONDITIONAL POSTERIOR DISTRIBUTION

We describe the conditional posterior distributions for the latent variable model denoted LVM model. (The conditional posterior distributions specific to the power and sample size calculations are presented in Appendix A of O'Malley, Normand, and Kuntz, 2002). The

LVM model is given by $f(Y_{1ij} \mid \pi_{ij}) = \text{Bernoulli}(\pi_{ij}), f(Y_{2ij} \mid \mu_{ij}, \sigma_i^2) = N(\mu_{ij}, \sigma_i^{\circ})$, where $\log\text{it}(\pi_{*}) = \theta_{1i} + \beta_1' x_{ij} + \gamma_1 b_{ij}, \mu_{ij} = \theta_{2i} + \beta_2' x_{ij} + \gamma_2 b_{ij}$, and $b_{ij} \sim N(0,1)$. The higher order components of the model are denoted as follows:

$\beta_k \sim N(b_k, V_k), \theta_{ki} \sim N(\mu_k, \tau_k^2), \ \gamma_1 = 1, \gamma_2 \sim N(g_2, w_2^2), \sigma_i^2 \sim IG(u_1, u_2), \mu_k \sim N(m_k, s_k^2), \tau_k^2 \sim IG(q_{k1}, q_2)$,

where N(.) denotes the normal density function, and IG(.) denotes the inverse-gamma density function. The Roman letters g_2, w_2^2, u_1, u_2 and $b_k, V_k, s_k^2, q_{k1}, q_{k2} (k = 1,2)$ denote parameters with assigned values.

Let $\tilde{X}_2$ be the matrix with rows $[e_i', x_{2ij}', b_{ij}](i = 2 \ldots, n; j = 1, \ldots, m_i)$, where e_i is the vector of length n-1 with (i-1)th element 1 and 0s elsewhere (recall that $\tilde{X}_2$ is devoid of data from the first trial because no patients were angiographically followed-up). Let $t_2 = (\mu_2 j', b_2', g_2)'$, where j is a vector of $n-1$ 1s, and $\tilde{V}_2$ be the block diagonal matrix defined by the n-1- dimensional identity matrix, V_2, and w_2^2. The conditional posterior distributions are given by

$$(\tau_1^2 \mid \cdot) \ \sim \ IG\left[q_{11} + \frac{n}{2}, \left\{\frac{1}{q_{12}} + \frac{1}{2}\sum_{i=1}^{n}(\theta_{1i} - \mu_1)^2\right\}^{-1}\right]$$

$$\left[q_{21} + \frac{n-1}{2}, \left\{\frac{1}{q_{22}} + \frac{1}{2}\sum_{i=2}^{n}\left(\theta_{2i} (\tau_2^2 \mid .) \ \sim \ \text{IG} - \mu_2\right)^2\right\}^{-1}\right]$$

$$(\mu_2 \mid .) \ \sim \ \text{N}\left(\frac{s_2^2 \sum_{i=2}^{n} \theta_{2i} + \tau_2^2 m_2}{(n-1)s_2^2 + \tau_2^2}, \frac{s_2^2 \tau_2^2}{(n-1)s_2^2 + \tau_2^2}\right)$$

$$(\sigma_i^2 \mid .) \ \sim \ \text{IG}\left[u_1 + \frac{m_{2i}}{2}, \left\{u_2 + \sum_{j=1}^{m_i}\left\{Y_{2i} - (\theta_{2i} + \beta_2' x_{2ij} + \gamma_2 b_{ij})\right\}^2\right\}^{-1}\right]$$

$$(\theta_2, \beta_2, \gamma_2 \mid .) \ \sim \ N\left[\left(\tilde{X}_2' \tilde{X}_2 + \tilde{V}_2^{-1}\right)^{-1}\left(\tilde{X}_2' Y_2 + t_2\right), \left(\tilde{X}_2' \tilde{X}_2 + \tilde{V}_2^{-1}\right)^{-1}\right]$$

$$(\theta_1, \beta_1 \mid \cdot) \ \propto \ \prod_{i,j}\left[\frac{\exp\{(\theta_{1i} + \beta_1^j x_{1ij} + \gamma_1 b_{ij}) Y_{1ij}\}}{1 + \exp(\theta_{1i} + \beta_1^j x_{1ij} + \gamma_1 b_{ij})}\right] \frac{\exp\{-(\beta_1 - b_1)' V_2 (\beta_1 - b_1)/2}{(\det V_2)^{1/2}}$$

$$\cdot \frac{\exp\left\{-\sum_{i=1}^{n}(\theta_{1i} - \mu_1)^2 / (2\tau_1^2)\right\}}{(\tau_1^2)^{n/2}}$$

$$(b_{ih} \mid .) \ \alpha \ \frac{\exp\left[(\theta_{1i} + \beta_1' x_{1ij} + \gamma_1 b_{ij}) Y_{1ij} - \left\{Y_{2ij} - (\theta_{2i} + \beta_2' x_{2ij} + \gamma_2 b_{ij})\right\}^2 / (2\sigma_i^2) - b_{ij}^2 / 2\right]}{1 + \exp(\theta_{1i} + \beta_1' x_{1ij} + \gamma_1 b_{ij})}$$

To maintain identifiability b_{ij} =0 if PDS is not measured for the jth patient in the ith trial.

APPENDIX B: NUMERICAL COMPUTATION ALGORITHM

The following algorithm outlines the simulation experiment used to produce the numerical results presented in this paper.

1. For simulation $s = 1,...S$:
   a) Select a positive integer m^s_{n+1} (determined from a designed experiment).
   b) Draw (i) X^s_{n+1} from $f(X_{n+1} \mid D_h)$, and (ii) (θ^s_h, ξ^s) from $f(\theta_h, \xi \mid D_h)$; followed by (iii) θ^s_{n+1} from $w(\theta_{n+1} \mid \theta^s_h)$; followed by (iv) y^s_{n+1} from $p(y_{n+1} \mid X^s_{n+1}, \theta^s_{n+1}, \xi^s)$.
   c) Compute $p^s = \Pr(\mathcal{H}_A \mid y^s_{n+1}, X^s_{n+1}, D_h)$, and record $u^s = I(p^s \geq 1\text{-}\alpha)$, $c^s = \theta^s_{n+1} - \theta^s_b$, and $t^s = \bar{Y}^s_{n+1}$.
2. Fit models to the simulated data $\{u^s, p^s, c^s, t^s, m^s_{n+1}\}_{1:S}$, and determine the optimal sample size or otherwise.

REFERENCES

ARMINGER G., KÜSTERS U. (1988). Latent trait models with indicators of mixed measurement level. In: Latent Trait and Latent Class Models (R Langeheine, J Rost, Ed.), New York: Plenum, 51-73.

ATKINSON D. (1997). Assessing non sampling errors in survey data through random intercept models. In: *American Statistical Association Proceedings of the Section on Survey Research Methods*, 401-406.

BAIM D.S., CUTLIP D.E., O'SHAUGHNESSY C.D., HERMILLER J.B., KEREJAKES D.J., GIANBARTOLOMEI A., KATZ S., LANSKY A.J., FITZPATRICK M., POPMA J.J., HO K.K.L., LEON M.B., KUNTZ R.E. (2001). Final results of a randomized trial comparing the NIR stent to the Palmaz-Schatz stent for narrowings in native coronary arteries. *American journal of Cardiology 87*, 152-156.

BAIM D.S., CUTLIP D.E., MIDEI M., LINNEMEIER T.J., SCHREIBER T., COX D., KEREIAKES D.J., POPMA J.J., ROBERTSON L., PRINE R., LANSKY A.J., HO K.K.L., KUNTZ, (2001). Final results of a randomized trial comparing the Multilink stent to the Palmaz-Schatz stent for narrowings in native coronary-arteries. *American journal of Cardiology 87*, 157-162.

BERGER JO (1985). Statistical Decision Theory and Bayesian Analysis, 2nd Edition. New York: Springer- Verlag.

CUTLIP D.E., LEON M.B., HO K.K., GORDON P.C., GIANBARTOLOMEI A., DIVER D.J., LASORDA D.M., WILLIAMS D.O., FITZPATRICK M.M., DESJARDIN A., POPMA J.J., KUNTZ R.E., BAIMS D.S. (1999). Acute and nine-month clinical outcomes after " suboptimal" coronary stenting: results from the Stent Anti-thrombotic Regimen Study (STARS) registry. *Journal of the American College of Cardiology 34*, 698-706.

DUNSON D.B. (2000) Bayesian latent variable models for clustered mixes outcomes,. *Journal of the Royal Statistical Society, Series B 62*, 355-366.

EFRON B (1979). Bootstrap methods: Another look at the jacknife, *The Annals of Statistic, 7*, 1-26.

FDA Pre-Market Approval P970020. ACS Multi-link TM coronary stent system (Guidant Corporation). http:// www.accessdata.fda.gov/scripts/cdrh/cdocs/cfPA/pma.cdm

FDA Pre-market Approval P970035. AVE Micro Stent II over-the-wire coronary stent system and AVE GFX (Medtronic AVE, Inc.). http//www.accessdata.fda.gov/scripts/cdrh/cfdocs/cfPMA/pma.cfm

FISCHMAN D.L., LEON M.B., BAIM D.S., SHATZ R.A., SAVAGE M.P., PENN I., DETRE K, VELTRI L., RICCI D., NOBUYOSHI M., CLEMAN M., HEISER R., ALMOND D., TEIRSTEIN P.S., FISH R.D., COLOMBO A., BRINKER J., MOSES J., SHAKNOVICH A., HIRSHFELD J., BAILEY S., ELLIS S., RAKE R., GOLDBERG S. (1994). A randomized comparison of coronary-stent placement and balloon angioplasty in the treatment of coronary disease. Stent Restenosis Study Investigators. *New England Journal oJ Medicine 331*, 496-501.

GELFAND A.E., SMITH A.F.M. (1990). Sampling based Approaches to calculating marginal densities. *Journa! of the American Statistica! Association 85*,398-409.

GEMAN S., GEMAN D. (1984). Stochastic relaxation, Gibbs distributions and the Bayesian restoration of images. *IEEE Transactions on Pattern Analysis and Machine Intelligence 6*, 721-41.

GERSH B.J., FISHER L.D., SHAFF H.V., RAHIMTOOLA S.H., REEDER G.S., FRATER R.W.M. MOGOON D.C. (1986). Issues concerning the clinical-evaluation of new prosthetic heart valves, *Journal oJ Thoracic and Cardiovascular Surgery 91*, 460-466.

GRUNKEMEIER G.L., STARR A., RAHIMTOOLA S.H. (1992). Prosthetic heart valve performance: Long term follow-up. *Current Problems in Cardiology 17*, 331-406.

GRUNKEMEIER G.L. (1993). Will randomized trials detect randorn valve failure? Reflection on a recent FDA workshop. *Jornal oJ Heart Valve Disease 2*,424-429.

HASTINGS W.K. (1970). Monte Carlo sampling methods using Markov Chains and their applications. *Biometrika 57*, 97-109.

HSIEH F.Y., BLOCH D.A., LARSEN M.D. (1998). A Simple Method of Sample Size Calculation For Linear and Logistic Regression, *Statistics in Medicine 17*, 1623-1634.

KEREIAKES D.J., LINNEMEIER T.J., BAIM D.S., KUNTZ R.E., O'SHAGHNESSY C., HER-MILLER J., FINK S., LANSKY A., NISHIMURA N., BRODERICK T.M., POPMA J.J. (1999). Procedural and Late Outcomes Following Multi-Link Duet Coronary Stent Deployment. *American Journal of Cardiology 84*, 1385-1390.

LAD F. (1996). Operational Subjective Statistical Methods. New York: Wiley.

LEON M.B., BAIM D.S., POPMA J.J., GORDON P.C., CUTLIP D.E., HO K.K., GIAMBARTOLOMEI A., DIVER D.J., LASORDA D.M., WILLIAMS D.O., POCOCK S.J., KUNTZ R.E., (1998). A clinical trial comparing three antithrombotic-drug regimens after coronary-artery stenting. *New England Journal of Medicine 339*, 1665-71

LINDLEY D.V. (1997). The Choice of Sample Size, *The Statistician 46*, 129-138.

METROPOLIS N., ROSENBLUTH A.W., ROSENBLUTH M.N., TELLER A.H., TELLER E. (1953). Equations of State Calculations by Fast Computing Machines. *Journal of Chemical Physics 21*, 1087-92.

MULLER P., PARMIGIANI G. (1995). Optimal Design via Curve Fitting of Monte-Carlo Experiments, *Journal of the American Statistical Association, 90*, 1322-1330.

O'MALLEY A. J., NORMAND S-L.T. AND KUNTZ R.E., (2003). Estimation of the Objective Performance Criterion for Medical Device Trials: Coronary Artery Stenting. To appear: *Statistics in Medicine 22*.

O'MALLEY A. J., NORMAND S-L.T. AND KUNTZ R.E., (2002). Sample Size Calculation for an Historically-Controlled Clinical Trial with Adjustement for Covariates, *Journal of Biopharmaceutical Statistics 12*, 227-247.

SAMMEL M.D., RYAN L.M., LEGLER J.M. Latent Variable Models for Mixed Discrete and Continuous Outcomes. *Journal o] the Royal Statistical Societ, Series B 59*, 667-678.

SELF S.G., MAURITSEN R.H.(1988). Power/sample size calculations for generalized linear models, *Biometrics 44*, 79-86.

SERRUYS P.W., DEJAEGERE P., KIEMENEIJ K., MACAYA C., RUTSCH W., HEYDRICKX O., EMANUELSSON H., MARCO J., LEGRAND V., MATERNE P., BELARDI J., SIGWART U., COLOMBO A., GOY J.J., VANDENHEUVEL P., DELCAN J., MOREL M.A. (1994). A comparison of balloon-expandable-stent implantation with balloon angioplasty in patients with coronary artery disease. Benestent Study Group. *New England Journal of Medicine 331*, 489-95.

SIGNORINI D.F. (1991). Sample size for Poisson regression, *Biometrika 78*, 446-50.

SPIEGELHALTER D.J., FREEDMAN L.S. (1986). A predictive approach to selecting the size of a clinical trial, based on subjective clinical opinion, *Statistics in Medicine 5*, 1-13.

WEISS R. (1997). Bayesian sample size calculations for hypothesis testing, *The Statistician 46*, 185-191

WHITTEMORE A.S. (1981). Sample size for Logistic Regression With Small Response Probability, *Joumal oJ the American Statistical Association 76*, 27-32.

Chapter 11

AN ADAPTIVE SIR ALGORITHM FOR BAYESIAN MULTILEVEL INFERENCE ON CATEGORICAL DATA

S. Pezzulli*
Department of Meteorology, The University of Reading, UK.

1. INTRODUCTION

To understand nature and causes of variation in natural populations, independent samples often review and integrate the findings of several research studies. In this case, we may expect some differences, but also some persistent patterns in the observed frequencies.

A way to represent such expectations is via Bayesian Multilevel (or Hierarchical) modelling. Generally, these models specify a common distribution (the *prior*) for the parameters of the populations. This prior, in turn, depends on some further parameters (the *hyperparameters*) that follow a known distribution (*the hyperprior*). The multistage process can also be extended to further levels, with the main advantage of allowing separate modelling for distinct sources of uncertainty (see Gelman *et. al.*, 1995 and Dey *et al.*, 2000).

Categorical (or compositional) samples are the most simple and common data in sciences and trace back a long history (Aitchinson, 1986). A sample composition into k categories: $A_1, A_2, \ldots, A_k$, is simply the data-count vector $y=(y_1, y_2, \ldots, y_k)$ of these attributes out of $n=\Sigma_i\, y_i$ observations, where $i=1,2,\ldots,k$. DNA fingerprint studies, for example, rely on increasingly large sets of compositions into a number of *allelic states* (depending on the locus under investigation).

* For correspondence: spezzulli@hotmail.com

The observational model for compositions is the Multinomial distribution. The Bayesian conjugate model is especially relevant in Population Genetics. Wright (1969) defined this model under a particular form, highlighing the role of inbreeding within populations. The inbreeding coefficients Fst are important to study the phylogenesis of species and the historical patterns of migration and interbreeding and were investigated at length (see e.g. Hartl and Jones, 1998). They were either derived theoretically under simple genetic models and estimated in real populations by using a variety of approaches.

Wright uses the inbreeding coefficient as a given scale for his prior distribution. In Section 2 we present the hierarchical extension of this coniugate model for compositional data. The Wright's form is retained and an hyperprior distribution is used by taking account of the genetical literature.

The sampling-importance-resampling (SIR) algorithm, introduced by Rubin (1987), can be opportunely defined in this case. The SIR algorithm generates values from some target density p, by extracting a random sample $\{x_t\}$ from an approximating distribution q and, then, by re-sampling a smaller data-set from the initial sample with probabilities proportional to the importance weights $w_t=p(x_t)/q(x_t)$.

The SIR method obviously relies for its efficacy on the approximating density. Here we use an adaptive form, because the approximation can be improved by a Monte Carlo step after the SIR iteration. It follows a recursive algorithm.

The iterated-SIR (or SIR-MC) algorithm is presented in Section 3 and finally shown at work with some diagnostics taken from our case studies. The method can be useful in different applications. We apply the method for a Forensic identification application (section 4) and for a study on colour-blindeness in North-East India (section 5).

2. THE HIERARCHICAL WRIGHT'S POPULATION MODEL

From now on, let us denote by i the category index (i=1,2,...,k). We start to set the notation for a generic sample. The distribution of a compositional vector **y**, given a fixed sample size n, is the Multinomial probability distribution on the (k–1)-dimensional simplex of nonnegative integers y_i such that $\Sigma y_i=n$:

$$\text{Mult}_n(\mathbf{y} \mid \pi) = \frac{n!}{y_1!y_2!\cdots y_k!}\pi_1^{y_1}\pi_2^{y_2}\cdots\pi_k^{y_k}$$

The conjugate distribution for the probability parameter $\pi=(\pi_1, \pi_2, ..., \pi_k)$ is the Dirichlet

$$\mathrm{Dir}(\pi \mid \alpha) = \Gamma(\alpha_1 + \alpha_2 + \ldots + \alpha_k) \prod_i \frac{\pi_i^{\alpha_i - 1}}{\Gamma(\alpha_i)}$$

defined on the $(k-1)$-dimensional simplex for π and depending on k nonnegative hyperparameters $\alpha=(\alpha_1,\alpha_2,...,\alpha_k)$. The vector α represents an *a priori* composition with *pseudo*-sample-size $A=\Sigma\alpha_i$. This is the ordinary parametrization, the most common in the statistical literature.

For Wright's parametrization, let $\theta=\alpha/A$ and $f=1/(1+A)$. We introduce the equivalent notation

$$\mathrm{Dir}(\pi \mid f, \theta) \equiv \mathrm{Dir}(\pi \mid \alpha=(1/f-1)\,\theta)$$

referring to a relative-scale hyperparameter $f\in(0,1)$ and a location hyperparameter θ in the $(k-1)$-dimensional simplex. Then

$$E(\pi \mid f, \theta) = \theta,\ \mathrm{Var}(\pi i \mid f, \theta) = f\, \theta i(1-\theta i),\ \mathrm{Cov}(\pi i, \pi i' \mid f, \theta) = -f\, \theta i\, \theta i' \ (i \neq i'). \tag{1}$$

We also need the following result (see e.g. Bernardo and Smith, 1994). Assume a parameters prior $p(\pi|f,\theta)=\mathrm{Dir}(\pi|f,\theta)$ with observational model

$$p(y \mid \pi) = p(y \mid \pi, \theta, f) = \mathrm{Mult}_n(y \mid \pi)\,.$$

Then the data distribution conditional to the hyperparameters is the Multinomial-Dirichlet mixture:

$$\mathrm{MD}_n\,(y \mid \theta, f) \equiv p(y \mid \theta, f) = \int \mathrm{Mult}(y \mid \pi)\ \mathrm{Dir}(\pi \mid f, \theta)\ d\pi_1 d\pi_2 \cdots d\pi_k$$
$$= \frac{\Gamma(A)n!}{\Gamma(A+n)} \prod_i \frac{\Gamma(y_i + A\theta_i)}{\Gamma(A\theta_i)y_i!}, \tag{2}$$

where the integral holds over the $(k-1)$-dimensional simplex and $A=f^{-1}-1$.

2.1 Model Assumptions

Let us introduce J populations, with population index $j=1,2,...,J$. When J *independent* $\mathrm{Mult}(y_j|\pi_j)$ has been sampled from, we use a compact notation in defining the data, the parameters and the hyperparameters through the lists

$Y=\{y_1,y_2,...,y_J\}$, $\Omega=\{\pi_1,\pi_2,...,\pi_J\}$ and $H=\{\theta,f\}$, respectively. The entire data collection follows the distribution:

$$p(Y \mid \Omega) = \Pi_j \operatorname{Mult}(\mathbf{y}_j \mid \pi_j)\,. \tag{3}$$

We assume a parameters prior

$$p(\Omega \mid H) = \Pi_j \operatorname{Dir}(\pi_j \mid f_j, \theta) \tag{4}$$

and a given hyperprior distribution, $p(H)$, to be specified in sub-section 2.3.

Note that the vector $f=(f_1,f_2,...,f_J)$ allows for different scales for the π_j, while their expectation is the same common vector θ.

A hierarchical model can be always seen as an ordinary Bayesian model with prior $p(H)$ and a mixture likelihood for the observational distribution. For the hierarchy defined here, by means of the result in (2), the latter is simply

$$p(Y \mid H) = \Pi_j \operatorname{MD}_{n_j}(y_j \mid \theta, f_j) \tag{5}$$

The definitions (3) and (4) alone, with known H, represent the Bayesian model used by Wrigth (1969) for allelic counts. In this case, the posterior update of (4) is the result of J independent updatings. That is:

$$p(\Omega \mid H, Y) = \Pi_j \operatorname{Dir}(\pi_j \mid \theta A_j + y_j)\,. \tag{6}$$

with $A_j = f_j^{-1} - 1$.

2.2 Genetical interpretation

Let the proportion of allele A be θ in an original population **P**, while in a sub-population **S** the same probability is π. Assuming random mating, the probability of an heterozygous individual in **S** is $2\pi(1-\pi)$. But what can be said if π is unknown and we can use θ only?

As a first answer, it depends on the degree of *inbreeding* within the sub-population. Intense or weaker forms of inbreeding are qualitatively similar. The principal consequence is that homozygous offspring in **S** is more frequent than in **P**. Biologists are familiar with this fact known as the *Wahlund effect.* In subdivided groups it is common to observe an excess of homozygotes and a corresponding reduction of eterozygotes, with respect to the original population.

In order to quantify this mechanism, Wright (1969) defined the inbreeding coefficient, $F_{ST} \in (0,1)$, as the proportionate reduction in subpopulation heterozygotes that would be expected with random mating from the original population. In other words, if E is the expected frequency of (A, not-A)-genes in **S**, then

$$F_{ST} = 1 - E/[2\theta(1-\theta)]$$

Wrigth's influential work was based on the Bayesian conjugate model for multinomial data. In fact in this case we have just one subpopulation and 2 categories. If we know the relative scale parameter f of **S** (and the relative frequency θ in **P**) then, by (1), the expected heterozygotes and homozigothes are respectively:

$$E = \mathrm{E}[2p(1\text{-}p)|f, \theta\,] = 2\theta(1-\theta)\,(1-f)$$

$$O = \mathrm{E}[p^2|f, \theta\,] = f\,\theta(1-\theta) + \theta^2$$

It also follows that $F_{ST} = f$. The relative scale coefficient of a subpopulation **S** measures the expected proportionate heterozigous reduction with respect to the original **P**.

2.3 Hyperprior choice

For the hyperprior distribution $p(H)=p(f,\boldsymbol{\theta})$, Balding and Nicholson (1996) consider an unknown hyperscale vector $\boldsymbol{f}$, but assume to know the hypermean $\boldsymbol{\theta}$. On the other hand Gelman et al.(1995) define the same hierarchy and allow for uncertainty on both $\boldsymbol{f}$ and $\boldsymbol{\theta}$, but inbreeding is the same over all the populations. The present approach keeps unknown all the hyperparameters without (deterministic) restrictions.

A simple choice for $p(H)$ is for example

$$p(H) = p(\boldsymbol{\theta}) \cdot p(f) = \mathrm{Dir}(\boldsymbol{\theta}|\mathbf{1}) \cdot \Pi_j\, h(f_j) \qquad (7)$$

where $h(f)$ is some *typical* inbreeding distribution. For $p(\boldsymbol{\theta})$ we use the uniform distribution on the simplex: $\mathrm{Dir}(\boldsymbol{\theta}|\mathbf{1})$, in which $\mathbf{1}$ is the k-dimensional vector (1,1,...,1). This choice represents an ignorance position on the hypermean and avoids expressing any prior preference.

For the inbreeding distribution, Balding and Nichols (1996) tailored an *informative*

$$p(f) = \Pi_j h(f_j).$$

by means of literature based information on Caucasian populations for the common Fst prior $h(f)$. More precisely, they set

$$\text{Fst} = (1 + e^Z + e^W)^{-1},$$

where Z and W are independent Normal variables with mean 3.5 and standard deviation 1.5.

In term of pseudo-sample size, the sum of two i.i.d. Lognormals $A = e^Z + e^W$ has about mean 200 and 9th decile 500. The density h(Fst) is shown in Figure 1. It has mode 0.0025, median 0.01 and about 95% of the probability accumulates on values lower than 0.06. (Note that among offspring of first cousins: $F_{ST}=1/16=0.0625$.).

In summary, for our genetical examples we use the *semi-informative hyperprior* (7), with the Balding and Nichols empirical prior for f and the uniform for θ.

The method presented in the next subsection 3.2 can be adapted to different choices of $p(H)$. We need to assume *prior conditional independency within the Fst* (e.g. within $(f_1, f_2, \ldots, f_J|\theta)$), that is the rather general expression

$$p(H) = p(\theta)\, \Pi_j h_j(f_j \mid \theta). \tag{8}$$

3. THE ADAPTIVE SIR ALGORITHM

Here we show a method to sample from the distribution of the hyperparameter list $H=(f,\theta)$, after observing the data Y from J sub-populations. This is all we need, because after having sampled H^*, say, from the marginal posterior distribution $p(H|Y)$, we can easily sample Ω^* from $p(\Omega|H^*,Y)$ by means of (6), to obtain the joint sample (H^*,Ω^*) from $p(H,\Omega|Y)$. Then the probability of any event of interest can be evaluated on these joint-posterior samples. We refer to standard texts (Gelman *et al.*, 1995; Ripley, 1986 and Ross, 1997) for standard simulation procedures.

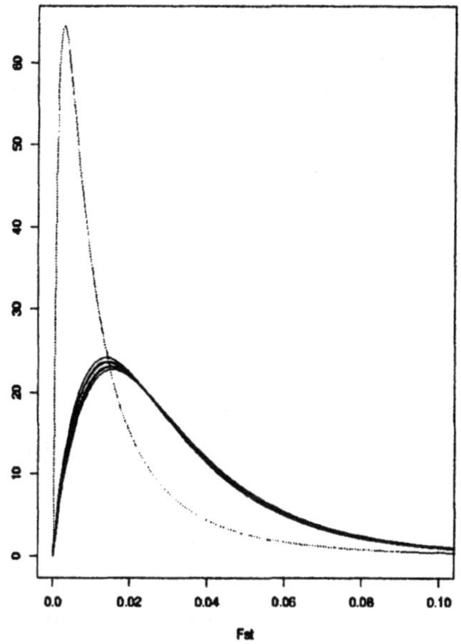

Figure 1. Approximating posterior distributions of the Sicilian inbreeding coefficient at the locus TH01, for the first ten iterations of the ISIR algorithm. The dotted curve on the left is the prior density h (used in the first iteration for rj, see section 3.3). The plot is limited to Fst in (0,0.1) for presentational purposes.

3.1 The SIR algorithm

Our target density is $p \equiv p(H \mid Y)$, the hyperparameters marginal posterior distribution. By (5) we obtain:

$$p \equiv p(\theta, f \mid Y) \propto p(\theta, f)\, \Pi_j \, \mathrm{MD}_{n_j}(y_j \mid \theta, f_j) \,. \tag{9}$$

For the approximating density:

$$q \equiv q_1(f)\, q_2(\theta \mid f). \tag{10}$$

we specify the conditional part as a mixture of Dir distributions:

$$q_2(\theta \mid f) = \Sigma \gamma_j \, \mathrm{Dir}(\theta \mid 1 + y_j) \tag{11}$$

with mixing probabilities $\gamma_j \propto (f_j^{-1} - 1)$. For the marginal approximation, we simply fix

$$q_1(f) = r_1(f_1) \cdot r_2(f_2) \cdot \ldots \cdot r_J(f_J) \tag{12}$$

where the probability density functions r_j are the current estimates of the univariate marginal posterior densities $p(f_j|Y)$.

The approximating distribution q depends on the densities r_j. For the starting choices we only have the prior itself, that is the same function h for all j. Hence we propose to use, at first, the SIR algorithm with: $r_j(f)=h(f)$ and $\gamma_j=1/J$.

It is relatively easy to sample from the approximation q. (Perform one independent extraction from each r_j, thus completing the vector $\boldsymbol{f}$. Then, compute the corresponding weights γ_j and select an index j in $\{1,2,...,J\}$ with probabilities $\{\gamma_1,\gamma_2,...,\gamma_J\}$ respectively. Finally, sample θ from the $\text{Dir}(\theta|\mathbf{1}+\boldsymbol{y}_j)$ corresponding to the selected index j).

The SIR algorithm can be summarized by the following 3 steps:

1. <u>Sampling</u> Sample T independent H_t from $q(H)$ (t=1,2,..,T).
2. <u>Importance weighting</u> Compute the weights $w_t \propto p(H_t|Y)/q(H_t)$ and their sum $W=\Sigma w_t$.
3. <u>Resampling</u> Sample H^* from $\{H_t\}$ with probabilities $\{w_t/W\}$.

Since q is strictly positive wherein p is, it can be show (see Ross, 1997, 10.5) that for $T\rightarrow\infty$ the distribution of H^* converges to p.

A number $\tau>1$ of values is usually resampled, with $\tau<<T$. Gelman et al. (1995) suggest a ratio $\tau/T\cong 1/20$ when moderately good approximations are thought to be available. The resampling step should be done without replacement, in order to avoid the worst cases, when the importance weights are strongly dominated by just one or very few of them. These cases indicate a poor approximation (see 3.3).

Finally, let us explain the choice of q as given by (10), (11) and (12). For the marginal posterior approximation (12) of $p(f|Y)$, we are simulating independence amongst the inbreeding coefficients. Posterior dependence is more difficult to model and to sample from.

For the mixture in (11), approximating the hypermean conditional posterior $p(\theta|\boldsymbol{f},Y)$, note that any component $Dir(\boldsymbol{\theta}|\mathbf{1}+\boldsymbol{y}_j)$ would be the posterior update of the uniform prior density $\text{Dir}(\boldsymbol{\theta}|\mathbf{1})$ if the data vector $\boldsymbol{y}_j$ was multinomial with parameter $\boldsymbol{\theta}$ *in place of* $\boldsymbol{\pi}_j$. By sampling from $Dir(\boldsymbol{\theta}|\mathbf{1}+\boldsymbol{y}_j)$, in other words, the *local* probability $\boldsymbol{\pi}_j$ is identified with the *global* one, $\boldsymbol{\theta}$, as it would be when generating from the target density, $p(\boldsymbol{\theta}|\boldsymbol{f},\text{Y})$, in the limiting case in which $f_j\rightarrow 0$ (and the other inbreeding coefficients remaining strictly positive, such that $\gamma_j\rightarrow 1$). It follows that the mixture will adapt the evidence provided by each data composition $\boldsymbol{y}_j$ accordingly to the sub-population's hyperscales, and the step-one-sampled hypermeans, $\boldsymbol{\theta}_t$ will explore the most important regions in the target domain.

3.2 Monte Carlo step to improve the approximating posterior

Note that, using (9), for any j we have:

$$p(f_j \mid \theta, Y) = C\, p(f \mid \theta)\, \mathrm{MD}_{n_j}(y_j \mid \theta, f_j)$$

where C depends on Y, θ and the remaining $f_{j'}$ (for $j' \neq j$), but does not depend on f_j. Since the likelihood factorises into the MD-mixtures, those univariate distributions can be easily computed if also the conditional prior factorizes, like we assumed in (8). In our simplest operational case (7) we can extract $h(f_j)$ from $p(f|\theta)$ and let C absorbing the residual factor, so that

$$p(f_j \mid \theta, Y) \propto h(f_j)\, \mathrm{MD}_{n_j}(y_j \mid \theta, f_j) \tag{13}$$

Let $\{\theta^*\}$ be the SIR sample. Conditionally on a resampled θ^* the univariate density kernels in (13) can be computed and normalized on a fine grid in (0,1). Because the θ^* are approximately sampled from $p(\theta|Y)$, it follows by Monte Carlo:

$$p(f_j \mid Y) \cong \Sigma_t p(f_j \mid \theta^*_t, Y) / \tau.$$

In this way, the SIR-sample provides a point-wise Monte Carlo approximation of each marginal posterior density $p(f_j|Y)$.

The SIR-sample can be seen as an improvement of the step-one sample $\{H_t\}$ from q. The importance-weights have this role of *adjusting the odds* to correct for the target. Therefore the Monte Carlo estimates will improve the components r_j of that approximation. For this reason, we propose to alternate SIR and Monte Carlo step above. This adaptive form of the SIR algorithm can be called iterated-SIR (ISIR) or also the SIR-MC algorithm, to emphasize the added step-four.

3.3 Further computations and diagnostics

The ISIR algorithm was implemented in Splus. We resampled τ=50 data out of T=10,000 initial generations, using a safe resampling ratio of 1/200. Severe looping can be avoided in the weights computation (by standard object-oriented manipulations on step-one-sampled hypermean and hyperscale *matrices*).

The convergence can be monitored on the most interesting quantities. In our practice, a few iterations are usually enough to adjust the approximating distribution, and the first one always provides the most drastic variation. For example, Figure 1 shows the first ten ISIR approximations of the Fst marginal posteriors for Sicilians (this study is discussed in the next section). The plot also illustrates the order of the MC approximation.

A syntetic convergence diagnostic is the concentration curve of the weights. Figure 2 shows this picture on the same data. The starting approximation (shadowed by vertical lines) illustrates a classical *bad* pattern for a sampling importance algorithm. When only very few H_t have been selected from the highest posterior region, those few samples possess all of the resampling-weights. Since the second approximation, instead, the highest 200 samples still possess less than 80% total importance, indicating that the sampler q is now much closer to the target.

Note that importance sampling is more efficient than the SIR itself. It follows that when the approximating posterior has been adjusted by the ISIR, then the relevant estimates can be more efficiently computed by importance sampling. This means to consider the initial (step-one) sample, weighted by the importance ratios and compute weighted expectations and frequencies of interest. For the latter, note that the relative importance frequency

$$f(B) = \frac{\sum_{H_t \in B} w_t}{W}$$

estimates the posterior probability $p(B|Y)$ for any borelian event B in the support of H. The histogram in Figure 3, for example (see section 5 for data discussion), was computed by aggregating these binned relative importance ratios over a 200,000 sample size.

The modifications for the general hyperprior case (8) are straightforward, like for example to use an informative Dir($\theta|\boldsymbol{u}$) instead of the uniform in (7). In this case, the approximating mixture (11) should also be subjected to the same variation (replacing **1** with $\boldsymbol{u}$) in order to mantain the perfect-approximation property for q_2 (when $\gamma_j \to 1$).

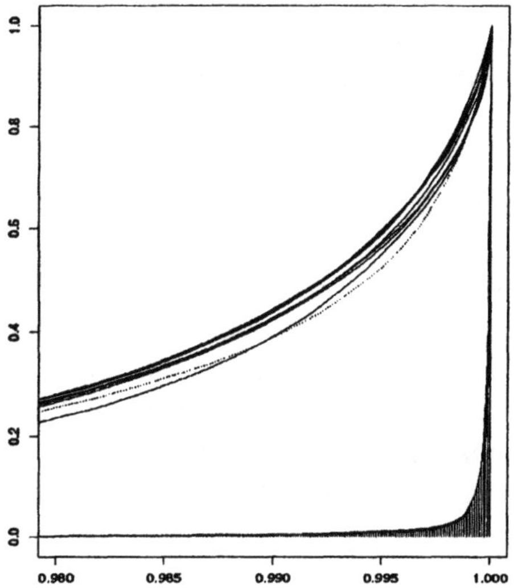

Figure 2. TH01 data. Concentration curves of the T=10,000 importance weights for the first ten iterations of the ISIR. The cumulated relative frequencies are restricted to the interval (0.98,1) in order to focus at the most important 200 weights (2% of 10,000). The first concentration curve is the lowest line (shown by verticals segments).

4. INBREEDING EFFECT ON FORENSIC IDENTIFICATION PRACTICE

The problem outlined in section 2.2 is a very common one; not only when dealing with extinct or rare populations. In a recurrent issue, the population originating the data is different from the one needed. Thus, in practice, one relies on samples from a larger group instead.

In forensic identification cases, for example, the data from a general population P are usually available, but the sub-population, S, from which defendant and crime perpetrator may both originate is scarcely known. Let us call G the event: "the defendant is the crime perpetrator". In comparing defendant and crime-scene fingerprints, the interesting case is when we observe a series $M=\{M_1, M_2, ...\}$ of matching evidences at a number of loci (because, of course, any mis-match would definitely disprove the identification and falsify G).

If we knew the subcomposition π it would be straightforward to proceed. The allelic states at the selected loci are independent (and in Court cases they also must not produce phenotipic expressions). Therefore the update of any initial probability $p(G)$ into the final $p(G|M)$ is done sequentially, until G can be accepted to be *practically sure* in Court. Often, in these cases, the bound for the practical certainty relies on the minimum number of digits that is necessary to round $p(G|M)$ up to one. Then the event G is considered sure. Otherwise, the evidence is inconclusive and more loci have to be analysed, if possible.

The Bayesian updating step is (essentially) provided by the so-called *product-rule*: π_i^2 (and $2\pi_i\pi_h$): the probability of homozigous (and heterozigous) matching-evidence under random selection from S, that is under the event *not-G*. (And an obvious observational model complete the likelihood conditionally to G). The product rules are unknown, however, and the current *plug-in* practice, of filling in the product-rules the general compositional vector θ, is tendencially unfair to the defendant. As shown in Section 2.2, more homozygotes are expected than in random mating from P and, in case of homozygote matching this directly results in overestimating $p(G|M)$.

Table 1. TH01 data (3486 total sampled alleles).

Allele	6	7	8	9	10	11	TOT
Region							
Lombardia	158	97	96	123	174	0	648
Friuli V. G.	41	35	26	39	49	0	190
Veneto	83	57	37	60	124	3	364
Emilia Romagna	154	74	54	82	125	3	492
Liguria	26	30	21	22	39	0	138
Toscana	78	60	45	51	94	0	328
Marche	105	68	65	79	113	0	430
Umbria	86	42	50	58	82	0	318
Lazio	119	79	63	107	139	3	510
Sicilia	20	2	8	22	16	0	68

Table 2. FES data (4348 total sampled alleles).

Allele	7	8	9	10	11	12	13	14	TOT
Region									
Lombardia	1	5	5	181	256	143	35	2	628
Friuli V. G.	0	4	4	60	89	45	8	0	210
Veneto	0	4	6	74	88	51	16	1	240
Emilia Rom.	0	3	1	129	228	138	32	3	534
Liguria	0	5	2	160	231	171	39	4	612
Toscana	0	1	2	142	200	144	32	3	524
Marche	1	2	0	134	179	102	27	1	446
Umbria	0	2	2	45	78	51	8	2	188
Lazio	0	5	1	134	200	143	29	4	516
Sicilia	0	2	5	110	185	104	41	3	450

In Pezzulli (2000), a forensic database at the loci TH01 and FES from ten Italian Regions is used to evaluate the bias against the defendant of the ordinary identification procedure. We give an account here and refer to the paper for more details. TH01 and FES data are shown in Table 1 and Table 2.

The traditional practice can be seen as using the Wright's formulas (E and O of section 2.2) with f=0. Given the marginal posterior distributions $p(f_j|Y)$, on the other hand, we can fix an Fst that is much more realistic and fair than the assumption of zero inbreeding. Likely, defendant and perpetrator belong to the same minority and even a generous *inbreeding allowance* does not necessarily spoil the weight of the evidence (see also Balding and Donnelly (1995) and references therein for this debate).

It follows that the identification probabilities $p(G|M)$ of any given evidence M can be computed by using the Wrigth's expected product rules (conditional to the chosen Fst) and then compared to the usual protocol (f=0). In our study we have chosen an inbreeding allowance, for each locus, equal to the maximum posterior expected values within the ten regions.

Table 3 shows the posterior expectations of the inbreeding coefficients for both the loci. These results agree in magnitude with other studies and confirm the observed variation between inbreeding across different loci (Balding and Nichols, 1996).

Table 3. Posterior expected Fst coefficients

Region	TH01	FES
Lombardia	0.6	0.3
Friuli V. G.	0.7	0.9
Veneto	0.8	0.7
Emilia Romagna	0.7	0.6
Liguria	1.1	0.4
Toscana	0.7	0.5
Marche	0.6	0.6
Umbria	0.8	0.5
Lazio	0.4	0.5
Sicilia	3.3	0.5

As expected, the effect of the adjusted formulas was found generally small and probably trascurable in many applications. But in Court cases the correction may be sensible, even when the matching evidence involves not-rare alleles. We found results reversed from "sure" to "inconclusive" either at 3, 5 and 7 digits (which is about all the usual rules).

In conclusion, the traditional practice uses the overall mean in place of θ and a zero inbreeding assumption between perpetrator and defendant. As shown here, a safer protocol can be suggested to allow for inbreeding, by updating our knowledge about Fst (and θ) at the investigated loci and then adopting an inbreeding allowance rule.

5. COLOUR-BLINDNESS IN NORTH EAST INDIANS

Colour-blindness is an x-linked recessive hereditary trait. Some authors have proposed relaxed selection to explain the variable rates found in different groups, but the hypothesis was criticized by others. For the colour-blind incidence in North-East India, Choudhury (1994) reported the sample frequencies on seven populations and accumulated other data from the literature. The whole collection regards 27 populations sampled in eight different surveys, for a total of 3998 individuals. In Table 4 we show these data (from Table 3 of the quoted paper). The relaxation selection hypothesis was found unsupported by these figures. At least for the economic conditions that were supposed to influence the differential operation of natural selection, the data show both high and low frequencies of colour-blindness with no clear pattern.

To explain variations in colour-blindness the Author was left to consider possible racial differences. He investigated the discrimination between Caucasoid and Mongoloid groups by means of the Pearson's Chi-Square test for comparing proportions, with 5% first-kind error.

Assamese and Bengali groups are prevalently Caucasoid and show 4.5% colour-blind incidence alltoghether, while the remaining populations are prevalently Mongoloid, with 2.9% rate. The Author compared Assamese only (4.1%) with Mongoloids, and found no significant difference. This is in contrast with the prevalent literature findings, quoted by the Author, wherein the rate in Caucasians is supposedly higher.

In Bengalis, on the other hand, the observed 8% incidence rate was found significantly higher than in both Assamese and Mongoloid people, and if Bengali and Assameses could be put together they would be significantly different from the Mongoloid. Thus the disputed discrimination, crucially, depends on the apparently outlying Bengali within the Caucasian populations.

In this (simultaneous) use of (marginal) tests it is not rare to obtain controversial results. Especially when the test is performed on different aggregations of the same data, the responses may be inconsistent. The main conclusion, in line with Choudhury (1994), is that the *p*-values are in a doubtful region and the tests remain inconclusive.

A less vague picture can be given by separate applications of our Bayesian Multilevel model on the Mongolian groups and the Assamese groups. The general Caucasian population (Assamese and Bengali) was also investigated. This is the hierarchical Beta-Binomial model with k=2 categories. We are interested in the hyper-mean $\theta=(b,1-b)$, where b van be seen as the colour-blind rate in the original population. In Figure 3 we compare the histograms of the marginal posterior distributions: $p(b|Y)$ in these three cases.

Table 4. Colour-blindness incidence rates in North East India

Population	Tested	Freq	Rate %
Caucasians	**1366**	**62**	**4.54**
Assamese caste Hindu	1217	50	4.11
Upper Brahmin	121	5	4.13
Upper Kalita	196	9	4.59
Upper Kaibarta	146	8	5.48
Lower Brahmin	145	6	4.14
Lower Kalita	330	12	3.64
Lower Kaibarta	101	2	1.98
Other castes	178	8	4.49
Bengali caste Hindu	149	12	8.05
Mongoloid populations	**2632**	**77**	**2.93**
Riang	195	3	1.54
Lushai	224	4	1.79
Naga	100	0	0.00
Khasi	495	19	3.84
Garo	136	4	2.94
Mikir	125	0	0.00
Miri	37	0	0.00
Rabha	131	4	3.05
Kachari	165	4	2.42
Kabui Naga	130	4	3.08
Meitei Manipuri	74	3	4.05
Bishnupriya Manipuri	120	4	3.33
Gallong	91	1	1.10
Nocte	78	0	0.00
Wancho	72	2	2.78
Tangsa	127	7	5.51
Digaru Mishmi	92	4	4.35
Idu Mishmi	87	4	4.60
Khampti	153	10	6.54

From fig. 3 it is evident that Caucasoid groups in North East India have an expected incidence rate of about 5%: with or without Bengali. The two distributions (in the two upper panels) are very close in shape and range. The Assameses (central panel) show just a minor leftward shift. This posterior invariance for the ancestor rates supports the hypothesis of a unique origin.

Finally, for the Mongoloids (lower panel), $p(b|Y)$ has a very different shape, more concentrated on smaller rates, with mode around 3%. The main part of the supported variability does not exceed the 5%-Assamese centre. Thus we found strong evidence to distinguish Assameses and Mongoloids.

In summary, Bengali and Assameses can be aggregated into a unique Caucasian population, while the incidence rate of their ancestors (or just of the original Assameses) stands quite apart from the original Mongoloid rate.

6. CONCLUSION

We proposed a model for data-counts among a set of attributes observed in different populations or groups. By allowing eteroscedastic groups the information about the common location can be processed simultaneously with the scales.

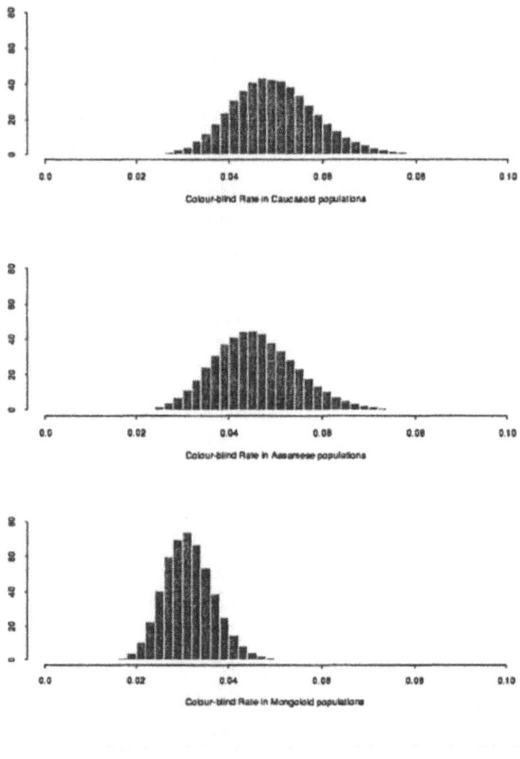

Figure 3. Histograms of the posterior distributions for the colour-blindness rates under three aggregations of the data from North East India.

An adaptive version of the SIR algorithm is defined for the Bayesian computations. The approximating posterior used by the SIR is improved by a Monte Carlo step, resulting in a fast and efficient iterative routine.

In a forensic application we illustrated a simple way to allow for inbreeding in identification cases. On our data, the correction is not dramatic but cannot be ignored. On the colour-blindness data in North-East India, classical testing gives controversial responses. More in line with literature findings, Assamese and Bengali can be seen, in our results, as originating from a unique (Caucasian) population, which stands far apart from the Mongoloids ancestral group.

REFERENCES

AITCHINSON, J. (1986). The statistical analysis of compositional data. Chapman and Hall: London.

BALDING, D. J. & DONNELLY P. (1995). Inference in Forensic Identification. *J. Roy. Stat. Soc.* A. 158: 21–53.

BALDING, D. J. & NICHOLS, R. A. (1996). Significant genetic correlations among Caucasians at forensic DNA loci. *Heredity 78*: 583–589.

BERNARDO, J. M. & SMITH, A. F. M. (1994). Bayesian Theory. Wiley: New-York.

CHOUDHURY, B. (1994). Variation in colour-blindness in North-East India. *Int. J. Anthrop. 9*: 303–308.

DEY, D. K., GHOSH, S. K. & MALLIK, B. K.(ed. 2000). Generalized Linear Models. A Bayesian Perspective. Marcel Dekker, Inc. New-York.

GELMAN, A. B., CARLIN, J. S., STERN, H. S. & RUBIN, D. B. (1995). Bayesian Yata Analysis. Chapman & Hall: London.

HARTL, D. L. & JONES, E. W. (1998). Genetics. Principles and Analysis. Jones and Bartlett Publishers: London (IV edition).

PEZZULLI, S. (2002). Bayesian multilevel modelling of compositional data for simultaneous inferences on allele compositions and inbreeding coefficients. *International Journal of Anthropology. 17 (3-4)*, 181-200.

ROSS, S. M. (1997). Simulation. Academic Press: San Diego.

RUBIN, D. N. (1987). A noniterative sampling/importance/resampling alternative to the data augmentation algorithm for creating a few imputations when fractions of missing information are modest: the SIR algorithm. Comment in the discussion of Tanner M. A. & Wong W. H. (1987). The calculation of posterior distributions by data augmentation. *J. Am. Stat. Ass. 82*, 528–550.

WRIGHT, S. (1969). Evolution and the genetic of populations. Vol. II: The theory of gene frequencies. Univ. Chicago Press.

Chapter 12

AGE AT DEATH DIAGNOSIS BY CRANIAL SUTURE OBLITERATION: A BAYESIAN APPROACH

A. Rinaldi,[1] E. Pacciani[2] and M. Di Bacco[3*]
Dipartimento di studi Geoec., Ling., Stat., Stor. per l'Anal. Reg., Università La Sapienza di Roma, Italy;[1] Soprintendenza ai Beni Archeologici della Toscana, Firenze, Italy;[2] Dipartimento di Scienze Statistiche, Università degli Studi di Bologna, Italy[3]

1. INTRODUCTION

In subadults and young adults, the bones of the cranial vault articulate by means of sutures, i.e. synarthroses (immovable or almost immovable joints). A suture consists of the edges of two adjoining bones, more or less serrate and fitting into each other, each one covered with a thin layer of fibrous connective tissue with the function of periosteum, which separates them and at the same time unites them. The appearance is that of continuous, sinuous, serrate lines, clearly delimiting the various cranial bones, along which growth of the cranial vault occurs; in fact, as long as the intervening connective membrane persists, the bone can continue to increase in surface area. This membrane can be more or less thick and thus the articulating bone surfaces can be more or less separated. The distance is usually greater in young individuals and decreases with age. In fact, starting at a certain age, ossification invades the sutural membrane and the sutures begin to disappear due to the progressive fusion of the bones (physiological synostosis).

The fusion occurs gradually, beginning at many different points along the sutural line and proceeding in tracts; thus it presents discontinuities that gradually increase in size until all traces of the suture disappear. Therefore, complete ossification of the sutures, which occurs infrequently, should only

* For correspondence: dibacco@stat.unibo.it

appear in the skull of elderly individuals. Ribbe (1885) divided the process into 5 phases:

Degree 0 - Open suture. There is a small separation between the two adjoining bones (which in life is occupied by the intervening connective membrane).

Degree 1 - Suture clearly visible as a continuous line with a zigzag course.

Degree 2 - Dashed sutural line, with intercalated tracts of complete fusion.

Degree 3 - Only traces of the suture remain, in the form of aligned dots.

Degree 4 - The suture is completely fused and no longer visible.

The ossification occurs first in the deep areas (endocranial side, i.e. on the inner table) and then superficially (ectocranial side, external table) where it begins at a mature age.

As early as the 19th century, the progressive degree of obliteration with age suggested that CSO could be used to determine the age at death. Indeed, it is still used as a diagnostic criterion, since - at least in the case of the archaeological excavations - cranial remains are among the most frequent skeletal specimens found. Nevertheless, the scientific debate about the efficacy of the diagnosis of age at death using CSO continues, with positions that are totally critical (see Hershkovitz et al., 1997 and the references cited there) and others that are more favorable (see Key *et al.*, 1994 and the references cited there).

Our aim is to contribute to the evaluation of the efficacy of CSO in diagnosing the age at death and to provide some general methodological suggestions which could be useful for other age indicators. We conducted an experimental control using a sample of skulls belonging to individuals of known age at death to investigate how CSO can be used to diagnose the age at death and whether it is a "good" way to make such a diagnosis.

2. MATERIAL AND METHODS OF DATA COLLECTION

The research was conducted on 198 skulls of adult individuals (from the age of 20), originating from various regions of Italy, who died around the end of the 19th century. The sample is housed in the Museo di Storia Naturale, sezione di Antropologia ed Etnologia, in Florence, Italy. The ages of the individuals were recorded in the catalogue of the Museum and were obtained from the Registry Office.

The methodology of data collection is the one proposed by Acsádi and Nemeskéri (1970) and later used by other authors (Perizonius, 1984). It is based on the subdivision of the main vault sutures (coronal, sagittal and lambdoid) into segments (sixteen segments on the ectocranial side based on detectable morphological differences, according to Vallois, 1937; sixteen segments of approximately equal length on the endocranial side) and on further evaluation of obliteration stage of each segment by Ribbe's scale (1885), modified by combining the first two degrees (0 and 1). In this way a scale of four degrees was obtained (1, 2, 3, 4). The reason for this modification is the difficulty in distinguishing between degrees 0 and 1 on the skull. In fact, we believe that the difference between them might not have a biological meaning but could be only a post-mortem accident.

3. BAYESIAN ANALYSIS

3.1 General description

Our statistical analysis follows a Bayesian-theoretic decision paradigm, which we will briefly outline. Let us start with some preliminary notation. Let us indicate by

$$\mathbf{x}^{(1)} = (x_1^{(1)},\ldots,x_{16}^{(1)}) \tag{1}$$

and

$$\mathbf{x}^{(2)} = (x_1^{(2)},\ldots,x_{16}^{(2)}) \tag{2}$$

the obliteration degrees of the endocranial sutures and ectocranial ones for a generic skull, and by a its age at death. Clearly each element in $\mathbf{x} = (\mathbf{x}^{(1)},\mathbf{x}^{(2)})$ can take one of the values in the set $\{1,2,3,4\}$, based on our previous classification. Moreover, for the i-th skull in our collection, let us specify by

$$\mathbf{x}_i^{(1)} = \left(x_{i,1}^{(1)},\ldots,x_{i,16}^{(1)}\right)$$

and

$$\mathbf{x}_i^{(2)} = \left(x_{i,1}^{(2)},\ldots,x_{i,16}^{(2)}\right)$$

the same quantities in (1) and (2), and by a_i its age at death. Hence we can denote by

$$\mathbf{X}=\{\mathbf{x}_i;i=1,...,198\}=\{(\mathbf{x}_i^{(1)},\mathbf{x}_i^{(2)});i=1,...,198\}$$

the set of the observed suture obliteration degrees for all the skulls in our collection and by $\mathbf{a}=\{a_i;i=1,...,198\}$ the corresponding set of ages at death.

To evaluate the reliability of CSO in estimating the age at death, we consider the age estimation problem for a new skull given our data in two different situations. In the first one, we assume that we know only the distribution of age at death *D*, while in the second we assume that we also know the skull's specific CSO information $\mathbf{x}=(\mathbf{x}^{(1)},\mathbf{x}^{(2)})$.

If we use a quadratic loss function, i.e. we define as

$$L(a,\tilde{a})=(a-\tilde{a})^2$$

the penalization suffered when estimating a real age at death a with the estimate $\tilde{a}$, then the optimal Bayesian estimates in the two previous cases are the means of the predictive distributions of age at death conditional to $\mathbf{E}_1=\{D,(\mathbf{X},\mathbf{a})\}$ and $\mathbf{E}_2=\{\mathbf{E}_1,\mathbf{x}\}$, respectively:

$$\bar{a}=\sum_{a\in\mathcal{A}} a\Pr\{a|\mathbf{E}_1\} \tag{3}$$

and

$$\bar{a}_{|\mathbf{x}}=\sum_{a\in\mathcal{A}} a\Pr\{a|\mathbf{E}_2\}. \tag{4}$$

where $\mathcal{A}$ is the set of all the possible ages at death (see, for example, Berger, 1988). Clearly $\bar{a}$ is the same for all the skulls, while $\bar{a}_{|\mathbf{x}}$ varies with $\mathbf{x}$. The Bayesian risks corresponding to (3) and (4) are

$$E[L(\bar{a})]=\sum_{a\in\mathcal{A}}(a-\bar{a})^2\Pr\{a|\mathbf{E}_1\}$$

and

$$E[L(\bar{a}_{|\mathbf{x}})]=\sum_{\mathbf{x}\in\mathcal{X}}\sum_{a\in\mathcal{A}}(a-\bar{a}_{|\mathbf{x}})^2\Pr\{a|\mathbf{E}_2\}. \tag{5}$$

where $\mathcal{X}$ is the set of all the possible values of **x**. Since $E\left[L(\bar{a})\right] \geqslant E\left[L\left(\bar{a}_{|\mathbf{x}}\right)\right]$, a natural way to measure the improvement in passing from the first situation to the second one, and thus to measure the usefullnes of the CSO information in the age diagnosis, is given by the normalized ratio

$$C_{\mathbf{x}} = \frac{E\left[L(\bar{a}_{|\mathbf{x}})\right]}{E\left[L(\bar{a})\right]}. \tag{6}$$

The case $C_{\mathbf{x}} = 0$ represents the situation where the suture information allows perfect estimates; the case $C_{\mathbf{x}} = 1$ represents the situation where the suture information is completely useless.

We use our data to define $\mathcal{A} = \{20,...,85\}$ and

$$\Pr\{a|\mathbf{E}_1\} = \Pr\{a|\mathbf{a}\} = \frac{\sum_{i=1}^{198}\{a_i = a\}}{198},$$

where $\{a_i = a\}$ is equal to one if $a_i = a$ and zero otherwise. In other words, we do not make an inference about the distribution of age of death. This choice is justified since the distribution of age at death in our collection is very similar to the one in the Italian population at the end of the 19th century, as shown by the demographic records of the time. On the other hand, the calculation of

$$\Pr\{a|\mathbf{E}_2\} = \Pr\{a|\mathbf{E}_1, \mathbf{x}\} = \frac{\Pr\{\mathbf{x}|a, \mathbf{E}_1\}\Pr\{a|\mathbf{E}_1\}}{\sum_{a' \in \mathcal{A}} \Pr\{\mathbf{x}|a', \mathbf{E}_1\}\Pr\{a'|\mathbf{E}_1\}} \tag{7}$$

depends on the predictive probability

$$\Pr\{\mathbf{x}_{199}|a_{199}, \mathbf{E}_1\} = \frac{\Pr\{\mathbf{x}_i|a_i; i = 1,...,199\}}{\Pr\{\mathbf{x}_i|a_i; i = 1,...,198\}}. \tag{8}$$

having defined, for notational convenience, $\mathbf{x}_{199} = \mathbf{x}$ and $a_{199} = a$.

3.2 The hierarchical model

Let us describe in detail the way we evaluate the conditional probabilities in the right hand side of (8) by means of a hierarchical model.

First, we notice that the classification method we follow does not distinguish between different segments. In other words, it assumes the exchangeability of both the endocranial sutures and the ectocranial ones, so that we can write for $v = 1, 2$ and any i

$$\Pr\left\{\mathbf{x}_i^{(v)} | \alpha_i^{(v)}\right\} = \int_{\Delta^4} \prod_{j=1}^{16} \left(\theta_{i1}^{(v)}\right)^{\left\{x_{i,j}^{(v)}=1\right\}} \dots \left(\theta_{i4}^{(v)}\right)^{\left\{x_{i,j}^{(v)}=4\right\}} dF\left(\theta_i^{(v)} \middle| \alpha_i^{(v)}\right) \tag{9}$$

for some $F(\cdot | \alpha_i^{(v)})$ with support in

$$\Delta^4 = \left\{\theta = (\theta_1, \dots, \theta_4) : \theta_k \geqslant 0 \text{ for any } k;\ \theta_1 + \dots + \theta_4 = 1\right\}.$$

The conditioning on $\alpha_i^{(v)}$ in (9) means that we have implicitly chosen a parametric form for the distribution function F characterizing our probability assignment about $\mathbf{x}_i^{(v)}$. Furthermore, the exchangeability assumption allows us to summarize our CSO data for each skull by the number of sutures having the four possible obliteration degrees. More formally, the set

$$\mathbf{s}_i^{(v)} = \left(s_{i,1}^{(v)}, \dots, s_{i,4}^{(v)}\right) = \left(\sum_{j=1}^{16}\left\{x_{i,j}^{(v)} = 1\right\}, \dots, \sum_{j=1}^{16}\left\{x_{i,j}^{(v)} = 4\right\}\right)$$

for every v and i forms a sufficient statistic for our inference (see, for example, Lad, 1995). In fact, since

$$\Pr\left\{\mathbf{s}_i^{(v)} \middle| \alpha_i^{(v)}\right\} = \frac{16!}{s_{i,1}^{(v)}! \dots s_{i,4}^{(v)}!} \Pr\left\{\mathbf{x}_i^{(v)} \middle| \alpha_i^{(v)}\right\}, \tag{10}$$

it is easy to show that we can refer to the predictive probability

$$\Pr\left\{\mathbf{s}_{199} \middle| a_{199}, \mathbf{E}_1^{\mathbf{s}}\right\} = \frac{\Pr\left\{\mathbf{s}_i \middle| a_i; i = 1, \dots, 199\right\}}{\Pr\left\{\mathbf{s}_i \middle| a_i; i = 1, \dots, 198\right\}} \tag{11}$$

with $\mathbf{E}_1^{\mathbf{s}} = \left\{(\mathbf{s}_i, a_i); i = 1, \dots, 198\right\}$ in place of (8) and write, in obvious notation,

$$C_{\mathbf{s}} = \frac{E\left[L\left(\bar{a}_{\mathbf{s}}\right)\right]}{E\left[L(\bar{a})\right]},$$

being $C_{\mathbf{s}} = C_{\mathbf{x}}$.

Second, we define the joint probability for the i-th suture set configuration s_i as

$$\Pr\left\{\mathbf{s}_i \,|\, \boldsymbol{\beta}_i\right\} = \int_{\mathcal{R}^k} \prod_{v=1}^{2} \Pr\left\{\mathbf{s}_i^{(v)} \,|\, \alpha_i^{(v)}\right\} dQ\left(\alpha_i^{(1)}, \alpha_i^{(2)} \,|\, \boldsymbol{\beta}_i\right) \tag{12}$$

for some parametric distribution function Q with support in $\mathcal{R}^k$, and where $\Pr\left\{\mathbf{s}_i^{(v)} \middle| \alpha_i^{(v)}\right\}$ for $v = 1,2$ is given by (10). Notice that representation (12) does not correspond to any exchangeability property, since the two factors inside the integral sign refer to different parameters. Indeed, its role is to admit that the pattern of CSO can vary depending on the cranial table (external or internal), even though knowledge of the CSO degrees on one table can obviously inform about the ones on the other table. To allow some dependence between $\mathbf{s}_i^{(1)}$ and $\mathbf{s}_i^{(2)}$, we have to consider a form of Q so that we can choose the measure of correlation between $\alpha_i^{(1)}$ and $\alpha_i^{(2)}$ by means of the value of the parameter vector $\boldsymbol{\beta}_i$.

Third, we assume the conditional exchangeability of the n suture sets s_i given the ages a_i, for any i, since we do not have any information that distinguishes our skulls, apart from their recorded ages at death. Therefore we can write, for $n = 198$ and $n = 199$,

$$\Pr\left\{\mathbf{s}_i \,|\, a_i; i = 1,\ldots,n\right\} = \int_{\mathcal{R}^m} \prod_{i=1}^{n} \Pr\left\{\mathbf{s}_i \,|\, \gamma, a_i\right\} dW(\gamma), \tag{13}$$

for some parametric distribution function W with support in $\mathcal{R}^m$. Setting n equal to 198 or 199 yields, respectively, the denominator and the numerator of (11). It is natural to link (13) to (12) by putting

$$\Pr\left\{\mathbf{s}_i \,|\, \gamma, a_i\right\} = \Pr\left\{\mathbf{x}_i \,|\, \boldsymbol{\beta}_i\right\},$$

and, at the same time, defining the parameter $\boldsymbol{\beta}_i$ as a function of γ and a_i. To denote that, we write, in short, $\boldsymbol{\beta}_i = \boldsymbol{\beta}(\gamma, a_i)$. The hierarchical model allows us to make our probability assignment about the conditional distribution of s_i given a_i for $i = 1,\ldots,n$, through elicitation of a distribution for the (hyper)parameter γ.

So far, we have described the general framework of our hierarchical model, as it results from our assumptions about the exchangeability of sutures and skulls and some generic parametric form for the prior distributions that we are going to detail.

In the choice of these distributions, we need to take into account two things: the ease of interpretation of parameters and hyper-parameters, and the feasibility of calculation of the posterior distributions. This suggests a complete reparametrization of the model which allows us to simplify its numerical computation. We begin by noting that it is convenient to merge the first two steps and write

$$\Pr\{\mathbf{s}_i|\boldsymbol{\beta}_i\} = \int_{\Delta^4\times\Delta^4} \prod_{v=1}^{2} (\theta_{i1}^{(v)})^{s_{i,1}^{(v)}} \cdots \left(\theta_{i4}^{(v)}\right)^{s_{i,4}^{(v)}} dV\left(\boldsymbol{\theta}_i^{(1)},\boldsymbol{\theta}_i^{(2)}|\boldsymbol{\beta}_i\right). \tag{14}$$

for some parametric distribution function V with support in $\Delta^4\times\Delta^4$. The reason is that there is no advantage in considering two integrations, specifying first a form for F, and then a form for Q, since (12) cannot in any case assume a tractable analytical form. In other words, solution (14) is computationally more convenient than the previous one since it avoids considering the parameters $\boldsymbol{\alpha}_i^{(v)}$ without reducing the flexibility of the model. Clearly, as before, we have to choose V so as to make $\boldsymbol{\theta}_i^{(1)},\boldsymbol{\theta}_i^{(2)}$ dependent. To do this, we consider the logistic transformation

$$\theta_{ik}^{(v)} = \theta_{ik}^{(v)}(\boldsymbol{\lambda}_i) = \frac{\exp\left\{\lambda_{ik}^{(0)} + \lambda_{ik}^{(v)}\right\}}{\sum_{d=1}^{4}\exp\left\{\lambda_{id}^{(0)} + \lambda_{id}^{(v)}\right\}} \tag{15}$$

for $k=1,\ldots,4$, $v=1,2$, where $\boldsymbol{\lambda}_i = \left(\lambda_{i1}^{(0)},\ldots,\lambda_{i3}^{(2)}\right)$, and with the convention, necessary for the identifiability of the model, that $\lambda_{04}^{(v)} = \lambda_{i4}^{(v)} = 0$ for any v. We specify for $\boldsymbol{\lambda}_i$ an independent components multinormal distribution, denoting by $\boldsymbol{\beta}_i = (\boldsymbol{\phi}_i,\boldsymbol{\delta}_i)$ its mean and variance vector. Notice that even if the components of $\boldsymbol{\lambda}_i$ are independent, the resulting compositional vectors $\boldsymbol{\theta}_{i1},\boldsymbol{\theta}_{i2}$ are correlated because of the common parameters $\lambda_{..}^{(0)}$. Then we define the transformation

$$\beta_i = \beta(\gamma, a_i) = \begin{cases} \phi_i = \gamma_0^{\{\mu\}} + a_i \gamma_1^{\{\mu\}} \\ \ln \delta_i = \gamma_0^{\{\sigma\}} + a_i \gamma_1^{\{\sigma\}} \end{cases}, \tag{16}$$

where $\gamma = \left(\gamma_0^{\{\mu\}}, \gamma_1^{\{\mu\}}, \gamma_0^{\{\sigma\}}, \gamma_1^{\{\sigma\}}\right)$ and with the notational convention that $\ln \delta_i = \left(\ln \delta_{i1}^{(0)}, ..., \ln \delta_{i3}^{(2)}\right)$. This parametric link is quite general and results in a CSO trend according to which the probability of the different obliteration degrees varies monotonically with age and whose precision also varies monotonically with age. Again, a convenient distribution for γ is an independent components multinormal distribution with vector mean μ^0 and variance vector σ^0.

We can summarize our hierarchical model with the following scheme:

1. Draw each component of γ from the normal distribution, the h-th component having mean μ_h^0 and variance σ_h^0. Then, for $i = 1, ..., n$:
   - 2.1. Compute $\beta_i = (\phi_i, \delta_i)$ by means of definition (16).
   - 2.2. Draw each component of λ_i from the normal distribution, the h-th component having mean ϕ_h^0 and variance δ_h^0.
   - 2.3. Compute $\theta_i^{(1)}, \theta_i^{(2)}$ by means of definition (15).
   - 2.4. Draw $s_{i,1}^{(1)}, ..., s_{i,4}^{(1)}$ from the multinomial distribution with size 16 and probability vector $\theta_i^{(1)}$ and draw $s_{i,1}^{(2)}, ..., s_{i,4}^{(2)}$ from the multinomial distribution with size 16 and probability vector $\theta_i^{(2)}$.

As usual, we use a very vague prior distribution, setting all the elements of μ^0 equal to zero and the elements of σ^0 quite large. By a well known argument, the large size of the data set should make our prior choice negligible.

We need an MCMC algorithm to yield a simulated sample from the updated distribution (11). The computational facilities offered by the WinBugs package allows us to code the algorithm simply by preparing a diagram specifying the relations between all the variables involved in the model, without having to worry about the more elaborated programming details (see, for example, Gilks et al., 1996, and the URL http://www.mrc-bsu.cam.ac.uk/bugs/ for all the informations about the Winbugs Project).

4. RESULTS

Because of the high number of parameters, the algorithm to handle our model turns out to be very time consuming. Hence, we require some criterion to simplify the numerical computation of index C_s, since it is not possible to consider all the possible configurations of s.

Our choice is almost compulsory. We could draw some configurations at random, but the number needed to obtain an acceptable estimate of C_s turns out to be quite large, and consequently the simulation time should be very great. Hence, we refer to the following estimate

$$\tilde{C} = \frac{\frac{1}{198}\sum_{i=1}^{198} L\left(\bar{a}_{s_i}\right)}{L(\bar{a})}$$

i.e., we restrict our evaluation of the Bayesian risk to the mean loss relative to the suture configurations appearing in our skull collection. This should provide some underestimation of the true value of C_s, since the same data is used twice, to build the model and to measure its efficacy. Nevertheless, we expect that the bias is very slight, and the simulation should provide a stable result in an acceptable time.

Our simulation yields a value for $\tilde{C}$ of about 0.65, a rather disappointing result: knowledge of CSO degrees decreases the risk in estimating age at death only by about 35%. To interpret this result pratically, we can say that if 10 years is the mean error estimate of age at death without CSO information, then the use of such information would reduce the error to $10 \times \sqrt{0.65} = 8.06$ years. This little difference suggests that to obtain an acceptable age at death estimator, it would be worthwhile looking for some other indicators besides cranial suture obliteration.

REFERENCES

ACSÁDI, G., AND NEMESKÉRI, J., 1970, History of human life span and mortality, Akadémiai Kiado, Budapest.

BERGER, J. O., 1988, Statistical Decision Theory and Bayesian Analysis - Second Edition - Spinger-Verlag, New York.

GELMAN, A., CARLIN, J. B., STERN, H. S., RUBIN, D. B., 1995, Bayesian Data Analysis, Chapman and Hall, London.

GILKS, W. R., RICHARDSON, S. & SPIEGELHALTER, D. J., 1996, Monte Carlo Markov Chain in practice, Chapman & Hall, London.

HERSHKOVITZ, I., LATIMER, B., DUTOUR, O., JELLEMA, L. M., WISH-BARATZ, S., ROTHSCHILD, C. Why do we fail in aging the skull from the sagittal suture? American Journal of Physical Anthropology, 1997; 103: 393-399.

KEY, C. A., AIELLO, L. C. AND MOLLESON, T., 1994, Cranial suture closure and its implications for age estimation. International Journal of Osteoarchaeology, 4: 193-207.

LAD, F., 1996, Operational Subjective Statistical Methods, John Wiley & Sons, New York.

PERIZONIUS, W. R. K. Closing and non-closing sutures in 256 crania of known age and sex from Amsterdam (A.D. 1883-1909). Journal of Human Evolution, 1984;13: 201-216.

RIBBE, F. C., 1885, Etude sur l'ordre d'oblitération des sutures du crâne dans les races humaines. Thèse de Médicine, Paris.

VALLOIS, H. V., 1937, La durée de la vie chez l'homme fossile. L'Anthropologie, 19: 499-532.

Chapter 13

BAYESIAN ESTIMATION OF RESTRICTION FRAGMENT LENGTH FROM ELECTROPHORETIC ANALYSIS

J. Shoemaker[1] and A. Rinaldi[2*]

Department of Biostatistics and Bioinformatics, Duke University Medical Center, Durham, NC, U.S.A.[1] *Dipartimento di Studi Geoec., Ling., Stat., Stor. per l'Anal. Reg., Università "La Sapienza" di Roma, Italy*[2]

1. INTRODUCTION

Treatment of DNA with a restriction enzyme yields fragments of variable length and number. Both the fragment number and fragment lengths are useful in several biological and genetic analyses, such as genomic mapping.

During electrophoretic analysis, the shorter fragments move faster through the electrophoretic gel, and thus travel further than the longer ones, i.e. the mobility of a fragment decreases with its length. By plotting the lengths of a standard set of fragments whose lengths are known, against their mobility, one can infer the length of an unknown fragment on the basis of the observed mobility. However, accuracy of this procedure is limited (see Elder, 1979 and Elder and Southern, 1987) and indeed, it is important to recognize that measurement error cannot be eliminated.

The length estimation problem can be formalized through a functional relationship between mobility and length using a set of standard fragments. A widely accepted model, whose theoretical justifications can be found, for instance, in Elder (1979) and Schaffer and Sederoff (1981), assumes that mobility m and length l are linked by the relation

$$(m - m_0)(l - l_0) = c \tag{1}$$

* For correspondence: antonio.rinaldi@unimi.it

where m_0, l_0 and c are parameters to be estimated using the observations obtained with the standard set of fragments.

In this paper we assume the validity of model (1) and investigate its use in estimating the unknow length of a fragment. Section 2 provides background on some previosly proposed methods. In Section 3 we describe a predictive Bayesian solution which tackles the problem in a probabilistic perspective. A numerical example in Section 4 illustrates our procedure.

2. SOME PREVIOUS PROPOSALS

Some methods to estimate the parameters in (1) have been proposed in the literature. Here we briefly discuss two of these methods

In the first method we discuss (Elder, 1979), only three pairs of observation are used to obtain the parameter estimates: (l_1, m_1), (l_2, m_2) and (l_3, m_3), where, for $i = 1,2,3$, l_i and m_i are the length and mobility of three standard fragments. This is achieved by writing:

$$(m_i - m_0)(l_i - l_0) = c \quad i = 1, 2, 3$$

and solving for m_0, l_0 and c. In his first development of the method, Elder (1979) suggests choosing three standard fragments spanning a wide range of lengths, but in a subsequent paper Elder and Southern (1987) follow a different procedure. They consider only standard fragments whose mobilities are closest to the mobility of the fragment whose length must be determined. Then two different estimates of the parameters of model (1) are computed. The first relies on the two closest standard fragment with higher mobility and the closest standard one with lower mobility. The second estimate relies on the closest standard fragment with higher mobility and the two closest standard ones with lower mobility. The final estimate is the arithmetic mean of the two preliminary estimates.

In the second method, Schaffer and Sederoff (1983) apply a version of the least squares. If n fragments form the standard set, and thus there are n pairs of observations (l_i, m_i), $i = 1, \ldots, n$, they write:

$$c_i = (m_i - m_0)(l_i - l_0) \quad \mathrm{i} = 1, \ldots, \mathrm{n}.$$

Then, after defining

$$\overline{c} = \frac{1}{n}\sum_{i=1}^{n} c_i ,$$

the two parameter estimates of m_0 and l_0, $\hat{m}_0$ and $\hat{l}_0$, are determined by minimizing the sum of the squares

$$Q=\sum_{i=1}^{n}(c_i-\overline{c})^2$$

Hence they are used to estimate of the last parameter in this way:

$$\hat{c}=\frac{1}{n}\sum_{i=1}^{n}(m_i-\hat{m}_0)(l_i-\hat{l}_0)$$

Then in both methods the parameter estimates are used to provide the unknown lengths via model (1). Schaffer and Sederoff suggest using the standard deviation

$$\left(\frac{1}{n-3}\sum_{i=1}^{n}(d_i-\overline{d}\right)^{\frac{1}{2}},$$

where $d_i=l_i-\hat{c}/(m_i-\hat{m}_0)+\hat{l}_0$ is the difference between the i-th real length and the i-th estimated length of the standard set and $\overline{d}=\sum_{i=1}^{n}d_i$, to describe the goodness of fit of the model in terms of the lengths being studied.

Using the same terms cited in Weir (1996, page 294), one can say that Schaffer-Sederoff's method is an example of global analysis, since all the observations have the same weight, while Elder-Southern's method is an example of local analysis, because it supposes that model (1) holds with the same parameter values only in the neighbourhood of the length to be determined.

Nevertheless both methods are questionable. The crucial point is that they yield only point estimates, without saying anything about the reliability of the estimates: there is no probabilistic evaluation of their precision.

3. A BAYESIAN PROPOSAL

To overcome the drawback just underlined, we propose to construct via Bayes' theorem the predictive distribution of l_{n+1} given m_{n+1} and the n pairs of length and mobility $D = \{(l_i,m_i),\ i = 1, \ldots, n\}$ of the standard set. This approach is essentially predictive, since it recognizes that the main aim of model (1) is to infer the unknown length of a fragment. Furthermore, it allows us not only to build a point estimate for the unknown fragmet length, but also to make statement about its precision.

We consider that, assuming its parameters are known, the relation (1) provides the value of the mobility corresponding to any possible length apart from an additive error. Moreover, we assume that the fragments in the standard set can be not all equally weigthed, but that their importance can depends on the distance from the length of interest: in other word, we expect that the more a fragment's length is near the one to be estimate, the more it is informative.

We do this by assigning to any mobility m_i a conditional normal distribution with mean

$$r_i = c/(l_i - l_0) + m_0$$

and variance given by

$$s_i^2 = s_m^2 + s_r^2 (l_i - l_{n+1})^2 .$$

This writing formally describes the fact that the variability of the observations depends additively on two factors. The first factor s_m^2 corresponds to the measurement error, the same one for whatever mobility, while the second factor s_r^2 interpretates the weakening of model effectiveness when we consider lengths farther off from the one we have to estimate.

Therefore, if we write the distribution of all the mobilities given the corresponding lengths as

$$f(m_1,\ldots,m_{n+1} \mid l_1,\ldots,l_{n+1}) = \int_\Theta \prod_{i=1}^{n+1} f(m_i \mid l_i, l_{n+1}, \theta) f(\theta) d\theta , \tag{2}$$

where we denote with $\theta = (c, l_0, m_0, s_m^2, s_r^2)$ the parameter vector and with Θ the parameter space, we obtain the predictive distribution of l_{n+1} given m_{n+1} and D,

$$f(l_{n+1} \mid m_{n+1}, D) = \frac{f(m_1,\ldots,m_{n+1} \mid l_1,\ldots,l_{n+1}) f(l_{n+1})}{\int_{\Re_+} f(m_1,\ldots,m_{n+1} \mid l_1,\ldots,l_{n+1}) f(l_{n+1}) dl_{n+1}} . \tag{3}$$

Notice that we use the same letter for all the densities in (2) and (3), even if it represents both the likelihood and different prior distributions. Moreover, notice that we work conditionally on the fragment lengths of the standard set, since they are not choosen at random but assigned before the electophoretical analysis. So, to complete our framework we need to specify the prior distribution for l_{n+1} and for the parameter vector θ.

With respect to the prior distribution for l_{n+1}, we assume that the occurrence of restriction sites follows a Poisson process. This reflects the idea that a chromosome can be divided into very many small intervals, and that the probability of observing a restriction site is the same in each interval, while the probability of observing two or more restriction sites in each interval is negligible, and the occurrence of rescriction sites in a certain interval does not depend from the occurrence of restriction sites in another non-overlapping interval. Under these assumption, it is known that the distribution of the length between two successive restriction sites follows the exponential law (see, for example, Karlin and Taylor, 1975, Ch.8).

As regard as the prior distribution for parameter vector θ, for the sake of simplicity we assume that its elements are a priori independent, so to write

$$f(\theta)=f(c,l_0,m_0,s_m^2,s_r^2)=f(c)f(l_0)f(m_0)f(s_m^2)f(s_r^2)$$

and we give to $\ln c$, l_0, m_0, $\ln s_m^2$ and $\ln s_r^2$ appropriate normal distributions. This choice is one of many equally acceptable solutions and it is suggested here mainly for convenience, since the elements of θ are only the parameters of an ideal relation and we cannot refer to some their physical properties; we need only to describe our opinions through some flexible distributions.

To summarize, we can write, with some obvious notation,

$$\begin{aligned}
&m_i \mid l_i,l_{n+1},\theta \sim N(r_i,s_i^2)\\
&l_{n+1} \sim Exp(\lambda)\\
&l_0 \sim N(\mu_{l_0},\sigma_{l_0}^2)\\
&m_0 \sim N(\mu_{m_0},\sigma_{m_0}^2)\\
&\ln c \sim N(\mu_{\ln c},\sigma_{\ln c}^2)\\
&\ln s_m^2 \sim N(\mu_{\ln s_m^2},\sigma_{\ln s_m^2}^2)\\
&\ln s_r^2 \sim N(\mu_{\ln s_r^2},\sigma_{\ln s_r^2}^2).
\end{aligned}$$

The parameter values of the prior distributions can reflect the knowledge acquired from previous similar experiments, or they can be assigned to specify vague distributions. Of note is that, if certain degenerate priors for s_m^2 or s_r^2 are used, different types of analysis are allowed. For instance, one can achieve a global analysis by setting $s_r^2 = 0$, since in this way all the observations in the standard set have the same weight. Indeed, this is equivalent to make the assumption of conditional independence of the n+1 pairs (l_i, m_i), that is to set $\prod_{i=1}^{n+1} f(m_i \mid l_i, l_{n+1}, \theta) = \prod_{i=1}^{n+1} f(m_i \mid l_i, \theta)$ under the integral signs of (2), as in the standard predictive inference (see Aitchison and Dunsmore, 1975, Ch.10). Otherwise, one can achieve a strictly local analysis setting $s_m^2 = 0$, assuming the measurement error is negligible. In fact, this behaviour is more reasonable than that prescribed by Elder-Southern method, since no information from the standard set is disregarded, each observation having a weight according to its importance as to the new fragment.

Once all its components are specified, the predictive distribution (3) remains well specified. Even if the analytical integrations are not feasible, it is not difficult to simulate a sample from it using a numerical tecnique such as importance sample algorithm (along the lines described in Gelman *et al.*, 1995, Ch.9 and 10) or a MCMC algorithm (see, for example, Gilks *et al.*, 1996). In this way we are able to draw the posterior distribution graph of l_{n+1} or, more simply, to calculate some of its quantiles and its mean, which is the best point estimate using a quadratic loss function (see, for example, Berger, 1988, Sec.4.3).

4. A NUMERICAL EXAMPLE

We now propose a numerical example to test the reliability of the described procedure. Table 1 (given in Weir, 1996, page 294), indicates the lengths and mobilities of six HINDIII restriction fragments.

Table 1. Migration and length of Hind III restriction fragments (data from Weir, 1996)

l_i	m_i
23.1	11.5
9.4	17.2
6.6	23.5
4.4	34.0
2.3	55.0
2.0	60.0

These data have been used to carry out a cross validation: each length of the standard set has been removed, one at a time, from the set of available data and the remaining data have been used to estimate it. Table 2 reports the results of the computation for our method and the two other ones described in Section 2, to facilitate the comparison of numerical values.

Table 2. Summary of length estimates obtained from cross validation for data in Table 1

l_i	Bayesian Estimates			Schaffer-Sederoff Estimates	Elder-Southern Estimates
	Mean	Standard Error	95% Probability Interval		
23.1	14.39	2.169	10.66 – 20.28	20.64	-
9.4	10.28	1.512	7.724 – 14.20	12.55	10.0
6.6	6.912	0.6333	5.434 – 8.459	7.41	6.49
4.4	4.247	0.2532	3.728 – 5.018	4.07	4.33
2.3	2.277	0.1096	2.011 – 2.521	1.69	2.3
2.0	2.021	0.1261	1.441 – 2.260	1.32	-

The real lengths are in the first column, while the following three columns show some features of the Bayesian posterior distributions: mean, standard error and a 95% probability interval. All the posterior distributions are unimodal with a very slight asymmetry. The last two columns indicates the point estimates of Schaffer-Sederoff least squares method and Elder-Southern method.

To obtain the Bayesian predictive distributions, we have used the computational facilities offered by the Winbug package (for details, see the web site http://www.mrc-bsu.cam.ac.uk/bugs/winbugs/contents.shtml), setting the prior distribution parameters to the following values:

$$\lambda = 0.125$$

$$\mu_{l_0} = 0,\ \sigma^2_{l_0} = 10$$

$$\mu_{m_0} = 0,\ \sigma^2_{m_0} = 10$$

$$\mu_{\ln c} = 3,\ \sigma^2_{\ln c} = 10$$

$$\mu_{\ln s^2_m} = -1,\ \sigma^2_{\ln s^2_m} = 10$$

$$\mu_{\ln s^2_r} = -1,\ \sigma^2_{\ln s^2_r} = 10$$

The value of λ is equal to the reciprocal of the mean of the standard fragments, in such a way that the mean of the prior distribution for l_{n+1} is equal to the mean of the lengths in the standard set, while the other parameter values specify vague distributions. With Elder-Southern method, the first and last estimates have not been computed, since there are no length in the standard set with a higher or lower mobility than that corresponding to the length to be determined. The second and penultimate estimates have been made using only one set of three standard fragments, instead of two, as suggested in Weir (1996, page 295).

For these data, Schaffer-Sederoff estimates seem to be better than Elder-Southern ones. Bayesian point estimates are quite good, except in the first case, which deserves separate consideration. It very bad, as is the probability interval, but we have to notice that the corresponding length is very far from the other ones. Indeed, both Elder (1979) and Weir (1996, page 295), prudently advise not to attempt a length estimation beyond the range of the standard fragments in order to avoid large errors. Furthermore, the size of the Bayesian probability intervals strongly increases with the distance between the length to be estimated and the closest lengths of the standard set. We have observed the same behaviour with other data sets, not shown here. Hence the Bayesian analysis suggests that it would be very advisable to choose the standard fragments so that their lengths are uniformly distributed along their whole variation range. On the contrary, no similar considerations are possible using Schaffer-Sederoff and Elder-Southern methods.

REFERENCES

AITCHISON J., DUNSMORE I.R., (1975), Statistical Prediction Analysis, Cambridge University Press, Cambridge.

BERGER J.O., (1988), Statistical Decision Theory and Bayesian Analysis - Second Edition -, Spinger-Verlag, New York.

ELDER J.K., (1979), Measurement of DNA length by gel electrophoresis, *Analytical Biochemistry, 100*, pp. 319-323.

ELDER J.K., SOUTHERN E.M., (1987), Computer aided analysis of one-dimensional restriction fragment gels, In Nucleic Acid and Proteine Sequence Analysis, d. M. J. Bishop and C. J. Rawlings, pp. 165-172, IRL Press, Oxford.

GELMAN A., CARLIN J.B., STERN H.S., RUBIN D.R., (1995), Bayesian Data Analysis, Chapman and Hall, London.

GILKS W.R., RICHARDSON S., SPIEGELHALTER D.J., (1996), Monte Carlo Markov Chain in practice, Chapman & Hall, London.

KARLIN S., TAYLOR H.M., (1975), A first course in stochastic processes, Academic Press, New York.

SCHAFFER H.E., SEDEROFF R.R., (1981), Improved estimation of DNA fragment lengths from agarose gels, *Analytical Biochemistry, 115*, pp. 113-122.

WEIR B.S., (1996), Genetic Data Analysis 2: methods for discrete population genetic data, Sinauer Associated, Sunderland.